Statistics in Medical Research

STATISTICS IN MEDICAL RESEARCH

Methods and Issues,
with Applications in Cancer Research

Edited by

VALERIE MIKÉ

Memorial Sloan-Kettering Cancer Center
and Cornell University

KENNETH E. STANLEY

Harvard University School of Public Health
and Sidney Farber Cancer Institute

JOHN WILEY & SONS
New York   Chichester   Brisbane   Toronto   Singapore

Library of Congress Cataloging in Publication Data:

Main entry under title: Statistics in medical research.

(Wiley series in probability and mathematical statistics.
Applied probability and statistics, ISSN 0271-6356)
   Includes index.
   1. Medical research—Statistical methods—Congresses.
2. Cancer—Research—Statistical methods—Congresses.
3. Biometry—Congresses. I. Miké, Valerie, 1934- . II. Stanley,
K.E. (Kenneth E.) III. Series. [DNLM: 1. Biometry—Methods—
Congresses. 2. Neoplasms—Congresses. 3. Research—Congresses.
QZ 206 C748s 1981]

R853.S7S78   1982   610'.7'2   82-10871

ISBN 0-471-86911-2

Printed in the United States of America

10 9 8 7 6 5 4 3 2 1

To the memory of Jerome Cornfield

From here on, as far ahead as one can see, medicine must be building, as a central part of its scientific base, a solid underpinning of statistical knowledge. Hunches and intuitive impressions are essential for getting the work started, but it is only through the quality of the numbers at the end that the truth can be told.

Lewis Thomas

Preface

There is a growing need in medical research for the contributions of professionals trained in biostatistics and epidemiology, and there is a nationwide shortage of adequate manpower. This was also a conclusion of recent studies carried out by the National Research Council of the National Academy of Sciences. Biostatistics and epidemiology were specifically identified as areas in which educational programs should be supported.

The subject was discussed at length in the course of a workshop on epidemiology and biostatistics organized by the National Cancer Institute in 1979. Since there are not enough professionals in these fields to meet the needs of medical schools and cancer centers around the country, the recommendation was made that special seminars and teaching materials be developed to enhance the effectiveness of individuals now filling many of the positions. The statisticians attending this meeting included Theodore Colton, Valerie Miké, and Marvin Zelen, who was then Chairman of the Biometrics Section of the American Statistical Association. In response to the general recommendation of the workshop, Marvin Zelen subsequently asked Valerie Miké to chair a new committee of the Biometrics Sec-

tion that was being established to plan a summer conference on statistics in cancer research. Theodore
Colton and Kenneth Stanley agreed to serve as committee members, and were later joined by David Braun,
Richard Gelber, and Martin Lesser. A grant proposal
for support of this activity was submitted to the NCI
in 1980 and it was awarded in early 1981.

The conference was held at Memorial Sloan-Kettering
Cancer Center during the week of June 22-26, 1981.
Lectures and panel discussions covered a broad spectrum of topics, from study design and statistical
methodology to medical ethics and aspects of teaching
and consulting in the medical community. In addition
to statisticians from major institutions around the
country, the faculty included an attorney and practic-
ing physicians representing the fields of medicine,
surgery, pathology, psychiatry, and medical ethics.

This book is based on the lectures and discussions
presented at the conference. Many participants expressed the view that the material covered would be
of interest to a wider audience and should therefore
be published as a volume.

The book offers a comprehensive overview of the
field of biostatistics. Although the emphasis of the
meeting was on cancer research, nearly everything discussed is applicable to other areas of medical investigation. Since there are currently many opportunities in biostatistics, this volume can provide useful
information for classically trained statisticians interested in entering the field, and it can help those
new to the field to become more effective collaborators. It can serve as stimulus for graduate students
in statistics, to nurture their interest and to prepare them for careers in biostatistics. It can also
be read with benefit by clinical investigators seeking
a better understanding of statistical concepts and related multidisciplinary aspects of medical research.

The chapters in the book have been grouped according to content. The introductory paper on the role

of statistics in medical research is followed by a
section on epidemiology. An overview is given of
both descriptive and analytic epidemiology in the
context of cancer research, and there is a thought-
provoking article concerned with analyzing recent
trends in cancer mortality and incidence.

The next section focuses on important issues pertaining to clinical studies. Chapter 4 presents a
historical perspective and reports on the results of
a survey in which senior investigators and statisticians were asked to assess the impact of statistics
on advances made in the treatment of cancer. An interesting outcome was the high response rate and the
nearly complete consensus of the respondents. Chapters 5 and 6 are edited transcripts of panel discussions exploring ethical, legal, and psychological
issues as well as statistical problems related to the
planning of clinical studies.

A section on practical considerations provides
"how-to" information for the newcomer to clinical research. Chapter 7 defines basic terms and outlines
procedures for the design of clinical trials; useful
tables for sample size calculations are also included.
Specific guidelines on data management and quality
control are offered in Chapter 8. Chapter 9 provides
the beginner with detailed instructions on acquiring
efficient and cost-effective computing capability.
It contains an annotated listing of major data base
management systems and statistical software and graphics packages, complete with addresses and telephone
numbers of vendors.

The papers dealing with statistical methodology
are grouped in Chapters 10-15. These are meant to
provide an introduction to the relevant material, with
an overview of current developments. The chapters
present basic concepts of the analysis of survival
data, starting with a discussion of survival curves
and progressing to group comparisons and model building. Two chapters are devoted to the analysis of

categorical data, using the approach of log-linear
and logistic models. The section concludes with an
assessment of methods for monitoring and stopping
clinical trials. This is the only part of the book
that contains material requiring more than an elemen-
tary background in statistics. But the definitions,
examples, and extensive bibliographies given in each
chapter offer worthwhile information for any serious
reader.

The final section contains two panel discussions
on communication, and these should be of equal interest to statisticians and biomedical investigators.
Chapter 16 explores problems of interaction with the
medical community in the statistician's triple role
as consultant, collaborator, and teacher. Chapter 17
is concerned with the interpretation and presentation
of statistical results.

The four multidisciplinary panel discussions help
to convey the full flavor of medical research, including the complex and essentially open-ended nature of
questions pertaining to research involving human subjects. Treatment of controversial matters is reported
as it took place in the various sessions. References
include guides to the vast literature of the new field
of bioethics. The texts of the Nuremberg Code and the
Declaration of Helsinki are reproduced in full at the
end of Chapter 5.

For simplicity of style the pronoun "he" has been
used throughout.

We would like to thank all those who contributed
to the preparation of this volume. In particular,
help with editing the panel discussions and reading
the papers was provided by Jenny Baglivo, David Byar,
Theodore Colton, Mitchell Gail, Edmund Gehan, Nancy
Geller, Susan Groshen, Martin Lesser, and Howard
Thaler. Blanche Sherman gave essential administrative
support. The most extensive contribution was made by
Larry Fishman, who first served as conference coordi-
nator and subsequently as editorial assistant. He

carried much of the overall responsibility for communicating with the authors and assembling the material;
he then also typed the camera-ready version of the
manuscript.

Finally, we would like to express our deep appreciation to Dr. Marthana Hjortland, Program Director
for Biometry, Special Programs Branch, Division of
Cancer Cause and Prevention, National Cancer Institute, who played a significant role in providing the
advice and encouragement needed to ensure the successful completion of this entire project. The work was
supported by NCI Grant CA-29801.

Valerie Miké
Kenneth E. Stanley

New York, New York
Boston, Massachusetts
April 1982

Contributors

GEORGE J. ANNAS, J.D., M.P.H.
Department of Social Medical Sciences
    and Community Medicine
Boston University School of Public Health
Boston, Massachusetts

JOHN C. BAILAR III, M.D., Ph.D.
U.S. Environmental Protection Agency
Washington, D.C. and
Department of Biostatistics
Harvard University School of Public Health
Boston, Massachusetts

DAVID W. BRAUN, JR., Ph.D.
Biostatistics Laboratory
Memorial Sloan-Kettering Cancer Center
    and Cornell University
New York, New York

BYRON W. BROWN, JR., Ph.D.
Division of Biostatistics
Stanford University School of Medicine
Stanford, California

DAVID P. BYAR, M.D.
Biometry Branch
National Cancer Institute
Bethesda, Maryland

ERIC J. CASSELL, M.D.
Department of Public Health
Cornell University Medical College
New York, New York

THEODORE COLTON, Sc.D.
Epidemiology and Biostatistics Section
Boston University School of Public Health
    and Hubert H. Humphrey Cancer Center
Boston, Massachusetts

JEROME J. DECOSSE, M.D., Ph.D.
Department of Surgery
Memorial Sloan-Kettering Cancer Center
New York, New York

MITCHELL H. GAIL, M.D., Ph.D.
Biometry Branch
National Cancer Institute
Bethesda, Maryland

EDMUND A. GEHAN, Ph.D.
Department of Biomathematics
The University of Texas System Cancer Center
Houston, Texas

RICHARD D. GELBER, Ph.D.
Department of Biostatistics
Harvard University School of Public Health
    and Sidney Farber Cancer Institute
Boston, Massachusetts

E. ROBERT GREENBERG, M.D.
Department of Community and Family Medicine
Dartmouth Medical School
Hanover, New Hampshire

LAWRENCE E. HINKLE, JR., M.D.
Department of Medicine
Cornell University Medical College
New York, New York

JAMES F. HOLLAND, M.D.
Department of Neoplastic Diseases
Mount Sinai School of Medicine
New York, New York

JIMMIE C. B. HOLLAND, M.D.
Psychiatry Service
Department of Neurology
Memorial Sloan-Kettering Cancer Center
New York, New York

STEPHEN W. LAGAKOS, Ph.D.
Department of Biostatistics
Harvard University School of Public Health
    and Sidney Farber Cancer Institute
Boston, Massachusetts

MARTIN L. LESSER, Ph.D.
Biostatistics Laboratory
Memorial Sloan-Kettering Cancer Center
    and Cornell University
New York, New York

ROBERT J. LEVINE, M.D.
Department of Internal Medicine
Yale University
The School of Medicine
New Haven, Connecticut

THOMAS A. LOUIS, Ph.D.
Department of Biostatistics
Harvard University School of Public Health
Boston, Massachusetts

VALERIE MIKÉ, Ph.D.
Biostatistics Laboratory
Memorial Sloan-Kettering Cancer Center
    and Cornell University
New York, New York

FREDERICK MOSTELLER, Ph.D.
Department of Health Policy and Management
Harvard University School of Public Health
Boston, Massachusetts

JUDITH R. O'FALLON, Ph.D.
Cancer Center Statistics
Mayo Comprehensive Cancer Center
Rochester, Minnesota

CARL M. PINSKY, M.D.
Department of Medicine
Memorial Sloan-Kettering Cancer Center
New York, New York

PAUL P. ROSEN, M.D.
Department of Pathology
Memorial Sloan-Kettering Cancer Center
New York, New York

MARVIN A. SCHNEIDERMAN, Ph.D.
Clement Associates
Arlington, Virginia

DAVID A. SCHOENFELD, Ph.D.
Department of Biostatistics
Harvard University School of Public Health
    and Sidney Farber Cancer Institute
Boston, Massachusetts

KENNETH E. STANLEY, Ph.D.
Department of Biostatistics
Harvard University School of Public Health
    and Sidney Farber Cancer Institute
Boston, Massachusetts

Contents

xix

Statistics in Medical Research

Part I
Introduction

CHAPTER 1

The Role of Statistics in Medical Research

FREDERICK MOSTELLER

Before giving you my views on the opportunities and obligations of statistics and statisticians in medical research, I had best outline my personal experience so that you can adjust for my biases and weaknesses.

Until about 1948, I did no medical research at all, my applied work falling instead primarily in industrial and engineering statistics and basic research in social science. In 1948, I became acquainted with Dr. Henry Beecher, of the Department of Anesthesia of Massachusetts General Hospital in Boston, and consulted with him and his co-workers for many years. His research was in analgesics -- studying drugs -- and in various aspects of the science of anesthesia. I had an opportunity to consult with many young anesthesiologists on their research problems.

These opportunities have led me to a wide acquaintance with biomedical researchers. Through one of these researchers, Dr. John Bunker, and the National

---

This work was supported by Rockefeller Foundation Grant RF#79026.

3

Research Council, I had the opportunity of participating in the National Halothane Study, a study of the safety of anesthetics where statistical collection and analysis played a big role. I learned a lot from this experience.

That study was an example of symbiosis between statistics and medicine in a public health issue. Although several methods of analysis were possible, the many variables and the many categories for each variable -- age, length of operation, kind of operation, anesthetic, sex, physical status -- forced us to consider multivariate approaches. We tried out many methods, but one stood out as especially natural -- the log-linear models for contingency tables. We used them in the study (3), and then over the next few years, we organized the methods systematically so that now they are widely available (1,5,7).

Along with Howard Hiatt at the School of Public Health at Harvard, I developed a Faculty Seminar in Health and Medicine which has run for a number of years, and there we studied intensively costs, risks, and benefits of surgery, again with John Bunker (2).

Through the Institute of Medicine of the National Academy of Sciences, and the Office of Technology Assessment of the Congress, I have had a chance to think about health policy and biomedical research policy as well as scientific research. I have discovered how few therapies, diagnostics, and preventive methods have been solidly evaluated (10).

During the past 4 years, I have chaired the Department of Biostatistics at Harvard. Through this activity, I have been concerned about the quantitative education of physicians and of other biomedical research workers.

IMPORTANCE OF VARIANCE

Why do statistics play a role at all in medical investigations? Generally because of the heavy role

of variation in medical work. In some areas of the
world's work, variation is not key to the events being
studied; for example, in chemistry we often have perfect mixing and the analysis of a drop is the same as
that of a bucket of the same substance. But in the
biological and social sciences and, of course, in engineering (and much medical work is like engineering
in the sense that we are more involved in technology
than with basic science), variation is the rule. In
engineering, we have the problems of the need for
quality control arising from troublesome variation.
In medicine, patients just are not all alike, nor are
physicians, hospitals, or communities. Under the
most carefully controlled conditions, patients do as
they please. In the main, our results are of the
form that more or fewer people respond to a new therapy than to the old one. We find tendencies, rarely
laws. Once we are far from the all-or-none situation,
measurement of uncertainty becomes important. Thus,
a fundamental idea from statistics is that we must
use probabilistic as well as deterministic thinking.
     In olden times, it was possible for one case study
to become the ruling event. It is still a great
source for hypothesis generation and the study of
process, but to reduce the excessively heavy impact
of the single case, we need statistics. The aston-
ishing fact is that if we have two equally likely
categories, then gathering 1000 cases does not lead
to half of each kind, but can produce numbers generally in the range of 47 to 53%. This is chastening
when we think of searching for gains among small differences. An improvement of 3% in death rate is a
lot. Worse yet, for samples of 100, the corresponding
variation is from 40 to 60%, yet 100 seems like a
great many cases to most clinicians, and rightly so
from the effort required. Thus, variation and its
control are fundamental to research in medicine.

PROBLEM FORMULATION

For me and many of my friends, the fundamental
role of the statistician in the consulting or collaborative relationship is that of problem formulation.
This requires a great deal of time and attention, and,
most difficult, open minds but not empty ones. To do
consulting well requires a great deal of good will on
both sides -- both on the part of the researcher with
the problem, and on the part of the statistician being consulted. A beginner might suppose that statisticians would come armed with a very large number of
methods and techniques (and they do) and that when
the investigator asks a question, the statisticians
merely thumb through an index of methods and produce
an appropriate one (they do not).

This idea is mistaken on several counts. First,
it assumes that all the statistical techniques that
are needed have already been invented, and second
that the statistician is in charge of them all. Neither concept is correct. The fact that a serious researcher comes to a statistician for help is already
a symptom that something unusual is afoot. The research worker will have had training in the methods
that are especially appropriate to the research, and
so something nonroutine must have come up or the research worker would not be consulting statisticians,
attractive as they are. Instead he or she would be
home running the experiment, analyzing the data, or
writing up the paper for publication. Thus, the
symptom that provokes the consulting relationship is
that something new has come to the attention of the
investigator, who is concerned to take care of it.

The standard approach by the research worker is,
"I have a 5-minute question." The statistician without an hour free at that point should make a future
appointment. Those 5-minute questions are just the
"come on." The investigator tells a short story
about the research and asks what to do, and it seems
clear that what is needed is, let us say, a simple

t-test for the difference between two means. Ha!   It
really was a 5-minute question. So the statistician
inquires, "Have you considered using the t-test?"
The answer will come back something like this, "Well,
yes, and we generally use Welch's approach for unequal variances, but something about this problem
makes us think that this approach won't do." The investigator was just trying the statistician out before offering the challenge of the actual problem.
Also, there is always concern that the consultant may
speak nothing but complex variables or matrix algebra.

The problem is then likely to begin tumbling out.
Some peculiar feature of the situation spoils certain
of the measurements, or a special index needs to be
constructed, or a new control group or design needs
to be created. This routine consulting problem has
become a research problem for the statistician. The
first step is to find out what the problem is; for
that, it usually needs to be gone over several times,
and the statistician needs to explain it in turn to
the investigator to make sure that everyone is in
agreement. As long as the investigator is not satisfied, the full complexity of the problem has likely
not been handled, and it needs to be at some stage.

Problem formulation, therefore, is one of the most
difficult and important jobs for the statistician,
and it must be done in collaboration with the research
worker.

Once the problem has been formulated, then a second role comes along, that of problem solver. Ordinarily we have many ways to solve a problem, and once
it is clearly stated, many people may be able to provide solutions of differing sorts. Many statisticians
enjoy working on well-posed problems, and those who
come to statistics through the mathematical route are
likely to find pleasure in this activity.

Let me mention a rather specialized topic: simulation. Sometimes we can use a mathematical model to
approximate what is likely to occur. If it has
stochastic or chance elements in it, we can run the

process through a mathematical simulation a few or a
great many times to get an idea of the distribution
of outcomes. Sometimes such simulations actually answer medical problems. Other times they may help
with the design or analysis of an investigation.

DESIGN OF INVESTIGATIONS

Because investigations are varied in their kinds,
I cannot treat all possible sorts today. Let me distinguish observational studies of the population as
it stands, such as sample surveys, from studies of
causation as in comparative experiments. In sample
surveys the purpose is to find what the situation is
in a population, as when a sample of the U.S. population takes a physical examination, and thus makes it
possible for the National Center for Health Statistics
to estimate the health status of the nation. In the
main, no action is taken toward members of the sample;
the purpose is to describe the population.

In comparative experiments, the purpose is to discover whether the "treatment" has an effect and how
much it is, as compared with some other treatment,
usually the standard one. We study causation here.
We change the treatment. Do not confuse the two. In
sample surveys, we change nothing, we observe. Thus,
when we observe a difference in health, say, between
rural and urban people, be careful not to attribute
the difference to the rural-urban division. We have
not changed people from rural to urban and observed
the effect on their health. Be wary of regression
and other related studies intended to prove causation
without actually changing the variables. These studies are suggestive, and sometimes valuable, but not
proof.

Sometimes observational studies take the place of
experiments because they are the only studies available and sometimes because they are so compelling.
Epidemiologists design studies to compare responses

of those in a control group with those exposed to
some treatment. The hope is that the association
with a group is not caused by the treatment or its
outcome. In other words, these observational studies
are designed to come as close as possible to being
randomized experiments.

In some instances, the effect of the treatment is
so unusual, severe, or sudden that its causative feature is compelling. In still other instances, the
evidence may come from a great variety of sources
with a common message. In both these instances, we
tend to accept causation, more gradually in the latter.

The main kinds of comparative experiments are:
(a) parallel studies where two or more independent
groups are compared using different treatments; (b)
crossover studies where the same individuals are studied more than once with different treatments; and (c)
sequential investigations where some sort of rules of
assignment may be applied that change as information
is acquired during the investigation. One of statistics' jobs is to explain the advantages and hazards
of the crossover design.

In both kinds of investigations, observational
studies and experiments, the control of sampling error is one of the primary efforts. Another important
one is to make sure that what we want to measure can
be deduced from the data. This problem is called the
problem of identifiability. Sometimes we measure
something in such a way that we cannot untangle the
components. Often the problem formulation requires
us to find a way out of this box. If we always measure the total x + y, we cannot get x without more information.

In the midst of variation from every possible
source, when studying a potential experimental design,
you can help yourself a great deal by stopping and
asking one question: "If I had all the data in the
world free of charge and measured without error, could
I answer my question?" Sometimes we get so wrapped

up in worrying about error and unreliability we forget the main issue.

NONSAMPLING ERRORS

In many investigations, though, it is the nonsampling errors that cause the most trouble. Consequently, many statistical devices have been introduced to help control the quality of the study as it
is executed and to strengthen the analysis once the
study has been carried out. We might list a few of
these devices, used largely in experiments.

Randomization is used in both experiments and sample surveys to allocate treatments to patients and to
select patients from populations. Part of the reason
for randomizing is to prevent bias on the part of the
person assigning the treatments or selecting people
for interview.

In experiments, blindness is also desirable when
it can be achieved. There are several kinds, and
among them, the blindness of the patient to the actual
treatment, the blindness of the investigator to the
treatment assignment, and the blindness of the evalua-
tor of the outcome of the investigation to the treatment assigned. All these maskings are intended to reduce the effects of prejudices in the evaluation -- to
improve objectivity.

Introduction of adjustment for outside variables
that add variability to an analysis, such as smoking,
is called covariance adjustment, a valuable way to
reduce unreliability.

ANALYSIS

In analyzing investigations, we have 3 main forms:
confirmatory, descriptive, and exploratory. Under
confirmatory, we include ideas relating to statistical
inference, such as tests of hypotheses and confidence

intervals. These have associated with them many special techniques, but the t-test and the chi-square
for a contingency table are popular examples. In
general, anything that leads to P-values is associated
with confirmatory analysis.

The ideal circumstance here is that a preplanned
analysis is carried out as intended, planned in advance of the experiment. Statistics is intended to
make you aware of the problems of multiplicity and
selectivity that arise when many tests are done on
the same data and selective reporting takes place.
In a few instances, we have remedies for going to the
well as often as we like, but in the main we are not
well defended against authors who do many analyses
and report only those that favor a particular position. This sort of activity, sometimes called data
dredging, makes a mockery of significance levels.
Thus, one role of a statistician is to help everyone
appreciate what is required for honesty in reporting.

You may ask, "Well, shouldn't the investigator be
allowed to analyze the data in depth?" The answer is
"yes" and that is the purpose of exploratory data
analysis. With no holds barred, you use any methods
you prefer to try to get the data to tell what they
are concealing. Such explorations are necessary and
laudable and we have many methods available, but they
should not be confused with confirmation of hypotheses. Explorations are hypothesis-generating efforts,
not hypothesis-confirming analyses. It is important
to carry out both kinds of activities, and important
to keep the results separate and distinct in their
reporting.

In the last few years, exploratory data analysis
has come into its own with many new and old methods
organized by John Tukey (11) and others (8,9,12) to
study data in such a way that the analysis is defended against outliers and so that the distributional assumptions are modest.

Generally, we distinguish between two desirable
properties: resistant methods and robust methods.

The sample median is a resistant estimator of the
population median. The resistance refers to the fact
that a large change in a small part of the data little affects the value of the estimate. On the other
hand, a large change in a small part of the data affects the sample mean a great deal. It is not resistant. Throw a millionaire's fortune into the income distribution of a college class, and you make a
substantial difference in the average, but not in the
median.

Resistance is desirable, but it can be overdone;
for example, a number that does not change at all,
like 100, is terribly resistant to changes in the
data. If you always answered 100 to every estimation
problem, you would have a resistant estimator. Thus,
an estimate can be too resistant. To the idea of resistance, we have also adjoined the idea of robustness. There are several kinds of robustness, but I
talk here about robustness with respect to outliers
and to the shape of the distribution. Certain statistics preserve almost all their good properties over a
large class of distributional assumptions, and are
also very strong when idealized assumptions such as
those of the normal distribution are met.

Many of these estimates are complex, but one that
is simple is called the trimmed mean. Chop a percentage of measurements off both ends of the ordered sample, and take the average of the middle values remaining. The median chops about 50% off each end. But it
turns out that for many purposes, chopping about 20%
off each end and averaging what is left in the middle
does a very good job of estimation for a very large
family of distributions including those that have outlier problems. Thus, the trimmed mean would be an
example of a robust estimate of the population mean.

Finally, another purpose of analysis is for description of the data. We will call it descriptive
statistics. These just summarize the data, usually
in simple ways as a prelude to presentation.

REPORTING

Statistics also tells us something about reporting. When we report an investigation, we should be telling its properties, and especially those properties that will help the reader know whether the investigation was well done. The knowledge of eligibility of patients for the study, of objectivity of assignment, of randomization and how the randomization was done, what blindness was used, whether informed consent was obtained, whether all patients were followed and if not why, what statistical analyses were carried out, and other things all should be reported. One of the least reported matters in comparative studies has to do with the power of the investigation. This is a statistical concept, and it measures how likely the study is to find an effect of a given size if it is present. It is closely related to sample size and precision of measurement.

Freiman et al. (6) reported in The New England Journal of Medicine that 50% of a collection of over 70 studies that reported that they had not observed a statistically significant difference had such low power that they would have had only a 50% chance of detecting an improvement of 50% in the patients.

We would like to think that when the result is not statistically significant, we are confident that there is not a large improvement available from the tested therapy. If the sample sizes are too small or the method of measurement too crude, then the investigation does not have much chance of detecting a difference even if it is present. This is what power is about. Thus, it is one thing to say that the result is not statistically significant and thus dismiss a new therapy, and quite another to add the statement, "By the way, we didn't have one chance in 10 of finding a large favorable effect, even if it were present." Thus, power analysis is a valuable adjunct.

Of course, it is possible to explain the weakness of an investigation in other ways -- for example, by giving confidence limits.

My own attitude toward confidence limits and tests of significance is that they represent ways of reporting the results of investigations. I do not think of them as decision devices but as conclusion devices. Lest you think this is a distinction without a difference, notice that a conclusion is a view held and subject to change with additional information. But a decision is oriented to direct action such as policy for treating the patient. We are distinguishing between thinking and action. It takes more than statistical significance to lead to medical action because there is so much to consider: training needed, costs, danger to the patient, potential gain.

What about statistical decision theory? This has its place in certain parts of clinical medicine, and also in medical policy, but this chapter is not long enough to include it. It would offer one way of actually deciding on a course of action as distinct from deciding what to believe. The complications such as cost, danger, and training requirements associated with a new therapy could lead one to a conclusion that the therapy was definitely preferable to the standard but that we were not ready to use it in practice.

SCHOOLS OF THOUGHT

In statistics, as in any field, we have various schools of thought. For example, we have the "frequentist" school, which bases much of its work on the Neyman-Pearson and Fisher approach to statistics with confidence intervals and significance tests, but they do not ordinarily employ prior distributions directly. They use prior information in the design of a study and in the interpretation, but usually not in the formal analysis.

Another school is the Bayesian school, which tries to take into account in the analysis the prior probabilities of various events.

These groups often have heated arguments about appropriate methods. I think that you can assume that both sides of such an argument have something useful to say. Indeed, over the last few years some methods called "empirical Bayes" have been introduced which allow frequentists to formulate some of their problems the way a Bayesian might, and still use only the data from the investigation.

You should not, however, suppose that these discussions are merely tempests in teapots. It is well known that the sensitivity and specificity alone do not determine the usefulness of a clinical test. We need also to know something of the prior probability of having the disease. If no one in the tested population has the disease, even sensitivity and specificity of 0.99 leave the test useless. And so, in even this little example we can see the merits of prior probabilities.

TABULATION

With respect to tabulation, we have a major issue. Is your reporting intended to memorialize your data or to help the reader understand it? If you measured a physical constant more accurately than others have, you do want to memorialize.

1. If memorializing is the goal, you keep as many significant figures as you own.
2. If understanding is the goal, report as few digits as you can and still communicate the message.

Furthermore, in a row-by-columns table, if you want to do a good job, take out the grand mean or median and the row and column effects and report them on the margin and the residuals in the cells. This would tell the reader what is going on. You may have to argue with the editor to get it published, but surely it is the wave of the future.

A custom has grown of reporting percentages based on counts to one decimal, for example, 73.4%. Sometimes this makes it possible to recover the counts, but it often just clutters up a table, especially if the sample sizes are small.

Let us illustrate how we might improve understanding of a two-way table by using the approach of effects: grand location plus row effect plus column effect plus residuals. Suppose Table 1 is a set of measurement data organized into a two-way table.

TABLE 1. Two-Way Table of Measurements

	U	V	W
A	9325	9361	9308
B	9331	9351	9320
C	9318	9348	9331
D	9310	9336	9325

The four digit numbers make it hard to look at. If we subtract 9300 from every entry, we already have improved the appearance a great deal, as Table 2 shows.

In Table 2, we have also indicated the row medians preparatory to removing their effect from the rows. Table 3 shows the results after subtracting the row medians from the numbers in the rows of Table 2. Finally, Table 4 gives the results when column medians are removed. Ehrenberg (4) gives a well-illustrated discussion of these ideas in his first two chapters.

All told, we see that the grand effect is about

9328, the row effects are slight, the column effects are larger, and the residuals vary a good deal.

TABLE 2. Table 1 after Removing 9300

	U	V	W	Row median
A	25	61	8	25
B	31	51	20	31
C	18	48	31	31
D	10	36	25	25

TABLE 3. Table 2 after Row Medians Are Removed

	U	V	W	
A	0	36	−17	−3
B	0	20	−11	3
C	−13	17	0	3
D	−15	11	0	−3
Column median	−6	18	−6	9328

TABLE 4. Table 3 after Column Medians Are Removed

	U	V	W	Row effects
A	6	18	-11	-3
B	6	2	-5	3
C	-7	-1	6	3
D	-9	-7	6	-3
Column effects	-6	18	-6	9328

TO SUM UP

Statistics has many roles. The first is to adjoin probabilistic thinking to deterministic thinking.

Second is problem formulation: How can you measure what you want to measure?

Third, experimental and study design including observational studies a la epidemiology, and sample surveys and experiments, as in biostatistics.

Fourth, quality control in the implementation of studies; here what we call methodology plays a major role.

Fifth, analysis, and the three main kinds are (a) confirmatory, (b) descriptive, and (c) exploratory. It is important to keep these distinct in reporting.

Sixth, reporting itself is a major statistical contribution with concern for multiplicity of end points, changing definitions, multiplicity of analysis, and selective reporting as well as clarity.

I have not dealt with graphics though these are important and crucial to communication, but they deserve a lecture of their own. Let me say that Edward Tufte at Yale University is developing an important work in this field and that we all await its appearance. I have discussed memorializing versus communicating data and the idea of presenting two-way tables as grand mean or median plus row and column effects plus residuals.

REFERENCES

1. Bishop, Y. M. M., Fienberg, S. E., and Holland, R. W. (1975), Discrete Multivariate Analysis: Theory and Practice, MIT Press, Cambridge, Massachusetts.

2. Bunker, J. P., Barnes, B. A., and Mosteller, F. (1977), Costs, Risks, and Benefits of Surgery, Oxford University Press, New York.

3. Bunker, J. P., Forrest, W. H., Mosteller, F., and Vandam, L. D., eds. (1969), The National Halothane Study, U.S. Government Printing Office, Washington, D.C.

4. Ehrenberg, A. S. C. (1975), Data Reduction: Analysing and Interpreting Statistical Data, Wiley, London.

5. Fienberg, S. E. (1980), The Analysis of Cross-Classified Categorical Data (2nd ed.), MIT Press, Cambridge, Massachusetts.

6. Freiman, J. A., Chalmers, T. C., Smith, H., Jr., and Kuebler, R. R. (1978), The importance of beta, the type II error, and the sample size in the design and interpretation of the randomized control trial, The New England Journal of Medicine 299: 690-694.

7. Haberman, S. J. (1974), The Analysis of Frequency Data, University of Chicago Press, Chicago.

8. Hoaglin, D. C., Mosteller, F., and Tukey, J. W., eds. (1982), Understanding Robust and Exploratory Data Analysis, Wiley, New York.

9. Mosteller, F., and Tukey, J. W. (1977), Data Analysis and Regression, Addison-Wesley, Reading, Massachusetts.

10. Office of Technology Assessment (1978), Assessing the Efficacy and Safety of Medical Technologies, Congress of the United States, U.S. Government Printing Office, Washington, D.C.

11. Tukey, J. W. (1977), Exploratory Data Analysis, Addison-Wesley, Reading, Massachusetts.

12. Velleman, P. F., and Hoaglin, D. C. (1981), Applications, Basics, and Computing of Exploratory Data Analysis, Duxbury Press, Boston, Massachusetts.

Part II
Epidemiology

CHAPTER 2
Cancer Epidemiology

THEODORE COLTON
E. ROBERT GREENBERG

INTRODUCTION

In contrast to the therapeutic clinical trials that
are the focal point of much of this volume, epidemiologic research relies on observational rather than
experimentally derived data. Consequently, the approach and statistical methods employed in epidemiologic studies differ somewhat from those of clinical
trials. Some purists have held that the results of
observational studies have little credence. Epidemiologists strongly disagree. There are many situations
where randomized clinical trials are not feasible,
yet where information is necessary and where firm conclusions can be drawn. For example, some of the major exposure/disease relationships elucidated by cancer epidemiology include smoking and lung cancer, diethylstilbestrol (DES) and vaginal cancer, ionizing
radiation and leukemia, and asbestos and lung cancer.
In each of these situations, randomized clinical trials would have been both infeasible and unethical.
Yet, firm, scientific conclusions resulted from a
chain of evidence established by observational, epidemiologic studies. One of the purposes of this chapter is to indicate the methodologic nature of these
observational studies and how they can culminate with

causal conclusions.

One often cited definition of epidemiology is "the study of the distribution and determinates of disease frequency in man" (15). A convenient dichotomization of epidemiology is descriptive and analytic. Descriptive epidemiology "describes" the distribution of the disease within the group under study. Analytic epidemiology examines specific etiologic or causal hypotheses, that is, the "determinates" of disease. One can view descriptive epidemiology as hypothesis generating while analytic epidemiology concerns hypothesis testing.

DESCRIPTIVE EPIDEMIOLOGY

Rates

The three descriptive measurements of chief concern for the cancer epidemiologist are incidence, mortality, and survival. The former two are often defined as:

$$\text{Incidence} = \frac{\text{New cases of cancer during a specified time period}}{\text{Population at risk (free of cancer at the start of the period)}}$$

$$\text{Mortality} = \frac{\text{Deaths from cancer during a specified time period (usually a year)}}{\text{Midperiod population}}$$

"Incidence" is defined somewhat differently depending on the context in which it is used. For most descriptive purposes the definition above is used and the population at risk is taken as the midperiod population. In the context of analytic studies one may encounter the "instantaneous incidence rate" or the "incidence density" (21). Mortality is, of course, the incidence of death. Survival is not as simply

defined in chronic diseases such as cancer because of
the variable and often long periods of observation
between case identification and death. The methods
of survival analysis are described in other chapters
in the context of clinical trials (Chapters 10-12)
and are applicable in epidemiologic studies.

Survival rates have been used to provide information on patient prognosis and to compare prognosis
among different demographic groups of cancer patients
(2). Some authors have used survival data as an indicator of progress (or lack of progress) in the "war
on cancer" (12), although the use of survival data
for this purpose has its critics (9).

Vital Statistics and Tumor Registries as Sources of Data

For cancer mortality estimation, the vital statistics system and the Census Bureau population counts
provide the necessary data. Incidence estimation requires either a special survey, such as occurred in
1937-1938, 1947, and 1969-1971, or a population-based
tumor registry. Few cases of cancer (except perhaps
for nonmelanoma skin cancers) escape hospitalization
or some form of recording in a cancer treatment facility. Consequently, by assembling data from hospital records and records in other cancer treatment and
diagnostic facilities one may obtain a reasonably
complete count of cancer cases. An objective of a
population-based tumor registry is to record all newly
diagnosed (or incident) cases of cancer occurring
among the population residing within defined geographic boundaries. This is done by reviewing and ab-
stracting records in all hospitals in the area, records in hospitals in adjacent areas (to locate cases
diagnosed outside their residence area), records of
private radiotherapy clinics and pathology laboratories, and information gathered from death certificates. Since a cancer patient is likely to receive
services and treatments in several facilities, there

are difficulties in reconciling duplicate entries
from the various record sources and determining which
episode constituted the initial diagnosis. Nevertheless, population-based tumor registries form the most
common source for obtaining cancer incidence rates.

A program supported by the National Cancer Institute and entitled SEER (Surveillance, Epidemiology,
and End Results) consists of 10 population-based tumor
registries. The populations covered by these registries are entire states (Connecticut, Iowa, Utah, New
Mexico, Hawaii, Puerto Rico) or large metropolitan
areas (Detroit, San Francisco-Oakland), sometimes with
neighboring counties (Seattle together with the Olym-
pic peninsula, Atlanta together with several neighboring rural counties). The SEER registries collect both
incidence and survival data on their respective populations. Connecticut, now among the SEER registries,
is the best known and oldest of population-based
tumor registries in the United States and has incidence data going back to 1935. Often, in epidemiologic studies where an investigator wishes to compare
cancer incidence in a particular group with general
population incidence (see below), the data from the
Connecticut Tumor Registry serve as the reference or
"control" group. Further details on SEER operations
are described in an evaluation report of the SEER Program (3), and in SEER publications (34).

There are a number of other population-based tumor
registries in the United States; two of the larger
ones cover New York State and Los Angeles County, respectively. Both these registries measure only incidence and not patient survival.

Three Questions

The three basic questions of descriptive epidemiology are when? where? who? In other words, descriptive cancer epidemiology concerns how cancer is dis-·
tributed in a population with regard to time, place,
and person and combinations of these characteristics.

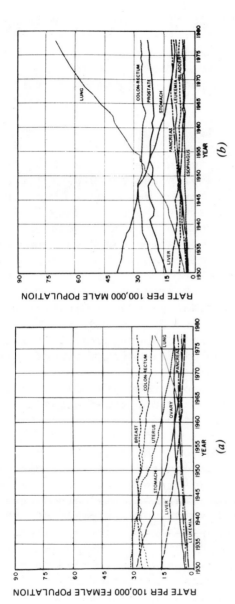

(a)

(b)

Figure 1a. Female cancer death
rates by site -- United States,
1930-1978. Rate for the female
population standardized for age
on the 1970 U.S. population.
Courtesy American Cancer Society,
Inc.

Figure 1b. Male cancer death
rates by site -- United States,
1930-1978. Rate for the male
population standardized for age
on the 1970 U.S. population.
Courtesy American Cancer Society,
Inc.

27

A fourth question, how?, is often the outcome of descriptive epidemiology and leads to the generation of
etiologic hypotheses to explain the findings concerning time, place, and person. Some examples of cancer
epidemiology dealing with each of these characteristics follow.

Time

Figure 1 displays trends in age-adjusted mortality
rates for cancers of several sites for U.S. males and
females, 1930-1978 (1). For males, the two most dramatic mortality trends are the sharp increase in lung
cancer and the steady decrease in stomach cancer.
For females, lung cancer mortality has been increasing, dramatically rising since about 1965. Mortality
from stomach cancer and uterine cervical cancer has
declined considerably. In Chapter 3 is an analysis of
time trends in cancer incidence rates. Clearly, the
correct analysis of these trends, in addition to suggesting etiologic hypotheses, is essential to answering the question, "Are we experiencing a cancer epidemic?" (6,24,29).

The one statistical method underlying Figure 1 is
age adjustment or standardization, a technique described in virtually all introductory biostatistics
and epidemiology texts (see Bibliography). Standardization entails adjustment by subclassification or
stratification and two methods are employed: direct
and indirect. The age adjustment in Figure 1 consists
of direct standardization, which is the method usually
employed in presenting a summary description of a
population's cancer incidence or mortality. The
choice of a reference population and the possibility
of using an age-truncated population (excluding data
from the elderly) are issues the statistician may
need to address (5). Indirect standardization is
usually employed in cohort studies (see below). In
working with the epidemiologist one will quickly gain
familiarity with both methods.

Figure 2 displays an analysis of time trends in age-specific incidence rates of cancer of the corpus uteri among U.S. women during 1970–1975 (32).

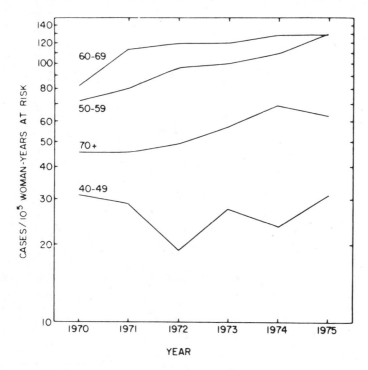

Figure 2. Incidence of cancer of the corpus uteri in the United States, corrected for the numbers of women with uteri intact, 1970–1975. Note that the vertical scale is logarithmic. Reproduced from Walker and Jick (32), "Cancer of the corpus uteri: Increasing incidence in the United States, 1970–1975." American Journal of Epidemiology 110: 47–51 (1979).

The results indicate that increasing incidence during this period was confined to women over age 50, namely, those who were postmenopausal. There was no apparent trend in incidence among women under age 50. The interesting statistical nuance in this analysis is that

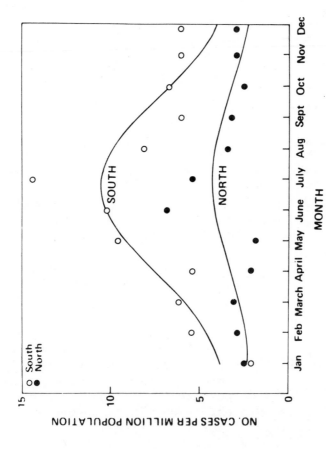

Figure 3. Incidence of skin melanomas of the upper and lower extremities in white females under age 55 years, by month of diagnosis and region. [South Region included: Atlanta, GA; Birmingham, AL; and Dallas-Ft. Worth, TX. North Region included: Detroit, MI; Iowa (entire state); Minneapolis-St. Paul, MN; and Pittsburgh, PA.] Reproduced from Scotto and Nam (28), "Skin melanoma and seasonal patterns." American Journal of Epidemiology 111: 309-314 (1980).

the denominators of women at risk of uterine cancer
have been adjusted to include only women with intact
uteri. Thus, women who have experienced a hysterec-
tomy have been excluded from the denominator since
they are, of course, not at risk of uterine cancer.
The proper statistical method for excluding hysterec-
tomized women from the denominators has been the subject of some controversy (18).

Occasionally with the analysis of disease trend
data over time, one encounters regression methods,
moving averages, or more sophisticated time series
analyses. Figure 3 also concerns effects over time
and is an analysis of seasonal incidence rates of
skin melanomas of the upper and lower extremities of
white females under age 55 in northern and southern
regions of the United States (28). The smooth, fitted curve was obtained by first-order harmonics (sine
curve models) with amplitude and phase angle estimated
by maximum likelihood. The fitted curves clearly
display a midsummer peak in incidence and the greater
amplitude in the South compared with the North. Visual inspection of Figure 3, however, indicates that
the model does not seem to fit the data particularly
well.

Place

Maps conveniently display geographic variation in
cancer rates. Figure 4 provides the distribution
among U.S. counties of mortality from cancer of the
rectum in white males for 1950-1969 (19). The counties with the highest rates (namely, the highest
decile) concentrate in New England and the mid-Atlan-
tic states. This is but one example from an atlas
prepared by NCI that depicts mortality by county for
each cancer site for U.S. white males and females
(19). There is a similar atlas of cancer mortality
for U.S. nonwhite males and females (20).

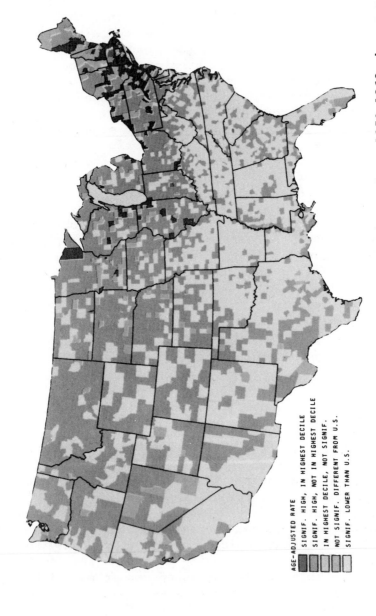

Figure 4. Mortality due to cancer of rectum for white males, 1950-1969, by county. Reproduced from Mason et al. (20).

Time and Place: Disease Clusters

The detection of clusters of disease in time and place has been of particular interest in cancer. Probably the most noted and researched cancer cluster is that of leukemia in Niles, Illinois (13). A more recently reported cluster is shown in Figure 5, which is a spot map of the occurrence of Hodgkin's disease in a rural, midwestern community of 1250 persons during the period of 1954 to 1973 (27). The striking feature of the map is the clustering of cases about a grain elevator which is the one industry of the town. The investigators concluded: "The data suggested that there was an environmental agent responsible for the elevated rates of Hodgkin's disease. ... We postulate that residents of the town are subject to chronic immune stimulation from mitogenic substances in this environment. These agents may alter immunity in the residents of this community and predispose them to acquiring Hodgkin's disease." Among the more widely employed statistical methods for analysis of a purported cluster are those of Knox (14), Mantel (17), and Ederer, Myers, and Mantel (8). A sizable literature on statistical methods for detecting disease clusters has grown. Walker (31), in a review of the history of clusters of leukemia cases, provides a useful summary of the methodology.

Person

It is difficult to undertake a descriptive analysis of cancer rates without taking into account some characteristic of person, at the least, sex and age. Figures 1 and 2, for example, each involved sex and age. Figures 3 and 4, as well as the results described in Chapter 3, involve rates specific for sex, age, and race.

Figure 6 shows variation by race in the incidence of ovarian cancer (33).

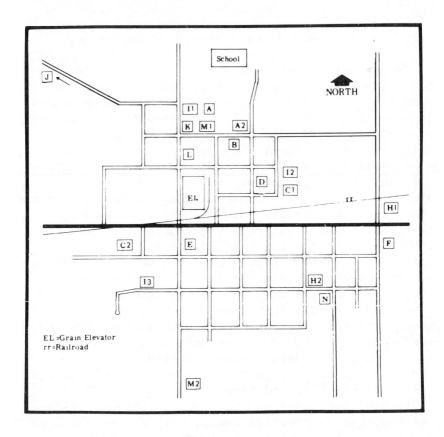

Figure 5. Schematic map of the town (total area represented, < 2.6 square kilometers). Each box indicates
a residence of a Hodgkin's disease (A-F, H-K) or lymphoma (L-N) case. Numbers to right of case letters
indicate successive residences subsequent to 1954.
(I3 and M2 are residence sites subsequent to diagnosis
of disease.) Reproduced from Schwartz et al. (27),
"A cluster of Hodgkin's disease in a small community:
Evidence for environmental factors." American Journal
of Epidemiology 108: 19-26 (1978).

The data for this analysis came from 4 population-
based tumor registries; these included 3 registries in

the SEER Program (Hawaii, New Mexico, and San Francisco-Oakland), and the Los Angeles County registry.

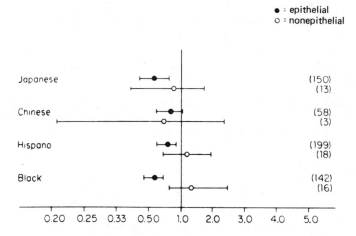

Figure 6. Ratio of incidence rate of epithelial and
nonepithelial ovarian cancer in women of 4 racial-
ethnic groups to rate in white women, standardized
for age and area, with 95% confidence limits. Number
of nonwhite cases in parentheses. Reproduced from
Weiss and Peterson (33), "Racial variation in the incidence of ovarian cancer in the United States."
American Journal of Epidemiology 107: 91-95 (1978).

The figure depicts for epithelial and nonepithelial
ovarian cancer the ratio of incidence rates in each
of Japanese, Chinese, Hispanic, and black women to
those in white women. The bars indicate 95% confidence limits on these summary ratios. For nonepithelial ovarian cancers there are no significant differences for each racial group compared with white women
since all the corresponding bars embrace a ratio of
1.0. For epithelial ovarian cancers, however, the
rate in each of Japanese, Hispanic, and black women
is significantly lower (P<.05) than in white women.

The rate in Chinese women is of borderline significance at the 5% level compared with whites.

The statistical analysis of these results is far
from trivial. The key results are the 95% confidence
limits on the summary ratio of the incidence rate in
each racial group to that of white women. Furthermore, as the legend indicates, the analysis was standardized for age and geographic area. Each point de-
picted in Figure 6 is a summary ratio of its several
component age-area specific ratios. What was required
was the sampling variation of a summary ratio that
consisted of a weighted average of several ratios of
random variables.

ECOLOGIC RELATIONSHIPS

Ecologic studies involve groups of groups rather
than individual persons. Cancer incidence and mortality data for various groups, usually geographically
defined, are available in published form or can easily
be derived from data files of tumor registries or
vital statistics offices. One can then relate these
cancer occurrence data to a wide variety of other data
available for these same geographic groups.

Figure 7 is an example of an ecologic correlation
where the groups consist of countries. The figure depicts the relation between age-adjusted breast cancer
mortality rates (ordinate) and per capita consumption
of dietary fat (abscissa) (4). The scatter diagram
clearly shows a strong correlation, a result that has
been used to support the notion that dietary fat consumption may be important in the risk of breast cancer.

Table 1 is another example of an ecologic relationship where the groups are 46 U.S. cities (10). The
dependent variable is cancer mortality rate (from all
cancers) while the independent variable is whether or
not the city had fluoridated water supplies during
the period 1969-1971.

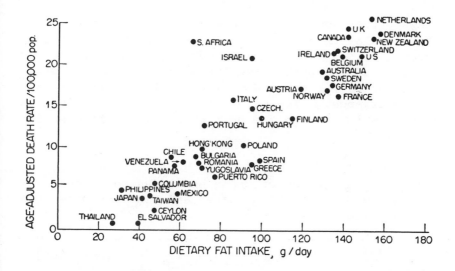

Figure 7. Correlation between age-adjusted death rates from female breast cancer and per capita consumption of fat. Reproduced from Carroll and Khor (4).

The first line in Table 1 shows the crude cancer death rates in the fluoridated and nonfluoridated cities. (The crude cancer death rates are simply the total numbers of cancer deaths divided by the respective total populations, without regard to any other factors such as sex, age, or race.) The overall crude cancer death rate in the fluoridated cities was 24% higher than in the nonfluoridated cities. Concerned about other factors that might distinguish fluoridated versus nonfluoridated cities, the investigator considered first the possibility of differences in age, race, and sex compositions of the two groups of cities and adjusted his results to remove the effects of these variables. (In this instance, he employed the indirect method of standardization.) This adjustment reduced the ratio to an 8% higher rate in the fluoridated cities. In addition, the investigator sought to investigate the effect of yet other factors on

this difference and, in particular, made adjustments
for population density, median education, median income, and, as a measure of industrialization, the percentage of the work force employed in manufacturing.
He adjusted for these 4 variables by weighted analysis
of covariance. (The weighting was necessary since the
cities which formed the unit of analysis differed in
size.)

TABLE 1. Comparison of Crude and Adjusted Cancer
Mortality Rates in Fluoridated and Nonfluoridated U.S.
Cities, 1969-1971[a]

Cancer mortality rate	Cancer mortality rates (per 1000)		
	24 fluoridated cities	22 non-fluoridated cities	Ratio (F/non-F)
Crude	206.6	183.0	1.24
Age, race, and sex adjusted	199.9	192.3	1.08
ANCOVA adjusted[b]	195.3	196.9	.99

[a]Data from Erickson (10). Reprinted, by permission of
The New England Journal of Medicine, 298: 1113 (1978).
[b]In addition to age, race, and sex, rates were adjusted for population density, median education, median income, and percentage of the work force employed in manufacturing.

The last line of Table 1 indicates that, with adjustment for these latter 4 variables, cancer mortal-

ity in the fluoridated cities was approximately the
same as that of the nonfluoridated cities. This example, in addition to illustrating an ecologic relation,
dramatically indicates the importance in observational
studies of accounting and adjusting for the effects
of disturbing, or as defined later, confounding variables.

A third example of ecologic correlation deals with
60 rural counties [i.e., non-SMSA (Standard Metropolitan Statistical Area)] in Iowa as groups where the
dependent variable is incidence of acute and chronic
lymphoid leukemia by sex and the independent variable
is density of various farm animals (7). Table 2
shows the results of tests of rank correlation. Acute
lymphoid leukemia in males exhibited significant correlation with density of cows, pigs, and chickens,
the strongest correlation being that with cows. In
further analyses, counties were grouped by thirds according to per capita total cattle population and
dairy cattle population. The gradient in incidence of
acute lymphoid leukemia was strongest for per capita
dairy cattle. From these results the authors generated 3 plausible etiologic hypotheses: consumption
of unpasteurized milk, direct occupational contact
with infected animals, and bites from hematophagous
insects.

Ecologic correlations, although often easily performed with readily available data, need cautious interpretation. One is tempted to draw conclusions
about individuals when, in fact, it is groups (and
rather large groups usually) that form the units of
observation and analysis. Individual effects are
easily masked by large group effects and inferences
regarding individuals are unwarranted. Furthermore,
ecologic correlations are particularly vulnerable to
the effects of intervening variables, as illustrated
by the data on fluoridation and cancer mortality.
Often the effects of important intervening variables
cannot be measured and taken into account in the
analysis. At best, ecologic correlations serve to

suggest hypotheses that might be better pursued by
analytic observational studies as described in the
following section.

TABLE 2. Rank Correlations between Incidence Rates of
Lymphoid Leukemia in Humans[a] and Farm Animal Densi-
ties[b] (by County) for the Rural Counties[c] in Iowa[g]

Farm animal species	Correlation coefficients by type of lymphoid leukemia			
	Acute		Chronic	
	Male	Female	Male	Female
Cows	0.36[d]	0.05	0.01	0.09
Pigs	0.23[e]	0.04	−0.05	0.14
Chickens	0.20[f]	0.09	−0.08	0.02
Turkeys	0.13	−0.01	−0.15	0.04

[a]Human data for 1969–1971.
[b]Animal density calculated for 1969 as animals per
person.
[c]Only the 84 rural and semi-rural counties are represented here (i.e., those counties with more than 30%
of the population living in rural areas).
[d]$P<.001$.
[e]$P<.01$.
[f]$P<.05$.
[g]Adapted from Donham et al. (7), "Epidemiologic relationships of the bovine population and human leukemia
in Iowa." American Journal of Epidemiology 12: 80–92
(1980).

ANALYTIC EPIDEMIOLOGY

Analytic cancer epidemiology involves hypothesis testing and purports to determine whether individuals who have experienced a particular exposure, compared with those unexposed, have greater risk of developing cancer. The exposure might result from a personal habit (e.g., cigarette smoking, coffee drinking, consumption of some dietary constituent), occupation (e.g., benzene, asbestos, ionizing radiation), some other aspect of the environment (e.g., passive smoking, residence proximate to a toxic waste dump site, some constituent of the water supply), or use of drugs or other medical procedures (e.g., stilbestrol during pregnancy, menopausal estrogens, mammography). In fact, although the term "exposure" is employed in this chapter, it could as well refer to an inherent personal characteristic (e.g., blood type, ethnic background, presence of a particular genetic marker). A more generic label is risk factor. Usually, the concern is with increased risk of a particular form of cancer although there are analytic studies that seek to examine increased risk for all forms of cancer.

Analytic epidemiologic studies seek to estimate relative risk, defined as the following ratio of incidence rates:

$$\text{Relative risk} = \frac{\text{Incidence rate among exposed persons}}{\text{Incidence rate among unexposed persons}}$$

The relative risk provides a measure of the strength of association between exposure and disease. In an analytic epidemiologic study, the pertinent null hypothesis is that the relative risk is unity, that is, there is no increased risk of disease associated with exposure. It is not enough merely to have a test of significance of this null hypothesis. One also wishes to know the magnitude of the effect and the sampling variation as represented by the point estimate of relative risk with a corresponding confidence interval statement.

In arriving at such estimates, one must be keenly aware of the observational nature of the approach, the fact that the groups one is comparing may differ in characteristics other than the independent variables chosen for study, and that the effects of these intervening variables need to be considered. Variates that are related both to the exposure and disease are termed confounding variables. For example, there are few situations particularly in regard to cancer, where age is not related both to exposure and disease. Hence, in an analytic study of cancer epidemiology, one would anticipate, at the least, some accounting or adjustment for the potential confounding effects of age. Often several potential confounding variables prevail and one would anticipate multivariate adjustments to account for the simultaneous effects of the several confounders. The previously mentioned study comparing cancer mortality in cities with and without fluoridated water supplies considered 7 potential confounding variables: age, sex, race, population density, education, income, and percentage employment in manufacturing. Adjustment for the confounding effects of the first 3 variables was by subclassification (i.e., standardization) and for the latter 4 variables by analysis of covariance. These are not the only two methods available for handling confounding. The main point here is not the method of adjustment but the principle that simultaneous adjustment for effects of several confounding variables underlies much of contemporary analytic epidemiologic research. The example cited of fluoridated water supply and cancer emphasizes the importance of confounding. The initial observed association among crude rates was entirely explained by the confounding variables examined and disappeared after adjustment. Epidemiologists employ methods to handle confounding in both the design and analysis of their analytic studies, more often in analysis.

In addition to interest in the effects of sampling

variation and errors, the epidemiologist is greatly
concerned with nonsampling errors. Of particular importance are selection (or ascertainment) bias and
observation bias. The former deals with how study
and comparison subjects are chosen and the extent to
which selective factors could distort sample results
and bias the ultimate estimate of relative risk. The
latter deals with how information is elicited during
an investigation and the extent to which, on the part
of observers, subjects, or data sources, misclassifi-
cations and recall errors might distort and bias the
results. In most contemporary reports of analytic
epidemiologic studies one can anticipate the "Discussion" section to contain speculation regarding the
potential impact on results of various possible selection and observation biases.

The two major research strategies of analytic epidemiology are cohort and case-control studies. In
both, the concept of time is essential. In chronic
diseases such as cancer, exposure may precede disease
by many years, sometimes even decades, as with occupational exposures. The key distinction between the
cohort and case-control strategies is that cohort
studies proceed forward in time from exposure to disease while case-control studies work backward in time
from disease to history of exposure. The simplest
and most clear-cut cohort study consists of two study
groups, a group of exposed individuals and a comparable control group of individuals who are unexposed,
with both groups followed forward in time to determine
disease incidence (or mortality). The simplest and
most clear-cut case-control study also consists of two
groups, a group of diseased individuals and a comparable group of individuals free of disease, with information for both groups garnered regarding history of
exposure. The following two sections elaborate, respectively, the features of cohort and case-control
studies and indicate their relative merits and
disadvantages.

COHORT STUDIES

Principles

There are two forms of cohort studies, <u>historical</u> and <u>prospective</u>, depending on whether the disease outcome events occur before or after the onset of the actual study. A prospective cohort study is one in which the investigation proceeds from current exposure to future disease. In a historical (or retrospective) cohort study, exposure occurred in the past and the disease or mortality end points have already occurred by the start of the study. The investigator uses historical information to reconstruct the disease experience of the exposed and unexposed subjects. In cancer epidemiology these circumstances pertain particularly to occupational forms of exposure where past records of employers, unions, or professional societies can be tapped to identify the exposed and unexposed groups. Even though the data are not collected concurrently, the historical cohort strategy still proceeds from exposure to disease. Some cohort studies involve both a historical and prospective component. That is, they deal with past exposures and disease outcomes up to the present time as well as with further follow-up from the present into the future to determine additional disease outcomes.

An important feature of cohort studies is the selection of the unexposed group for comparison with the exposed. <u>Internal</u> comparisons employ a group of unexposed individuals, chosen from analogous sources as the exposed, and followed in a similar manner as the exposed. With an internal comparison, results for both exposed and unexposed are subject to sampling variation. Sometimes, however, a cohort study consists only of follow-up of an exposed group, and the investigator wishes to compare the cohort's experience with that of the general population. This situation describes an <u>external</u> comparison group. If the outcome is mortality, one may wish to compare with the

mortality experience of the total U.S. population or
the total population in some particular U.S. region.
Here, published vital statistics data would serve as
the external reference. If cancer incidence is the
outcome, figures from the SEER registries, or with a
historical cohort study that predates SEER, the Connecticut Tumor Registry, would serve as the external
reference. With an external comparison group, only
the results in the exposed cohort are subject to sampling variation; the reference figures are population
data. Clearly, despite the deceptive statistical advantage with external comparisons in which only one
set of results is subject to sampling variation, well-
chosen internal comparisons provide a firmer scientific basis for drawing conclusions. With an external
comparison group there remain lingering doubts regarding comparability with the exposed and whether, in
fact, it is the exposure itself responsible for any
estimated risk or some intervening variables whose
effects could not be taken into account when making
the comparisons.

As an aid to an adequate understanding of a cohort
study, Appendix 1 presents a set of minimal questions
one might direct to an investigator who is planning
such a study, or, alternatively, that one might pose
when reading the report of a completed study. The
first 6 questions deal generally with design (prospective or historical cohort), definitions of terms
(exposures, outcomes, follow-up), choice of controls
(internal or external), and study procedures (enrollment of exposed and controls, nature of follow-up,
and outcome determination). Question 7 deals with the
issue of choosing confounding variables and Question 8
reiterates the concern for possible distortions resulting from selection and observation biases. Satisfactory answers to these latter two questions depend
on one's substantive knowledge of the exposure and
disease. The experienced cancer epidemiologist will
know the pertinent confounding variables to examine
and will be cognizant of what specific aspects of

selection and observation bias require consideration.

Finally, Question 9 elaborates those major statistical issues in a cohort study that may require the
aid of a biostatistician: What sample size is needed
for the study; how should one best summarize results;
how can one estimate relative risk and its confidence
limits; and what methods should one employ to handle
confounding variables and calculate adjusted relative
risks with the corresponding confidence interval. In
some situations, exposed subjects can be broken down
into graded categories based on their amount and/or
duration of exposure. Here, the epidemiologist has
particular interest in determining whether the
strength of association increases with the intensity
of exposure, and may seek the biostatistician's help
in exploring these dose-response relationships. The
statistically oriented sources listed in the Bibliography provide an introduction to the armamentarium of
methods available to deal with the above statistical
issues.

Example

The National Institute of Occupational Safety and
Health (NIOSH) undertook a cohort study at the Portsmouth Naval Shipyard (PNS) to determine whether occupational exposure to low-level radiation was associated with increased risk of cancer, particularly hematologic malignancies (25). The motivation for the
study was an earlier analysis of proportional mortality (see textbooks listed in Bibliography for description of proportional mortality) that suggested that
nuclear workers at PNS had increased risks of cancer
death, particularly from leukemia and other hematopo-
ietic malignancies (22). The Navy made available to
NIOSH its employment records as well as its records
of radiation exposure obtained from readings of film
badges and dosimeters worn by those qualified for radiation work. The total study cohort consisted of
all white males ever employed at PNS between January

1, 1952, and August 15, 1977, and numbered 24,545
workers. Since the study commenced in 1978, it is
clearly of the historical cohort type with variable
lengths of follow-up and a common closing date of
August 15, 1977.

An exposed worker was defined as any man who worked
at the shipyard during this period and who had a recorded occupational cumulative radiation exposure of
.001 rem or more; 7615 men met this criterion. There
were two unexposed groups. First, there were 15,585
shipyard workers who did not wear badges and for whom
there was no record of their ever having been assigned
radiation work. Second, there were 1345 men qualified
to undertake radiation work, monitored for radiation,
but whose total recorded occupational radiation exposure was less than .001 rem. To simplify the presentation, results only for the second comparison
group are presented. (The published report indicates
that the first unexposed group, those who never undertook radiation work, is not as comparable with the exposed as is the second group, radiation-qualified
workers who remained unexposed.)

Death was the outcome under study. Once the exposed and unexposed cohorts had been assembled from
the employment and radiation records, the investigators faced the formidable task of determining the vital status as of August 15, 1977 for each of the
nearly 25,000 men in the total cohort. Many men, of
course, were no longer employed by PNS and, subsequent
to termination of their PNS employment, their wherea-
bouts were unknown. Through a variety of sources
NIOSH investigators attempted to trace these men. At
the time of report preparation (December 1980), 4% of
the total cohort remained untraced and were deemed
lost to follow-up. Among exposed and unexposed radiation-qualified workers, losses to follow-up were 2
and 3%, respectively.

Once a subject was identified as deceased, the investigators sought a copy of the death certificate
and determined the date of death. A nosologist,

TABLE 3. Results of Cohort Study of Radiation: Qualified Workers at Portsmouth Naval Shipyard and Cancer Mortality[a]

	Unexposed <.001 rem	Exposed ≥.001 rem	Exposed	
			.001-.999 rem	≥1.000 rem
N	1,345	7,615	*	*
Person-years	24,232	98,223	65,326	32,897
Deaths:				
All cancer	50	201	133	68
All hematologic cancer	2	15	7	8
Leukemia	1	7	3	4
Death rate (per 1000 person-years):				
All cancer	2.06	2.05	2.04	2.07
All hematologic cancer	0.08	0.15	0.11	0.24
Leukemia	0.04	0.07	0.05	0.12
Relative risk:				
All cancer	1	0.99	0.99	1.00
All hematologic cancer	1	1.73	1.30	2.95
Leukemia	1	1.85	1.11	2.95

[a]Data from Rinsky et al. (25).

48

unaware of the decedent's exposure status, coded the causes of death on all certificates and followed standard coding procedures (i.e., the version of the International Classification of Diseases in effect at time of death).

The first 2 columns of Table 3 display the results for the unexposed and exposed cohorts of radiation workers. The second line in the table indicates the total person-years observation in each cohort at the end of the closing date, August 15, 1977. (An assumption was made that those lost to follow-up were alive; thus, the person-years totals are somewhat inflated.) The 3 following lines indicate the numbers of deaths due to all cancers, all hematologic cancers, and leukemia. Below the deaths appear the corresponding death rates (per 1000 person-years). Finally, the last set of figures are relative risks of cancer mortality. For all cancers combined there is no increased mortality risk with exposure. For hematologic cancers and leukemia, however, exposed workers have somewhat less than double the risk of mortality.

The last 2 columns in Table 3 indicate what results would obtain with application of a more stringent definition of exposure. Exposure defined as $\geq .001$ rem encompasses persons whose occupational exposures were so minimal that they were essentially unexposed. Inclusion in the exposed group of those with infinitesimal exposures would, of course, tend to blur and obliterate any real effects of exposure. One might draw an analogy to a smoking and health study where a smoker could be defined as any person who had ever smoked a cigarette in his lifetime.

A more stringent and perhaps more useful definition of occupational radiation exposure is a cumulative lifetime record of 1 rem or more. The last column in Table 3 indicates the results of this more stringent definition. For all hematologic cancers and leukemia, radiation workers with cumulative exposure of 1 rem or more had roughly 3 times the mortality of those with no exposure. (If, in fact, the definition of exposure

had been 1 rem or more, the unexposed group would actually be the combination of columns 1 and 3 in Table
3 and the relative risks of mortality for all cancers,
all hematologic cancers, and leukemia would be 1.01,
2.72, and 2.42, respectively.)

Since information on dosage groups was available,
yet another approach is to seek a dose-response relationship. Does the risk of mortality increase with
increasing levels of cumulative recorded lifetime radiation exposure? The NIOSH investigators state, "In
the PNS radiation workers, we found no positive dose-
response relationships between ionizing radiation dose
and mortality from any cause reported," but the report
does not describe the method employed to undertake
this analysis. One of us (TC), using the published
NIOSH data, conducted a weighted regression analysis
(weights were the person-years observation in each
dosage category) of hematologic cancer death rates on,
essentially, log(cumulative lifetime dosage) and found
a slope of borderline statistical significance (P=
.067, one-tailed test). This has resulted in a controversy with NIOSH regarding the interpretation of
their data and some dispute over a variety of technical, statistical issues (23). At this writing, the
controversy has not been settled.

The results in Table 3 and those cited above are
all crude in that no account has been taken of the effects of potential confounding variables. By subclassification, the NIOSH investigators considered the
following confounding variables: age, calendar time,
time since initial PNS employment, and duration of
employment. The method of analysis employed, however,
did not permit calculation of adjusted mortality rates
per person-year observation among exposed and unexposed. The NIOSH investigators employed an external
control, U.S. white male cause-specific mortality, to
each of their exposed and unexposed cohorts and, using
indirect standardization, calculated standard mortality ratios (SMRs) in each group. As a rough indication of the effect of adjustment for confounding on

the estimate of relative risk one may calculate the ratio of the SMRs in the exposed and unexposed cohorts. This yields ratios of SMRs for total cancer, hematologic cancers, and leukemia of 1.09, 2.06, and 1.94, respectively. These are larger than the unadjusted relative risks at the foot of column 1 in Table 3, indicating that adjustment for confounding effects of these 4 variables seems to enhance rather than moderate the unadjusted relative risks previously discussed. Other potential confounding variables one might wish to consider include smoking and occupational exposure to known carcinogens such as asbestos and benzene. Unfortunately, this information was not available for the cohort so adjustments for these possible confounding effects could not be undertaken.

Features of Cohort Studies

The relative merits of the cohort strategy emerge distinctly from the example of the NIOSH study of PNS workers. Cohort studies tend to be large, time consuming, and expensive. The NIOSH study involved tracking and determining the vital status of some 25,000 men, a task that required considerable staff effort and took nearly 3 years to complete. Although no specific budget items have been published, estimates in excess of $1 million have been mentioned at various meetings.

Cohort studies are particularly difficult when the disease is rare. The NIOSH study illustrates this clearly with regard to leukemia or even all hematologic malignancies. Among the total cohort of 25,000 the investigators found only 39 leukemia deaths and 84 deaths from all hematologic malignancies. The exposed cohort (i.e., $\geq$.001 rem cumulative lifetime dose), consisting of over 7500 men, yielded only 7 leukemia deaths and 15 deaths from all hematologic malignancies. Clearly, even under the circumstances of a possible threefold increase in relative risk, death from leukemia and hematologic malignancies remains a rare event.

Among the advantages of a cohort study is its provision of a direct estimate of rates, particularly within the exposed group. With an internal control group, one can examine relative risk by direct calculation of the ratio of two incidence rates. This was clearly evident in Table 3 with the NIOSH study.

The above circumstances provide cohort studies with the distinct advantage of greater intuitive appeal, particularly for those who are unfamiliar with epidemiologic methods. The cohort strategy of exposure to disease and the direct calculation of incidence or mortality rates are features easily comprehended by those familiar with the experimental method but with little background in epidemiology. As will be seen later, both the strategy and end results of case-control studies require greater knowledge of epidemiologic methods and are not as clear to the uninitiated as are cohort study methods and results.

Cohort studies of the historical type are often ideal when a reasonably large exposed group can be readily assembled from records. Accordingly, this study method has been used frequently to elucidate the relationship between occupational exposure and cancer risk. In general, cohort studies are best suited to situations where the exposure is relatively rare and the disease is relatively common.

CASE-CONTROL STUDIES

Principles

The case-control study starts with identification of a case group with the disease in question, and a control group without the disease. Controls may be individuals with other diseases or may be apparently healthy individuals selected from the general population. The study strategy proceeds "retrospectively" to determine history of exposure among cases and controls.

Case-control studies may use a matched or unmatched control group. In matched studies, control subjects are paired with cases, with each control selected to be similar to a case with regard to predetermined matching characteristics, (e.g., sex, race, age, and other potential confounders). If the disease is particularly rare and cases are scarce, study power may be increased by selecting more than 1 control for each case (although the law of diminishing returns begins to operate early and little is gained beyond a 4:1 control to case ratio). In unmatched studies controls are selected only in accordance with general criteria, such as a specified age range, residence, or medical facility. The methods of analysis for matched and unmatched studies differ somewhat, but the principles of analysis are the same.

Appendix 2 contains a series of pertinent questions for assessment of a case-control study. These questions deal with design (source and selection of cases), choice of controls, definition of terms (disease, exposure), study procedures (enrollment of cases and controls, nature of solicitation of information regarding history of exposure), choice of pertinent confounding variables, and possible distortions resulting from potential selection and observation biases. The major statistical concerns are choice of controls, matching cases and controls as a means of controlling confounding (what factors to match, the effect on validity and statistical efficiency, possible adverse consequences of overmatching), methods for estimating relative risk and its confidence limits, methods for handling confounding variables and calculating adjusted relative risks and their confidence limits, sample size determination, and, when appropriate, methods to explore dose-response relationships (i.e., whether the estimate of relative risk increases with increasing level and/or intensity of the history of exposure).

The result of a case-control study is an estimate

of relative risk obtained in an unmatched study from
calculation of the odds ratio. A discussion of the
basis for the odds ratio as an estimate of relative
risk appears in virtually every introductory epidemiology text (see Bibliography). In simplest terms, if
among cases $\underline{a}$ provide a history of exposure and $\underline{b}$ do
not while among controls $\underline{c}$ have a history of exposure
and $\underline{d}$ do not, then

$$\text{Odds ratio = Estimate of relative risk} = \frac{ad}{bc}.$$

If the study has employed one to one matching, then
the estimate of relative risk is given by the ratio
of untied pairs, that is, the number of matched pairs
where case has history of exposure and control does
not, divided by the number of matched pairs where control has history of exposure and case does not. If
more than one control is matched for each case, analogous methods are used.

   Methods for handling confounding in the analysis
of case-control studies as well as the means for determining corresponding confidence limits have been
the foci of a considerable amount of statistical investigation. In fact, there is an extensive literature on the statistical aspects of the case-control
study including both its design and analysis. A good
starting place for the reader who wishes to explore
these methods for case-control studies is one of the
more statistically oriented texts listed in the Bibliography.

Example

   A case-control study that has garnered considerable
public attention is that associating coffee drinking
with pancreatic cancer (16). The study's initial aim
in regard to pancreatic cancer was to reevaluate the
role of cigarette smoking (which had emerged as a risk
factor in previous studies), "to examine alcohol consumption as a possible confounding variable," and to

consider tea and coffee as "factors that have not been
adequately investigated in this disease."

Cases consisted of "patients with histologic diagnoses of cancer of the exocrine pancreas who were in
any of 11 large hospitals in the Boston metropolitan
area and Rhode Island between October 1974 and August
1979." Of 578 patients identified, 405 were interviewed and 38 subsequently excluded (nonwhite,
non-U.S. resident, over 79 years old, or interview information judged to be of questionable reliability),
leaving 367 as the total number of cases for the study
in relation to coffee.

For selection of controls,

"interviewers also attempted to question all other
patients who were under the care of the same physician in the same hospital at the time of an interview with a patient with pancreatic cancer. Either
before the interview (if the information was known)
or afterward, patients with diseases of the pancreas or hepatobiliary tract or diseases known to be
associated with smoking or alcohol consumption were
excluded."

Of 1118 eligible patients, a group of 700 was interviewed, and further winnowed down (employing the same
criteria above as with cases) to yield 643 total controls for the study. Controls in this study consisted
of patients with cancer other than that of the pancreas and biliary tract and a variety of other noncancer
conditions.

With regard to soliciting information on exposure
by personal interviews of cases and controls,

"Several questions in the interview probed the duration and intensity of smoking of cigarettes, ci-
gars, and pipes. Questions on alcoholic beverages
asked about the frequency of use before the onset
of illness, the age span over which such use occurred, and the type of beverage used most

frequently. The questions on tea and coffee were limited to the number of cups consumed in a typical day before the current illness was evident."

A coffee drinker was defined as someone who responded that his daily coffee consumption was one or more cups. Table 4 shows the results in the form of a fourfold table for all subjects and separately for men and women.

TABLE 4. Results of Case-Control Study of Coffee Drinking and Pancreatic Cancer[a]

	Total		Men		Women	
	Cases	Con-trols	Cases	Con-trols	Cases	Con-trols
Coffee drinker						
Yes	347	555	207	275	140	280
No	20	88	9	32	11	56
Total	367	643	216	307	151	336
Crude relative risk	2.75		2.7		2.5	
Relative risk adjusted for age[b]			2.6		2.3	
(95% conf. lim.)[b]			(1.2-5.4)		(1.2-4.6)	

[a]Data from MacMahon et al. (16). Reprinted, by permission of The New England Journal of Medicine, 304: 632, (1981).
[b]Not available for total group from published report.

Below each table crude relative risk appears, as calculated by the odds ratio estimate (ratio of cross products). Below the crude relative risks, the relative risks adjusted for age appear along with their corresponding 95% confidence limits. Note that each of the relative risks for men and women is elevated and statistically significant, at least at the 5% level. Further analyses indicated increased relative risk with increasing coffee consumption, a gradient that was highly statistically significant (P<.001).

Since the investigators found a positive association with smoking, they were concerned with the effects of smoking as a possible confounding variable in the relationship with coffee drinking. It certainly seems plausible that smoking would likely be associated with both pancreatic cancer and coffee drinking and thus indeed constitute a confounding variable. Analysis of the gradient with coffee consumption was conducted within each of 3 smoking categories (those who never smoked, exsmokers, current smokers) and overall with adjustment for smoking (as well as adjustment for age and sex as in previous analyses). The investigators found "a consistent association of pancreatic cancer with coffee drinking within each category of smoking and ... a consistent trend with coffee drinking after adjustment for smoking."

Thus, there remained a significant relationship of coffee drinking with pancreatic cancer, even after adjustment for the confounding effects of sex, age, and cigarette smoking. Furthermore, there was a gradient in the adjusted relative risk: As the amount of current coffee consumption increased, the estimated relative risk of pancreatic cancer increased.

The investigators recommended caution in interpretation of this finding, particularly since the association was unexpected and was not an a priori hypothesis underlying the investigation. They state that "the positive association with coffee consumption that we observed must be evaluated with other data before

serious consideration is given to the possibility of
a causal relation."

Among the considerable discussion and reaction this
report received, one group of investigators raised a
number of possible selection and observation biases
that would tend to make the reported association spurious (11). We leave it to the interested reader to
peruse this critique to judge the plausibility of the
specific selection and observation biases raised.

Features

Compared with cohort studies, case-control studies
tend to be smaller in size, relatively rapidly completed, and relatively inexpensive. They are suited
particularly to circumstances where the exposure is
common and the disease is rare. This was clearly the
situation with the study of coffee drinking and pancreatic cancer. Certainly, in the United States, exposure to coffee is quite common: In the study, 86%
of the controls reported coffee consumption of a cup
or more per day. Likewise, pancreatic cancer is quite
rare: Results from the SEER tumor registries indicate
an average annual incidence rate (age-adjusted) for
pancreatic cancer of 10 per 100,000 per year (34).

Consider the size of an analogous cohort study to
examine this relationship. With specification of a
5% significance level (two-sided) for testing the null
hypothesis of a relative risk of unity and a power of
80% of an alternative relative risk of 2.5, and with
an assumed follow-up of 10 years per subject, one
would have to enroll over 12,000 coffee drinking subjects and a like number of non-coffee drinkers.
[These calculations obtain from a method of sample
size determination in cohort studies provided by
Schlesselman (26).] In total this would entail
roughly 500,000 person-years of follow-up. The advantages of the case-control study in this particular
situation are evident.

Case-control studies, as exemplified by the data

and calculations in Table 4, do not yield absolute
rates but do permit accurate estimation of relative
risk. Relative risks from case-control studies depend
on the calculation of an odds ratio and the knowledge
that, under certain conditions, this yields an estimate of relative risk. Interpretation of results of
case-control studies requires a degree of epidemiologic knowledge and sophistication. For those unfamiliar
with epidemiologic methods, the case-control study requires more thought and explanation and lacks the simple, intuitive appeal of the cohort study.

Finally, as a corollary to the above-mentioned circumstances favoring the case-control approach, a circumstance unfavorable to the case-control approach is
rare exposure.

ASSOCIATION TO CAUSATION

Whether one can deduce causal relationships from
associations found in epidemiologic studies has been
a subject of much controversy over the years. In one
sense, this involves basic philosophical perspectives,
one's personal definition of "cause," and one's standards for what constitutes adequate proof. Results of
analytic epidemiologic studies have been dismissed at
times by the pejorative, "After all, it's only a statistical association found in an observational study."

There are strong contrary arguments that when results of observational studies meet certain requirements, they can indeed culminate in causal inferences.
Causal conclusions are best assessed with collation of
results from a variety of studies conducted with differing groups of subjects under different circumstances and with somewhat different methods of investigation. A set of requirements for inferring causal-
ity from observational studies that has received considerable use appears in Appendix 3, with some elabo-
ration of each.

An excellent illustration of the application of

these requirements is the original Surgeon General's
report in 1964 on smoking and health and, in particular, the strong causal conclusion regarding cigarette
smoking and lung cancer (30). The report contains one
of the earlier published versions and discussions of
the requirements listed in Appendix 3. With regard
to analytic epidemiologic studies, the committee members who prepared the report reviewed 7 studies of the
cohort type and 29 of the case-control type. These,
together with the results of laboratory experiments,
other basic science data, pathologic data, and clinical information, satisfied the requirements in Appendix 3 (except for item 6) and led to the causal conclusion of smoking and lung cancer that few, if any,
now dispute.

APPENDIX 1. QUESTIONS FOR ASSESSMENT OF A COHORT STUDY

1. Is the design a prospective cohort, historical cohort, or some combination?

2. What is the definition of exposure? Is it clear,
   workable, and applicable in identifying exposed individuals?

3. How are exposed subjects ascertained? What are the
   sources and over what period of time? What specific procedures and criteria are employed to enter
   exposed subjects into the study?

4. What is the nature of the unexposed group? Is it
   an external or internal comparison? If internal,
   what matching criteria with exposed, if any, are
   employed in selecting unexposed? What specific
   procedures and criteria are employed to enter unexposed subjects into the study?

5. What is the main outcome variable? Is it incidence, mortality, or something else? Is the

definition of outcome clear, workable, and applicable in determining equivalently, among exposed and unexposed, which subjects have reached end points?

6. What is the nature of follow-up? Is the duration of follow-up a fixed time period or variable time (e.g., common closing date)? Is active or passive (i.e., death clearance) follow-up employed? If active, what specifically constitutes follow-up, how frequently, and does it apply equally to exposed and unexposed?

7. What potential confounding variables are considered? Are any possible important confounding variables neglected?

8. What are potential selection and observation biases and what possible distorting effects might they have on results?

9. Statistical considerations:

a. How are results presented? Rates per person-year observation, ratios of observed to expected numbers resulting from indirect standardization (i.e., Standardized Morbidity or Mortality Ratios), or some other method?

b. What method is employed for estimating relative risk and determining its confidence limits?

c. What method is employed to make adjustments for confounding variables?

d. What is the rationale for choice of sample size or what power considerations have been employed?

e. If applicable, what method is employed to explore a dose-response gradient with exposure?

APPENDIX 2. QUESTIONS FOR ASSESSMENT OF A CASE-CONTROL
STUDY

1. What is the definition of "disease"? Is the definition clear, workable, and applicable in identifying cases?

2. How are cases ascertained? What are the sources,
over what period of time, for identifying cases?
What specific procedures and criteria are employed
to enroll cases into the study?

3. What is the nature of the control group free of the
"disease"? What are the sources for selecting controls (hospital with or without restriction to certain control-disease categories, neighborhood, or
some other type)? What matching criteria or other
criteria to ensure comparability are employed in
selecting controls? What specific procedures and
criteria are employed to enroll control subjects
into the study?

4. What is the definition of exposure? Is the definition of exposure clear, workable, and applicable
in determining equivalently among cases and controls who might have been exposed?

5. How is the history of exposure determined among
cases and controls? Is it gathered by review of
past records, respondents' self-reporting by questionnaires, interviews of respondents by telephone
or in person, or some other means? Is the respond-
ent the identified case or control or some proxy
(e.g., family member or neighbor)?

6. What potential confounding variables are considered? Are any possible important confounding variables neglected?

7. What are the potential selection and observation

biases and what distorting effects might they have
on results?

8. Statistical considerations:

  a. How should controls be selected? What, if any,
     matching criteria should be applied in selecting
     controls? How many controls per case should be
     selected?

  b. What method is employed for estimating relative
     risk and determining its confidence limits?

  c. What method is employed to make adjustments for
     confounding variables?

  d. What is the rationale for choice of sample size
     or what power considerations have been employed?

  e. If applicable, what methods are employed to ex-
     plore a dose-response gradient with exposure?

APPENDIX 3. REQUIREMENTS FOR ESTABLISHING CAUSATION
        FROM ANALYTIC OBSERVATIONAL STUDIES

1. Strength of the association.

   How large is the estimated relative risk?

2. Consistency of the association.

   Is the association found consistently with different studies of different populations using different methods of investigation?

   Are the estimated relative risks from different
   studies reasonably homogeneous?

3. Biologic credibility.

Is the association compatible with existing scientific knowledge both in the basic and clinical sciences?

Do the results dovetail with current theories of biologic mechanisms?

4. Time sequence: Exposure precedes disease.

Is there evidence that the exposure precedes the disease sufficiently in time in accord with the biologic credibility of the causal relationship?

5. Dose-response gradient.

Does the strength of the association increase as the amount, duration, or intensity of exposure increases?

6. Specificity of the association.

Is the association specific for a particular disease or some group of diseases?

Note. In practice, this requirement often fails to be satisfied; for example, cigarette smoking, which is causally related to lung cancer, is also causally related to a number of other cancers as well as to cardiovascular and respiratory diseases. With cancer, a more plausible causal relationship prevails when particular cancers are involved. One would be skeptical of a proposed causal relationship for an exposure associated with an increase in all forms of cancer.

REFERENCES

1. American Cancer Society (1982), Cancer Facts and Figures, American Cancer Society, New York.

2. Axtell, L. M., and Myers, M. H. (1978), Contrasts in survival of black and white cancer patients, Journal of the National Cancer Institute 60: 1209-1215.

3. Bagne, C., Fayen, E., et al. (1978), Evaluation of the Surveillance, Epidemiology and End Results Program of the National Cancer Institute, National Technical Information Service PB-80-105082.

4. Carroll, K. K., and Khor, H. T. (1975), Dietary fat in relation to tumorigenesis, Progress in Biochemical Pharmacology 10: 308-353.

5. Doll, R., and Cook, P. (1967), Summarizing indices for comparison of cancer incidence data, International Journal of Cancer 2: 269-279.

6. Doll, R., and Peto, R. (1981), The causes of cancer: Quantitative estimates of avoidable risks of cancer in the United States today, Journal of the National Cancer Institute 66: 1191-1308.

7. Donham, K. J., Berg, J. W., and Sawin, R. S. (1980), Epidemiologic relationships of the bovine population and human leukemia in Iowa, American Journal of Epidemiology 12: 80-92.

8. Ederer, F., Myers, M. H., and Mantel, N. (1964), A statistical problem in space and time -- Do leukemia cases come in clusters? Biometrics 20: 626-638.

9. Enstrom, J. E., and Austin, D. F. (1977), Interpreting cancer survival rates, Science 195: 847-851.

10. Erickson, J. D. (1978), Mortality in selected cities with fluoridated and nonfluoridated water

supplies, The New England Journal of Medicine,
298: 1112-1116.

11. Feinstein, A. R., Horwitz, R. I., Spitzer, W. O.,
and Battista, R. N. (1981), Coffee and pancreatic
cancer: The problems of etiologic science and epidemiologic case-control research, Journal of
the American Medical Association 246: 957-961.

12. Greenberg, D. S. (1975), Progress in cancer research -- Don't say it isn't so, The New England
Journal of Medicine 292: 707-708.

13. Heath, C. W., Jr., and Hasterlik, R. J. (1963),
Leukemia among children in a suburban community,
American Journal of Medicine 34: 796-812.

14. Knox, G. (1964), Epidemiology of childhood leukemia in Northumberland and Durham, British Journal
of Preventive and Social Medicine 18: 17-24.

15. MacMahon, B., and Pugh, T. F. (1970), Epidemiology: Principles and Methods, Little, Brown,
Boston.

16. MacMahon, B., Yen, S., Trichopoulos, D.,
Warren, K., and Nardi, G. (1981), Coffee and can-
cer of the pancreas, The New England Journal of
Medicine 304: 630-633.

17. Mantel, N. (1967), The detection of disease clustering and a generalized regression approach,
Cancer Research, 27: 209-220.

18. Marrett, L. D. (1980), Estimates of the true population at risk of uterine disease and an application to incidence data for cancer of the uterine
corpus in Connecticut, American Journal of Epidemiology 111: 373-379.

19. Mason, T. J., McKay, F. W., Blot, W. J., and Fraumeni, J. F., Jr. (1975), Atlas of Cancer Mortality for U.S. Counties: 1950-1969, U.S. Department of Health, Education and Welfare [DHEW Pub. No. (NIH) 75-780], Washington, D.C.

20. Mason, T. J., McKay, F. W., Hoover, R., Blot, W. J., and Fraumeni, J. F., Jr. (1976), Atlas of Cancer Mortality among Nonwhites: 1950-1969, U.S. Department of Health, Education and Welfare [DHEW Pub. No. (NIH) 76-1204], Washington, D.C.

21. Morgenstern, H., Kleinbaum, D. G., and Kupper, L. L. (1980), Measures of disease incidence used in epidemiologic research, International Journal of Epidemiology 9: 97-104.

22. Najarian, T., and Colton, T. (1978), Mortality from leukemia and cancer in shipyard nuclear workers, The Lancet 1: 1018-1020.

23. National Institute of Occupational Safety and Health (1981), Progress report of CDC/NIOSH study of nuclear propulsion and other shipyard workers -- period of January 1 to March 31, 1981, unpublished memorandum, National Institute of Occupational Safety and Health, Cincinnati, Ohio.

24. Pollack, E. S., and Horm, J. W. (1980), Trends in cancer incidence and mortality in the United States, 1969-1976, Journal of the National Cancer Institute 64(5): 1091-1103.

25. Rinsky, R. A., Zumwalde, R. D., Waxweiler, R. J., Murrary, W. E., Jr., Bierbaum, P. J., Landrigan, P. J., Terpilak, M., and Cox, C. (1981), Cancer mortality at a naval nuclear shipyard, The Lancet 1: 231-235.

26. Schlesselman, J. J. (1974), Sample size require-
    ments in cohort and case-control studies of
    disease, American Journal of Epidemiology 99: 381-
    384.

27. Schwartz, R. S., Callen, J. P., and Silva, J., Jr.
    (1978), A cluster of Hodgkin's disease in a small
    community: Evidence for environmental factors,
    American Journal of Epidemiology 108: 19-26.

28. Scotto J., and Nam, J. M. (1980), Skin melanoma
    and seasonal patterns, American Journal of Epide-
    miology 111: 309-314.

29. Smith, R. J. (1980), Government says cancer rate
    is increasing, Science 209: 998-1002.

30. United States Public Health Service (1964), Smok-
    ing and Health: Report of the Advisory Committee
    to the Surgeon General of the Public Health Serv-
    ice, U.S. Government Printing Office, Washington,
    D.C.

31. Walker, A. M. (1981), The clustering of leukemia:
    A review of history, strategies and results, un-
    published manuscript, Sidney Farber Cancer Insti-
    tute, Boston.

32. Walker, A. M., and Jick, H. (1979), Cancer of the
    corpus uteri: Increasing incidence in the United
    States, 1970-1975, American Journal of Epidemiol-
    ogy 110: 47-51.

33. Weiss, N. S., and Peterson, A. A. (1978), Racial
    variation in the incidence of ovarian cancer in
    the United States, American Journal of Epidemiolo-
    gy 107: 91-95.

34. Young, J. L., Jr., Percy, C. L., and Asire, A. J.
    (1981), Surveillance, Epidemiology and End

Results: Incidence and Mortality Data, 1973-77,
National Cancer Institute Monograph 57 [DHHS Pub.
No. (NIH) 81-2330], Washington, D.C.

BIBLIOGRAPHY

The following sources are for those readers who wish
to delve further into principles of epidemiology in
general, cancer epidemiology in particular, and statistical methods in epidemiology.

General Epidemiology Texts

Friedman, G. D. (1980), Primer of Epidemiology (2nd
ed.), McGraw-Hill, New York.

Lillienfeld, A. M., and Lillienfeld, D. E. (1981),
Foundations of Epidemiology, Oxford University Press,
New York.

MacMahon, B., and Pugh, T. F. (1970), Epidemiology:
Principles and Methods, Little, Brown, Boston.

Mausner, J. S., and Bahn, A. K. (1974), Epidemiology:
An Introductory Text, Saunders, Philadelphia.

Texts Specializing in Cancer Epidemiology

Fraumeni, J. F., Jr., ed. (1975), Persons at High
Risk of Cancer, Academic Press, New York.

Lillienfeld, A. M., Pederson, E., and Dowd, J. E.
(1967), Cancer Epidemiology: Methods, Johns Hopkins
Press, Baltimore.

Schottenfeld, D., and Fraumeni, J. F., Jr., eds.
(1981), Cancer Epidemiology and Prevention, Saunders,
Philadelphia.

Texts with Orientation to Statistical Methods in
Epidemiology

Anderson, A., Auquier, A., Hauck, W. W., Oakes, D.,
Vandaele, W., and Weisberg, H. (1980), Statistical
Methods for Comparative Studies, Wiley, New York.

Breslow, N. E., and Day, N. E. (1980), The analysis of
case-control studies, Statistical Methods in Cancer
Research, Vol. 1, International Agency for Research on
Cancer, World Health Organization, Lyon, France.

Fleiss, J. (1981), Statistical Methods for Rates and
Proportions (2nd ed.), Wiley, New York.

Ibraham, M., ed. (1979), The case-control study:
Consensus and controversy, Journal of Chronic Diseases
32: 1-144.

Kleinbaum, D. G., Kupper, L. L., and Morgenstern, H.
(1982), Epidemiologic Research: Principles and Quantitative Methods, Lifetime Learning Publications,
Belmont, California.

Rothman, K., and Boice, J. D. (1979), Epidemiologic
Analysis with a Programmable Calculator, U.S. Public
Health Service [DHEW Pub. No. (NIH) 79-1649],
Washington, D.C.

Schlesselman, J. J., and Stolley, P. (1981), Case-
Control Studies: Design, Conduct, Analysis, Oxford
University Press, New York.

CHAPTER 3

Trends in Cancer Mortality and Incidence in the United States: Is the Future Clear or Clouded?

MARVIN A. SCHNEIDERMAN

INTRODUCTION

The National Center for Health Statistics (24) has reported that cancer is among the very few diseases that have shown consistent increases in age-adjusted mortality rates in the last decade. These recent increases have come about despite reported improvements in survival (and treatment), some of which have been quite large (9,22).

It is the purpose of this review to look at the trends in cancer mortality to see if they can be accounted for, even in part, by trends in incidence. None of the existing data, incidence or mortality, is wholly satisfactory for examining cancer trends in the United States. Mortality is a resultant of incidence and failed treatment. The costs, the trauma, and the pain of cancer are usually more related to incidence (new cases diagnosed), persons hospitalized and treated, and families disrupted. Death is only the last step in the painful process. There is some evidence that deaths from cancer may, in the past, have been understated (27). Cancer was (and is) a loathsome disease and earlier thinking about cancer often looked on the disease as evidence of some stigma, or possibly even divine retribution for past foul behavior. There

71

seems to have been far less of this attitude prevalent
in the last few decades. Cancer mortality in total is
now probably rather accurately reported despite the
evidence that the site-specific reporting of cancer
may be in error, for some rather important sites (28).
   Incidence reporting may also be nonrepresentative.
In the United States, incidence statistics exist
mainly for a limited number of urban areas (36). Urban areas usually show higher cancer rates than rural
areas. Thus, incidence reporting may overstate the
total cancer burden even though the reporting of
trends will be more accurate.* Compared with more
recent data, cancer incidence reporting prior to the
1950s in the United States included a larger proportion of "death certificate only" reporting, that is,
including a case as "incident" when only a death certificate had been filed. If any portion of cancer is
curable, then "death certificate only" reports may imply cases missed who did not die; the rates will then
understate total cancer incidence (35). In the reports of the Third National Cancer Survey (covering
the years 1969-1971) and the more recent reports of
the National Cancer Institute's SEER program (1973 to
the present), "death certificate only" reporting has
been very low (35).
   The possibility exists that incidence reports and
mortality reports could show opposite trends, with incidence reports showing increases and mortality decreases. This could come about if incidence reporting
reflected earlier diagnosis of disease with consequent
increased probability of cure. Thus, greater physician (and public) awareness of cancer could lead to

---

*A comparison of the mortality rates for the areas
used by NCI for incidence reporting and mortality for
the United States as a whole shows the rates for the
"incidence areas" approximately 2% higher than for the
total United States (34).

increased diagnosis and reduced death. This may be
the case in breast cancer, where a surge in diagnosis
in 1974 and 1975 (30) followed the reports of breast
cancer in the wives of both the President and the
Vice-President of the United States. In 1981, the
National Center for Health Statistics (24) reported a
small decline in breast cancer mortality of 12.7 to
12.3 per 100,000 from 1979 to 1980. A similar pattern
may be developing for cancer of the prostate. In addition, there were reports of substantial increases
in incidence of cancer of the endometrium in the late
1960s and early 1970s (18,34) without a corresponding
increase in mortality. Case-control studies (19,21,
26,33) showed an association with postmenopausal estrogen use; both the use and incidence have since declined. This decline in incidence has not been followed by a change in mortality.

MATERIALS AND METHODS

The data in this paper derive from reports of the
National Center for Health Statistics (mortality) and
the National Cancer Institute (incidence). Where appropriate, the data are age adjusted. The overall
mortality data (for the entire century) are age adjusted to the U.S. population as of 1940. Where recent trends are compared in incidence and mortality
data, the data are age adjusted to the U.S. population
in 1970. Incidence data are confined to data from the
Second National Cancer Survey (1947-1948) (12) and
the special survey in Iowa (1950) (13),* the Third National Cancer Survey (1969-1971) (2), and the SEER
program of the NCI (1973-1977) (34). The data are

---

*The tabulations used here are from preliminary data
assembled in May 1981. Some minor subsequent refine-
ments changed the rates only slightly.

given for whites only, and are from the 4 reporting areas (Atlanta, Detroit, San Francisco-Oakland, Iowa) that contributed to all 3 sets of reports and from Connecticut. (The state of Connecticut has maintained its own tumor registry since the 1930s; the latter is now included among the SEER registries.) The data given here are confined to whites because the populations of nonwhites in these areas were too small for meaningful analysis. This is unfortunate because reported increases in mortality from cancer have been substantially greater in blacks than in whites (23,34), even in recent years, long after the introduction of Medicare, which may have led to a greater relative improvement in medical care for blacks than for whites.

For computation of the relative changes the appropriate rate at the first time period was used as the base to calculate the ratios for subsequent time periods. Data on incidence when given for age-specific groups (usually <15, 15-44, 45-64, 65-74, $\geq$75) have been age standardized within these age groups using the 1970 population of the United States as the standard. The incidence data exclude all reported skin cancers. This is unfortunate because, according to other reports (20,32), skin cancers, including melanoma, have increased rapidly in the last 10 years, in ways that do not seem to be related solely to ultraviolet ray exposure (32). Skin cancers were omitted because of differences in reporting and coding rules in the various surveys which make the skin cancer data not strictly comparable.

This chapter presents a different way of observing cancer trends than have other and earlier works (7,8, 11,25). The difference lies in looking at the data from an "index-number" point of view, considering the rates from 1947 to 1950 to be the base (100%) from which to compute percent changes for later time periods. This approach has the advantage of putting all the changes on the same scale, allowing easy visual examination of trends. Because of the substantial

interest that appears to exist over cancer trends
(leading to such extreme assertions that there have
been no increases in incidence in 50 years to assertions of an "epidemic"), I think that any newer or
simpler way of looking at the data is likely to help
resolve some of the issues.

The index-number approach has the disadvantage of
being anchored on one set of data (12), so that any
defects in those data are carried forward into all
the comparisons. For example, the late 1940s data
had a higher percent of cases reported as "death certificate only" (DCO) than did the later incidence surveys, thus raising the possibility that the true rates
may be understated in the late 1940s collection. If
this is true (and if the underestimation is serious)
then all the lines in the incidence figures shown here
would need to be rotated clockwise -- perhaps a few
degrees. The relationships among the lines on the
incidence figures would be preserved, however, unless
there were differential errors by age in the completeness of reporting.

A counter-problem exists. Four of the 5 contribu-
tors to the 1947-1950 data were one-time surveys, the
only exception being the Connecticut Tumor Registry.
One-time surveys may include prevalent cases as well
as incident cases, thus leading to overstatement of
rates. Thus there are two effects in the 1940s surveys that tend to push the rates in opposite direc-
tions. Whether the pushes balance or not I do not
know. Persons who are convinced that the 1940s data
should not be taken at face value may wish to look at
only the changes in the 1970s, when very little of the
data was reported as DCO and the surveys were not one-
time. The mortality data are all DCO, of course.

RESULTS

Figure 1 shows the age-adjusted mortality trends
for all cancer for the United States for all of the

twentieth century.[*]   Three features of these data are
of consequence:

1. There has been an increase throughout the century, greater in the early part of the century.
2. A leveling off appeared to be developing in the
   decade 1950-1960.
3. Since 1960 the rates have increased once again,
   although not as rapidly as in the first 4 decades of the century.

Figure 2 gives mortality data for the more recent
time period 1950-1978 by major age groups, <15, 15-44,
45-64, 65-74, and 75+. The relative trends (setting
1950 equal to 100 as a starting point) are sharply
different for different age groups. For the younger
persons (<45), there have been substantial declines,
reflecting in large part improvements in treatment for
such young persons' cancers as acute leukemia in children and Hodgkin's disease in young adults and the reduction in incidence of cancer of the uterine cervix.
The proportional reported increases in mortality for
older persons were nearly as great for the 45-64 age
group as for the 65-74 age group. The increases occurred both before and after the introduction of Medicare, making it unlikely that the reported increases
were solely artifacts of improved diagnosis and treatment. For the over 75 age group, there were small declines in cancer mortality until about 1970, and then
rather substantial increases.
Figure 3 shows relative incidence data similar to
the mortality data given in Figure 2. These data are
for whites only, and exclude all forms of skin cancer.

---

[*]Full reporting of mortality for all of the United
States did not begin until 1933. The earlier data
are estimates and reconstructions by the National
Center for Health Statistics from available data (6).

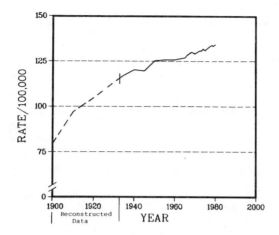

Figure 1. Cancer mortality in the United States, age adjusted using 1940 population.

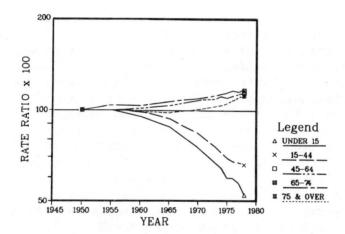

Figure 2. Mortality trends among all races, both sexes, all sites combined.

The relative decreases in incidence for younger persons (under 45) are not as great as the decreases in mortality, further supporting the observation that substantial improvements in treatment have taken place

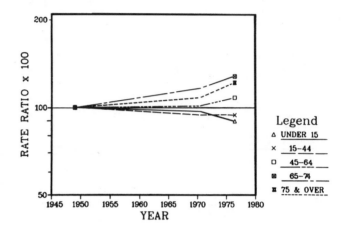

Figure 3. Incidence trends among whites, all sites excluding skin.

for cancers affecting younger persons (9). Unlike
the mortality data, the incidence data show substantial increases for persons over 75. If these increases reflect better access to medical care, leading to
earlier diagnosis of less rampant or rapidly fatal
cancer, then these incidence and mortality data are
not at odds with each other or with the mortality data
reflecting generally improved survival at all ages.
   The data shown so far have been combined for males
and females. If there are exposures to carcinogens
that are different for males and females, then the
patterns of incidence, over time, should be different.
Figure 4 shows the incidence trends separately for men
and women. Except for males under 15, the reported
declines in incidence have occurred only in women.
As with the mortality data, the greatest declines are
among the youngest persons, and the greatest increases
among persons 65-74. The recent (1970-1977) increases
in incidence in women were relatively uniform for all
ages over 45, while for men the changes were directly
age related, the greatest increases in men over 75 and
the greatest (and only) decrease for males under 15.

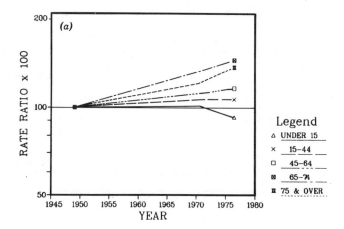

Figure 4a. Incidence trends among white men, all sites excluding skin.

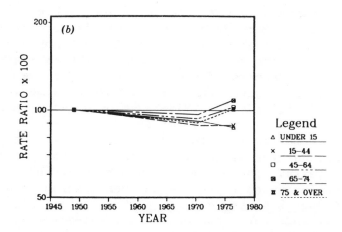

Figure 4b. Incidence trends among white women, all sites excluding skin.

A further examination of trends (giving data in units of new cases per 100,000 per year) is shown in Figure 5. The patterns for men and women are different at different ages. In persons age 15-44, cancer

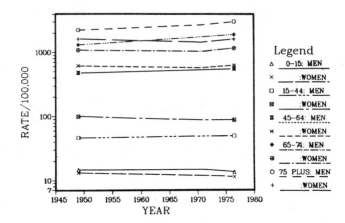

Figure 5. Incidence trends among w .tes, by age group.

is substantially more common in women than in men.
Among the older age groups, cancer is more common in
men. The differences lie largely, but not exclu-
sively, in the age distribution of the sex-related
cancers. Cancers of the uterine cervix, ovary, and
breast often occur in somewhat younger women. Median
age at diagnosis (in 1973-1977) of women with breast
cancer was 60.3 years, for ovarian cancer 60.0 years,
and for cervical cancer 52.7 years (34). For men,
median age for diagnosis of cancer of the prostate was
73.1 years. The one major cancer occurring among both
sexes for which there was an overwhelming male pre-
dominance was lung cancer, although males also have
higher incidence (and mortality) rates for almost every other form of non-sex-specific cancers. The median ages at diagnosis of lung cancer were: men,
65.4; women, 62.8.
    The incidence changes have not been uniform across
the major site groups (Figure 6). Since the late
1940s, the major (percentage) increases have occurred
in men in the urinary tract cancers (bladder and kidney), the respiratory cancers (mostly, but not exclu-
sively, lung cancer), the genital cancers (prostate),

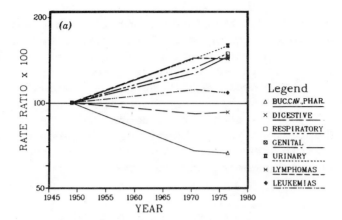

Figure 6a. Incidence trends among white men, major site groups.

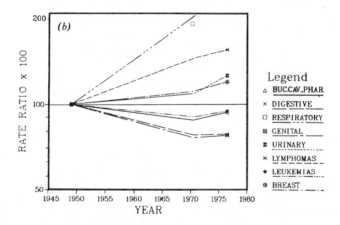

Figure 6b. Incidence trends among white women, major site groups.

and the lymphomas. The patterns in women show several interesting divergences. Great relative increases were seen in lung cancer, which may soon displace breast cancer as the leading fatal cancer among women.

(Breast cancer incidence is still much greater than lung cancer incidence.) There were steady increases in the lymphomas; substantial increases in the urinary cancers (as in men), and, as noted before, increases in breast cancer, mostly during the mid-1970s. While men showed increases in the genital cancers, among women there were reported decreases. The trend in the leukemias, as in the buccal cavity cancers, was opposite in women compared with men in recent years (men, down; women, up).

TABLE 1. Cancer Mortality-Incidence Ratios for Whites (1969-1978)[a]

	Men	Women
TNCS		
1969	.56	.56
1970	.58	.59
1971	.60	.60
SEER		
1973	.57	.56
1974	.57	.56
1975	.56	.55
1976	.56	.55
1977	.55	.55
1978	.55	.54

[a]Excluding breast and uterine corpus cancers in women.

There appears to be evidence, summarized above, that the incidence reporting may not have been of

uniform quality for all 3 years of the Third National
Cancer Survey (TNCS). In Table 1 are the mortality/
incidence ratios (for whites) by separate years for
1969-1971 (TNCS) and 1973-1978 (SEER) (30,34). For
women the data on cancer of the uterine corpus (incidence rapidly increasing in 1969-1971 and rapidly decreasing in 1973-1977) and breast cancer (rapid increase in incidence reported in 1974 and 1975) were
excluded from both the incidence and mortality data.
There is an apparent increase in the M/I ratio for
both men and women from 1969 through 1971, and then a
general, slow decline in this same ratio in the 6-year
period 1973-1978. The increase probably is not explainable by external factors such as worsening treatment or reduced medical care. On the other hand, the
general decline in the M/I ratio for the period 1973-
1978 is consistent with reported improvements in survival (22).

At least two possibilities exist to explain the an-
omalous M/I ratios: (a) The incidence data for 1969
are correct and 1970 and 1971 are both underreported;
and (b) the data for 1970 are correct, 1969 was over-
reported, and 1971 was underreported. If possibility
(a) is true, then the increasing trend in incidence
from the average of 1969-1971 to the average of 1973-
1977 will be overstated. However, if it is assumed
that the M/I ratio should have remained constant, the
observed rate for 1969-1971 would appear to underestimate the true rate by about 3%. If it is assumed that
the M/I ratio is decreasing, as suggested in the years
1973-1978, then it is more likely that possibility (b)
is correct. The trends for the average of 1969-1971
to 1973-1977 are then more likely to be correct. As
pointed out earlier, the data for 1947-1950 may also
misstate incidence because the percentage of cases reported as "death certificate only" was larger in 1947-
1950 than in the later surveys. Overstatement would
be due to the inclusion of cases (deaths) that were
actually prevalent (diagnosed in a prior year) whereas understatement would be due to the missing of

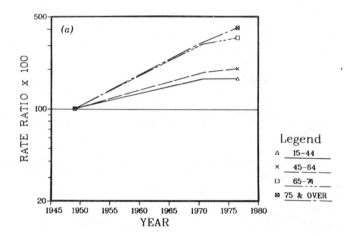

Figure 7a. Incidence trends among white men, respiratory system.

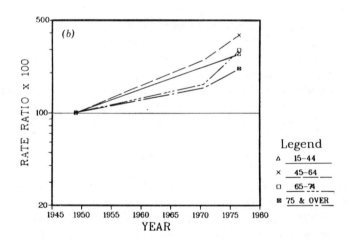

Figure 7b. Incidence trends among white women, respiratory system.

incident cases who did not die during the year. These possibilities further complicate trend considerations. Because large increases have occurred in the respiratory cancers, looking at the age-specific changes may be instructive (see Figure 7). In men, the increases are directly age related, the greatest increases occurring in the oldest men and the smaller increases in the younger men, with evidence of flattening out in the men under 45. In women the pattern is not so simple. Increases have occurred at all ages, with the greatest recent increase in women 45-74, but with substantial increases in both younger and older women.

The pattern of change in respiratory cancers and their reported strong association with cigarette smoking makes it worthwhile to examine other cancers believed to be associated with cigarette smoking. Among these are the urinary system cancers, cancers of the bladder and kidney. Bladder cancer has been reported as more likely to be related to cigarette smoking than kidney cancer (14). Figure 8 shows the changes in incidence of the urinary tract cancers in white men and women. Two things are of interest. The increases in men are substantially greater proportionally than the increases in women, and the proportional increases in kidney cancer have been greater than the increases in bladder cancer, the cancer reported to be more likely related to cigarette smoking.

The age-specific changes in the urinary system cancers are also of consequence (Figure 9). In both men and women, there were large increases in the youngest age groups (under 45). This, too, is in contrast to the respiratory cancer patterns, where the greatest increases were in the oldest age group in men and in intermediate age groups in women. Except for the youngest age group, the increases in men are directly related to age, with the greatest increases occurring at the oldest ages. Among women the age pattern is reversed. Increases are inversely related to age with the greatest increase occurring in the youngest age groups.

Figure 10 shows the age-specific increases in male genital system cancers. Increases have occurred at

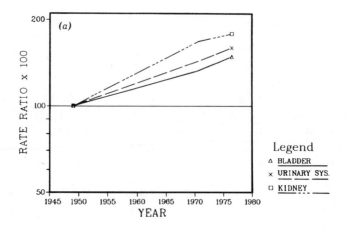

Figure 8a. Incidence trends among white men, urinary
system by site.

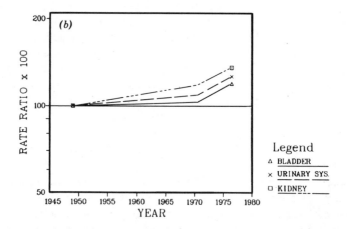

Figure 8b. Incidence trends among white women, urinary
system by site.

all ages, but no consistent pattern appears. In the
roughly 30 years covered, the age group 65-74 shows
the greatest relative increase while the age group 75
and over shows the smallest relative increase. The

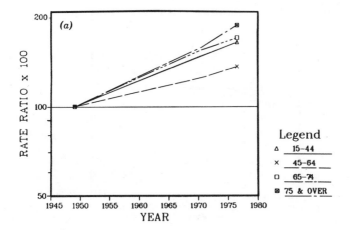

Figure 9a. Incidence trends among white men, urinary system.

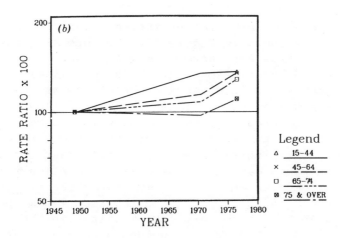

Figure 9b. Incidence trends among white women, urinary system.

two other age groups, 15-44 and 45-64, show intermediate relative increases which are similar.

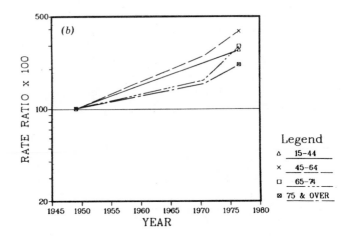

Figure 10. Incidence trends among white men, male genital system.

The peculiar behavior of the sex-specific cancers of women is shown in Figure 11. For breast cancer sharp increases are shown in women 45 and over for the most recent time period. This very likely reflects the surge in diagnosed breast cancer in the mid-1970s which, as mentioned earlier, followed the diagnosis of breast cancer in the wives of both the President and the Vice-President of the United States. However, this increased awareness of breast cancer in American women cannot be the sole explanation for the changes, because an increase in breast cancer among women under 65 is seen between the late 1940s and 1970, with by far the greatest increase in the age group 45-64. The data on incidence of cancer of the female genital organs are made up of diseases showing opposite trends. For the younger women, those under 45, a sharp decline in incidence is reported for the entire 30-year period 1947-1977. This reflects mainly the reductions in cancer of the uterine cervix. For the other age groups, the increases between the early and mid-1970s reflect the substantial increases, now

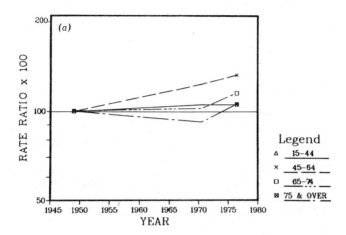

Figure 11a. Incidence trends among white women, breast cancer.

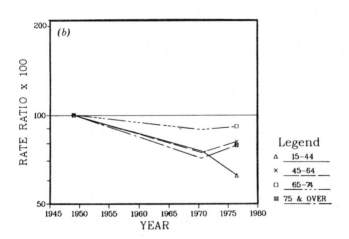

Figure 11b. Incidence trends among white women, female genital system.

ended, in cancer of the uterine corpus.

The greatest relative decreases in reported cancer

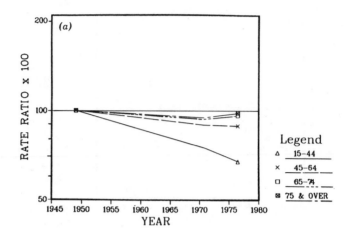

Figure 12a. Incidence trends among white men, digestive system.

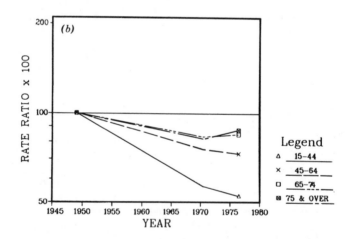

Figure 12b. Incidence trends among white women, digestive system.

incidence have occurred in the digestive system cancers taken as a whole (Figure 12). In both men and

women the decreases are inversely age related, with
the youngest persons showing the greatest proportional
decreases. In both men and women, small increases are
reported between the early and mid-1970s for persons
over 65. Since Medicare was already in effect in the
early 1970s it is possible that these increases might
reflect underreporting among the older age groups in
the earlier time period as suggested by the Mortality/
Incidence ratios given in Table 1.

When one looks at the age-specific changes for
stomach cancer and the remainder of the digestive system in parallel, two interesting facts emerge. First,
for stomach cancer, the percentage decreases in incidence are almost identical for all persons over 45,
and are about twice the decreases seen in the persons
under 45. Second, for all other digestive system cancers (combined) the pattern is reversed. Changes are
still age related, with decreases in the younger persons and increases in the older persons. In women the
decreases are greater and extend up to age 64. In
men, the decreases occur in the under-45-year age
range with progressively greater increases with increasing age. If one visualizes the age-specific
lines as representing the spread fingers of the left
hand, pivoting at the wrist, the hand representing
women's changes is tipped down (rotated clockwise)
about 20 degrees more than the hand representing men.

Figures 13 and 14 are reexaminations of the mortality trends first shown in Figure 1. Figure 13 is Figure 1 redrawn to include a second-degree mathematical
function fitted to the cancer mortality data, age
adjusted to 1940, for this century. The fitted curve
has a negative second-degree term, which implies that
a maximum rate exists, in time. This maximum was computed to come at roughly 1984 or 1985 and to be at a
rate of 132.2 deaths per 100,000. This rate, however,
was exceeded in 1976, and again in 1978, 1979, and
1980.

Because of the changes in rates that appeared to
be developing beginning around 1960, 3 other

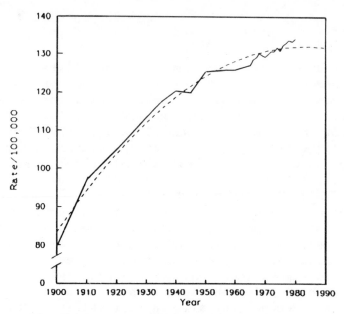

Figure 13. Cancer mortality, United States, 1900–1980, all races, both sexes (age adjusted to 1940).

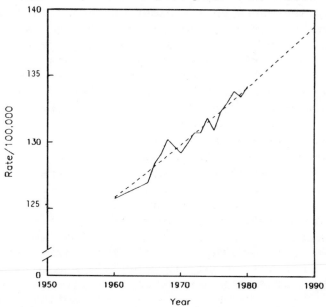

Figure 14. Cancer mortality, United States, 1960–1980, all races, both sexes (age adjusted to 1940).

second-degree curves were also fitted to the data.
Table 2 gives the results.

TABLE 2. Equations of Fitted Cancer Mortality Curves

| Period covered | Fitted curve | Computed Maximum | |
		Year	Rate
1900-1950	$80.9 + 1.48(yr-1900)$ $-.0124(yr-1900)^2$	1959-1960	124.7
1900-1960	$81.1 + 1.44(yr-1900)$ $-.0116(yr-1900)^2$	1962-1963	125.8
1960-1980	$142.0 - .783(yr-1900)$ $+.00802(yr-1900)^2$	None	

Figure 14 shows the data and the fitted second-
degree curve for the period 1960-1980 and shows no
maximum in the foreseeable future.

DISCUSSION

The likelihood that the trend in cancer mortality,
which was increasing at a decreasing rate for the
first half of this century, has changed direction and
appears to be increasing in the second half of the
century makes it worthwhile to examine the specific
trends by disease, sex, and age group. Because improved treatments since the 1960s should have the effect of reducing mortality, this apparently different
trend since 1960 takes on even more importance. In
order that the trend information not be confounded because of treatment improvements, I have looked at

incidence data where they are available.

Incidence data for the United States have some deficiencies. They cover about a 10% sample of the United States. The sample is not a random sample but is made up of reporting groups that have been able to gather reasonably good data for a defined population. This means that the data are derived more from urban than rural areas, and that they are better for areas with better or older established medical care systems. That the data reflect urban patterns more than rural patterns is both a blessing and a bane. It is a blessing because as the United States becomes more urbanized [over 80% of the population now lives in what the Census Bureau (31) defines as urban areas] these data become more representative of the country as a whole. It is a bane because, in general, urban areas have higher cancer rates than rural areas; thus, estimates of absolute rates derived from these incidence data will tend to overstate cancer incidence for the country as a whole. (Cancer mortality is about 2% higher for these areas than for the United States as a whole.) It is a further bane because as persons move from rural to urban areas the higher urban rates tend to be diluted by the lower rural rates that these persons may sustain. Thus, the possibility exists that increasing trends in reported incidence could underestimate the incidence trends among long-term residents of the urban areas. Migration in the opposite direction and migration of older, usually healthier, persons to retirement areas (which are not among the incidence reporting areas for the data given) will also perturb incidence trend data.

Mortality data (i.e., "death certificate" data) are at times not accurately reported, particularly with respect to specific primary site of cancer. For example, the mortality reports on cancers of the colon and rectum appear to grossly overstate one and understate the other (28). These misclassification problems are minimized when incidence data including information derived from hospital charts are used.

As there is geographic variation in cancer rates
as well as for the above reasons, I have chosen to
confine my examination of the trends in the age-,
sex-, and site-specific cancers to the incidence data
as reported in the 4 registries that were included in
the historical surveys system and in the SEER program,
plus the Cancer Registry of Connecticut, which is the
oldest continuous population-based cancer registry in
the United States. I had to restrict myself further
to considering the data for whites only (despite the
fact that the reported increases in mortality among
blacks have been substantially greater than among
whites).

Although these data are not included here, the reporting of illness for nonwhites suffers from several
problems. Sample sizes are often small, leading to
erratic statistical fluctuations. The quality of medical care for blacks, at least in the past, and perhaps even at present, is likely to have been poorer
than for whites, making reported diagnoses more questionable. If medical care has improved over time,
then trend data in nonwhites will be subject to more
error than trend data for whites, although reporting
of cancer has been considered to be less affected by
moderate changes in medical care than reporting for
other diseases, such as sudden deaths attributed to
heart disease or stroke (15).

Two issues seem to me to be of some consequence
here. First, have the reported increases in both cancer mortality and incidence seen since 1950-1960 been
"real," or can they be explained away as some arti-
fact? Second, if we conclude that the increases have
been real, to what factors can these increases be attributed?

In the mid-1970s there was a substantial increase
in breast cancer awareness, following the diagnosis of
breast cancer in Mrs. Ford and Mrs. Rockefeller. It
is possible that this increased awareness may have
spilled over into a general increased cancer awareness, leading to higher incidence rates for some other

cancers as well. If this is the case, some small declines may be expected for the later years of the
1970s, in contrast to 1974-1977.

The data here strongly support the idea that, in
whites at least, the increases in incidence (and
therefore, the likely increases in mortality) are
largely real. Because of the different patterns in
men and women it is unlikely that some generalized,
across-the-board reporting error, census undercount,
or change in medical care is responsible for this reported overall increase. This argument is supported
by the observation that increases are different for
different sites, and that for some sites important decreases have been seen. Because overall increases are
seen in both men and women in the 45-64 year old age
group as well as for the persons over 65, the reported
increases cannot be attributed solely to the greater
availability of medical care to persons over 65
through Medicare. Nor is it likely, on the other
hand, that the data for persons over 65 are grossly
untrustworthy because older persons underutilize medical care facilities (10) or get poorer medical care
than younger persons, now that Medicare and Medicaid
have been available for over a decade. This conjec-
ture cannot be verified by direct observation of incidence data, there being too few data points. However,
examination of Figure 2, mortality trends by age
group, shows essentially parallel trends for persons
45-64 (no Medicare) and persons 65-74 (Medicare starting in the 1960s). The increases for persons 65-74
were seen as early as 1955, preceding both Medicare
and the increases in the 45-64 year old persons.
(Increases in persons 75 and over came later, following some small, earlier declines.) The curves are
smooth, and show no abrupt increases as might be found
if Medicare had made observable changes in cancer
death rates for older persons. The Medicare effects
could be conceived of as operating in two opposite di-
rections with respect to reported cancer mortality.
Improved diagnosis could lead to cancer being identi-

fied more often as a cause of death. Earlier diagnosis could lead to improved treatment, and thus reduce
cancer mortality. To translate these observations to
incidence data it is necessary to assume that mortality follows incidence, which, as Table 1 shows, it
clearly does.

Examination of the age-specific trends for many of
the sites (or systems) leads to the observation that
many of the sites (often unrelated) show the "spreading fingers" pattern. The "spreading fingers" pattern
refers to the trends in age-specific rates. The
younger persons show decreasing rates while the older
persons show increasing rates. These divergent age-
specific trends deserve some attention and research.
I have suggested earlier (3) that the declines in cancer rates in young persons are consistent with 2 general patterns that have occurred since 1920: The reduction in mortality from viral (and other infectious)
diseases and the increased availability of fresh and
frozen foods made possible by improvements in trans-
port and refrigeration since the 1940s. If infectious
diseases act as promoters (or some other form of incomplete carcinogen), then reduction of infectious diseases should lead to reductions in cancer. This reduction should be seen first as those portions of the
population in which infectious diseases were first reduced, some 40 to 50 years ago, reach ages at which
significant cancer incidence occurs. Similarly the
greater availability of fresh and frozen foods
throughout the year since World War II with consequent
increased vitamin intakes (17) should also have the
effect of reducing cancer, again in the younger persons.

The reductions seen in younger persons should probably also appear first in those diseases with the
shortest latent periods, diseases often thought of as
childhood cancers. A preliminary examination of the
data supports this expectation.

The best-identified cause of cancer is cigarette
smoking. Cigarette smoking has been associated with

several forms of cancer: lung, head and neck, and
esophagus, larynx, pancreas, bladder, and perhaps kidney. Examination of trends for these several and different diseases should indicate whether the recent
trends in cancer incidence and mortality can be solely
(or largely) associated with cigarette smoking, as
some authors have suggested (11), or whether it is
meaningful to look for other causes and/or mechanisms
of disease causation that are different for the different diseases. It seems that there are sufficient
differences in trends from site to site that one must
conclude that important influences in addition to
smoking must be at work.

Similarly male-female differences in trends for
the non-sex-related sites should provide some clues
to etiology. Trends by age provide some evidence as
to whether reported increases may be artifactual such
as may be associated with changes in medical care. An
example would be the introduction of Medicare in July
1966, which provided government-supported medical care
assistance for persons over 65, and Medicaid, which
provided access to medical care for the indigent.

Several important facts emerge from the examination
of these data. First, the decreasing ratio of increase in cancer mortality seen after World War II has
turned around. Cancer mortality rates are once again
increasing. Decade by decade since 1900 the increases
in age-adjusted cancer mortality were (see Figure 1):

1900–1910	22%*	1940–1950	4%
1910–1920	8%*	1950–1960	0.3%+
1920–1930	8%*	1960–1970	2.7%
1930–1940	6%	1970–1980	3.9%

The data prior to 1930 are "reconstructions," and

---

*"Reconstructed" data.
+Smallest increase.

probably not worth as much attention as the later
data.

Similar nationwide data do not exist for incidence,
but the data reported here for a limited number of
population-based registries (all the data available
for the period 1947-1977) show a pattern similar to
the mortality.

The mortality trends are different for the different age groups. Greatest declines are for persons
under 45. There have been smaller incidence declines
in these younger persons, lending strong circumstan-
tial evidence to the claims for improvements in survival. There have been, overall, reported mortality
and incidence increases in persons over 45, lending
credence to the argument that not all the overall increase can be due to increased availability of medical
care for persons over 65. Persons 65-74 showed increases in mortality rates from cancer from 1950 on.
From 1955 until 1970 the rates for persons 75 and over
were below the 1950 mortality level. They have increased rapidly since.

Incidence patterns by age are different for (white)
men and women. Among males, in only the under-15 age
group were there decreases in total cancers. The
changes from 1969-1971 to 1975-1977 were directly age
related in men, but not in women. The relative increases were almost identical for all women over 45,
despite substantial decreases in cancers of the stomach and the uterine cervix. Overall, cancer in women
appeared at an earlier age than in men, perhaps reflecting a more substantial change in life-style, including patterns of employment, in women than in men
since World War II. On the other hand, the earlier
age at diagnosis of lung cancer among women is directly related to differences in smoking patterns for
men and women.

By major site group, the greatest percentage increases in incidence in men were in the urinary tract
cancers, with greater relative increases reported in
kidney cancers than in bladder cancers. These trends

raise questions as to the role of cigarette smoking
versus other environmental agents in the development
of these cancers, bladder cancer being considered more
likely to be associated with cigarette smoking than
kidney cancer. Patterns among women are similar, with
greater proportional increases in kidney cancer than
bladder cancer, despite the fact that the prevalence
of cigarette smoking, having earlier increased sharply, has remained relatively stable in recent years in
women while decreasing in men. Mortality from nonma-
lignant kidney diseases has also been reported to be
increasing within the past decade (24), suggesting
that perhaps some new kidney toxicants may have been
introduced into our environment in the recent past.
Other possibilities are that some new definitions or
patterns in reporting urinary tract disease have been
introduced.

The greatest proportional increases in cancer incidence in women have been in the respiratory tract cancers, which is clearly consistent with cigarette smoking patterns since 1940 among women. Also consistent
with the changing male-female cigarette smoking patterns have been the reduction in buccal cavity cancers
in men and the initial decline followed by a more recent increase in these cancers in women. Whatever the
general changes are that reduced buccal cavity cancers
in the 1950s and 1960s, the trend in women has been
offset since 1970, perhaps related to recent cigarette
smoking.

Increases have been reported in the lymphomas,
which, as far as is known, are not related to cigarette smoking. Some authors have speculated that this
is due to greater diagnostic acumen developing over
the last 30 years (29).

The increase in genital cancers in men in contrast
to the decrease in women is of substantial interest.
The increase in men has occurred at all ages and thus
is clearly not due only to improved diagnosis of prostate cancer in old men. Some industrial exposures
[e.g., cadmium (4,16)] have been associated with

cancers of the prostate. In women, decreases in genital tract cancer (mainly cancer of the uterine cervix) have occurred at all ages, since 1947, with the
greatest decrease reported in the youngest women.
This is in contrast to at least one report from Australia (1), which showed increases in cervical cancer
incidence in young women, ostensibly associated with
changing sexual mores, early sexual experiences, and
more sexual partners. The possibility exists, of
course, that the changes in sexual behavior have not
been as great in the United States as in Australia.
Increases in genital cancers in older American women
since 1969-1971 are due to increases in cancer incidence of the uterine corpus, probably associated with
postmenopausal estrogen use; as the use decreases, one
may expect declining rates (18).

Overall, then, it appears that (within whites) the
age, sex patterns of cancer incidence and the trends
in the cigarette-related cancers are sufficiently different to raise serious questions about some of the
explanations offered to account for the data. If new
hazards have entered our environment since World War
II, possibly related to our large increases in production and use of synthetic organic chemicals (5), they
could be responsible, in part, for the increased rate
of increase in cancer mortality (and incidence) since
the 1960s; this still needs to be evaluated. It is
important to isolate the reasons for the reduction in
buccal cavity and digestive tract, particularly stomach, cancers. These changes, as well as changes in
cigarette smoking, sexual behavior, and possibly diet,
deserve careful consideration and research so that
cancer might be prevented in the future. Prevention
might be successful in leading to a flattening, once
again, of the mortality curves that seemed to be developing in the 1950s.

If the dietary and infectious disease changes during this century have really been responsible for decreased cancer incidence in younger persons, these
patterns should move forward in time, leading

eventually to reductions at all ages. Reduced smoking
in men should have a similar effect. It now appears
that respiratory cancers in women will continue to increase for some time (probably through the end of the
century) and then eventually level off, if interactions with other environmental exposures are not
large. The increased production and use of synthetic
organic chemicals, many of which have been shown to be
carcinogens, will provide stimuli that increase cancer
rates. The answer to my question in the title is:
"Partly clouded, with some possibilities for clear-
ing."

ACKNOWLEDGEMENT

Many people including several former colleagues at
the National Cancer Institute helped in the development of this paper. I am particularly grateful to
Dr. Susan Devesa whose thoughtful professional collaboration cannot be acknowledged enough. Mr. John Horm
assembled the incidence data. Dr. David Levin oversaw
the computer graphics. Several senior scientists at
NCI reviewed the manuscript in detail, but wish to be
treated as anonymous referees. Dr. Harry Rosenberg of
the National Center for Health Statistics helped with
the mortality statistics. Dr. Mortimer Mendelsohn and
his associates provided helpful criticism when this
paper was given in a somewhat different form as the
Distinguished Scientist Lecture at the Lawrence
Livermore Laboratories in California. Dr. Valerie
Miké and her staff provided excellent scientific and
editorial assistance. Mrs. Ilene Fingerman and Ms.
Mary Reardon of Clement Associates guided the manuscript with care through several rewritings. The accuracy and the completeness of the data presented here
are due to the help of these and many other people.
All opinions, surmises, extrapolations, and errors are
mine.

REFERENCES

1. Armstrong, B. (1980), Changes in cervical cancer in Australia, paper presented at 1980 annual meeting, Clinical Oncological Society of Australia, 27 November 1980, Sydney.

2. Cutler, S. J., and Young, J. L., Jr., eds. (1975), Third National Cancer Survey: Incidence Data, National Cancer Institute Monograph 41, Department of Health, Education and Welfare [DHEW Pub. No. (NIH) 75-787], U.S. Government Printing Office, Washington, D.C.

3. Davis, D. L., Bridbord, K., and Schneiderman, M. (1981), Estimating cancer causes: Problems in methodology, production, and trends, in: Peto, R., and Schneiderman, M., eds., Quantification of Occupational Cancer, Banbury Report 9, Cold Spring Harbor Laboratory, Cold Spring Harbor, New York.

4. Davis, D. L., Bridbord, K., and Schneiderman, M. (1982), Cancer prevention: Assessing causes, exposures, and recent trends in incidence and mortality, Teratogenesis, Carcinogenesis, and Mutagenesis. (In press.)

5. Davis, D. L., and Magee, B. (1979), Cancer and industrial chemical production, Science 206: 1356-1358 (letter).

6. Department of Health, Education and Welfare, National Office of Vital Statistics (1958), Vital Statistics Special Reports, 43: October.

7. Devesa, S. S., and Silverman, D. T. (1978), Cancer incidence and mortality trends in the United States: 1935-1974, Journal of the National Cancer Institute 60: 545-571.

8. Devesa, S. S., and Silverman, D. T. (1980), Trends in incidence and mortality in the United States, Journal of Environmental Pathology and Toxicology 3: 127-155.

9. DeVita, V. T., Henney, J. E., and Hubbard, S. M. (1981), Estimation of the numerical and economic impact of chemotherapy in the treatment of cancer, in: Burchenal, J. H., and Oettgen, H. F., eds., Cancer: Achievements, Challenges, and Prospects for the 1980s, Vol. 2, Grune and Stratton, New York, pp. 859-880.

10. Doll, R. (1970), Cancer and ageing: The epidemiological evidence, Dorn Memorial Lecture, 10th International Conference of the UICC, May, Houston.

11. Doll, R., and Peto, R. (1981), The causes of cancer: Quantitative estimates of avoidable risks of cancer in the United States today, Journal of the National Cancer Institute 66: 1191-1308.

12. Dorn, H. F., and Cutler, S. J. (1955, Part I; 1959, Part II), Morbidity from Cancer in The United States, Part I, Public Health Monograph 29 and Part II, Public Health Monograph 56, U.S. Government Printing Office, Washington, D.C.

13. Haenszel, W., Marcus, S. G., and Zimmerer, E.G. (1956), Cancer Morbidity in Urban and Rural Iowa, Public Health Monograph 37, U.S. Government Printing Office, Washington, D.C.

14. Hammond, E. C. (1975), Tobacco, in: Fraumeni, J., Jr., ed., Persons at High Risk of Cancer, Academic Press, New York, pp. 131-138.

15. Heasman, M. A., and Lipworth, L. (1966), Accuracy of Certification of Cause of Death, H. M. Stationery Office, London.

16. International Agency for Research on Cancer (IARC) (1973; 1976), Monographs on the Evaluation of the Carcinogenic Risk of Chemicals to Humans, No. 2, p. 74; No. 11, p. 39, Lyons, France.

17. International Cancer Research Data Bank (ICRDB) (1981), Chemoprevention of carcinogenesis (oncology overview); Vitamin A in Cancer Biology (oncology overview), NCI, NIH, Bethesda, Maryland.

18. Jick, H. (1980), The epidemic of endometrial cancer: A commentary, American Journal of Public Health 70: 264-270.

19. Jick, H., Watkins, R. N., Hunter, J. R., Dinan, B. J., Madsen, S., Rothman, K. J., and Walker, A. M. (1979), Replacement estrogens and endometrial cancer, The New England Journal of Medicine 300: 218-222.

20. Lee, J. A. H., and Carter, A. P. (1970), Secular trends in mortality from malignant melanoma, Journal of the National Cancer Institute 45: 91-97.

21. Mack, T. M., Pike, M. C., Henderson, B. E., Pfeffer, R. I., Gerkins, V. R., Arthur, M., and Brown, S. E. (1976), Estrogens and endometrial carcinoma in a retirement community, The New England Journal of Medicine 294: 1262-1267.

22. Myers, M., and Hankey, B. (1980), Cancer Patient Survival Experience, [USDHHS Pub. No. (NIH) 80-2148], June.

23. National Center for Health Statistics (NCHS/DHHS) (1980), Monthly Vital Statistics Report 28(13): 4-5, November 13.

24. National Center for Health Statistics (NCHS/DHHS) (1981), Annual summary of births, deaths,

marriages, and divorces: United States, 1980,
Monthly Vital Statistics Report 289: 18, September
17.

25. Office of Technology Assessment (1981), Assessment
of Technologies for Determining Cancer Risks from
the Environment (Doll, R., and Peto, R., principal
contractors), Congress of the United States, U.S.
Government Printing Office, Washington, D.C.

26. Paffenbarger, R. S., Fasal, E., Simmons, M. E.,
and Kampert, J. B. (1977), Cancer risk as related
to use of oral contraceptives during fertile
years, Cancer 39: 1887-1891.

27. Percy, C., and Dolman, A. (1978), Comparison of
the coding of death certificates related to cancer
in seven countries, Public Health Reports 93: 335-
350.

28. Percy, C., Staneck, E., and Gloeckler, L. (1981),
Accuracy of cancer death certificates and its ef-
fect on cancer mortality statistics, American
Journal of Public Health 71: 242-250.

29. Peto, R. (1981), Recent trends and the 1978 estimates in quantification of occupational cancer,
in: Peto, R., and Schneiderman, M., eds., Quantification of Occupational Cancer, Banbury Report 9,
Cold Spring Harbor Laboratory, Cold Spring Harbor,
New York.

30. Pollack, E., and Horm, J. (1980), Trends in cancer
incidence and mortality in the United States,
1969-1976, Journal of the National Cancer Institute 64: 1091-1103.

31. U.S. Department of Commerce (1980), Statistical
Abstract of the United States (101st ed.), Washington, D.C., pp. 16-18.

32. Urbach, F. (1979), Potential effects on humans of alteration of the stratospheric ozone layer, A review of a report prepared for the National Academy of Sciences, The Skin and Cancer Hospital, Temple University, Philadelphia.

33. Weiss, N. S., Szekely, D. R., English, D. R., and Schweid, A. I. (1979), Endometrial cancer in relation to patterns of menopausal estrogen use, Journal of the American Medical Association 242: 261-264.

34. Young, J., Percy, C., and Asire, A. J., eds. (1981), Incidence and Mortality Data: 1973-1977, National Cancer Institute Monograph No. 57: Surveillance, Epidemiology and End Results Program, [DHHS Pub. No. (NIH) 81-2330], Washington, D.C.

35. Young, J., and Pollack, E. (1981), The incidence of cancer in the United States, in: Schottenfeld, D., and Fraumeni, J., eds., Cancer Epidemiology and Prevention, Saunders, Philadelphia.

36. Young, J., and Schneiderman, M. (1975), Cancer information subsystems in the United States of America, World Health Organization, DSI/CAN/WP/76.11, Geneva, Switzerland.

Part III
Issues in Clinical Studies

CHAPTER 4

Clinical Studies in Cancer: A Historical Perspective

VALERIE MIKÉ

The history of medicine is a rich and fascinating field, and its study is for me a pleasant avocation. I am especially interested in the interplay between the emergence of statistical ideas and advances in clinical medicine, including the impact of these ideas on the progress being made against cancer. It is probably premature to consider writing this particular chapter in the history of science, but I have a special reason for focusing on it today.

For the past 8 years I have been engaged in the development of a department of statistics at this medical center, and much of our work here pertains to research in cancer. A great deal of our time is spent on the many grant applications, site visits, and progress reports required to obtain the necessary government funds to support our activities. And now, on the tenth anniversary of the National Cancer Act, there are Congressional investigations of the cancer program and frequent critical and defeatist statements in the

---

This work was supported by National Cancer Institute Grant CA-08748.

111

news media. A recent editorial in The New York Times
asks: "Has the decade-long 'war on cancer' brought
real progress against the dread disease, or has it
been an extravagant $7.5 billion misfire?" (33). This
seems like a good time to pause and reflect on what we
are doing.

In the course of preparing this talk I sent letters
to some 50 senior clinical investigators and statisticians involved in cancer research, asking for their
comments. Specific issues of interest included the
following: the role of statistical methodology in
the advances made; the relevance of statistics to
Phase I-II trials; the respective contributions of
randomized versus historical controls; the impact of
single center versus cooperative group studies; major
problems; the role of regulatory agencies; and areas
most in need of further development. Without any
follow-up on my part, the response rate to the letter
was over 80%. The thoughts and views of my respondents are incorporated in this perspective.

An important first point is that our scope is much
broader than cancer research and biostatistics. It
is well known that the development of the classical
theory of statistics coincided with the birth of modern biology and was largely motivated by it; one need
only mention the names of Galton and Fisher (7,38,98).
It is probably also correct to say that within the
past two decades one of the most active research areas
in statistics has been that of biomedical applications. Biostatistics has come into its own as a
strong discipline. There has been extensive emphasis
on the design and analysis of clinical trials, the
handling of censored observations, the assessment of
covariates, and other related problems. The impetus
for this has come largely from research in clinical
oncology. The initial studies were undertaken and
much of the subsequent work carried out under sponsor-
ship of the National Cancer Institute (87).

Thus, while one may ask what statistics has done

for the cancer program, one need not ask what the
cancer program has done for statistics.

EARLY HISTORY OF MEDICINE

Concern with approaches to the treatment of disease
dates back to antiquity, and has produced insights
and tenets that are still valid today. The statement,
"One must attend in medical practice not primarily to
plausible theories, but to experience combined with
reason" is found in the Hippocratic writings (57).
These documents give evidence of close clinical observation and careful deduction concerning disease;
achievements were high in the diagnosis of many ail-
ments and the assessment of their prognosis. As far
as treatment was concerned, however, reliance on tra-
dition and authority was so strong that it generally
prevented recognition of the value of impartial observation. Thus, in spite of this precept of Hippocrates, therapy in ancient Greece was nearly always determined by a priori theories (11).
Similar exhortations appear in the writings of major figures of the Middle Ages and Renaissance, such
as Avicenna, Roger Bacon, and Leonardo da Vinci. Yet
in their advice on medical treatment these men also
generally gave the popular remedies of their own day
(11).
There was little systematic development of clinical
investigation even in the 17th century. Francis Bacon
proposed that more emphasis be placed on experience
in the selection of treatments, and that learned physicians contribute information on remedies "tried and
approved by experiment for the cure of particular diseases." And he cautioned: "This part therefore,
which treats of authentic and positive medicines, I
set down as wanting. But it is a thing that should
not be undertaken without keen and severe judgment,
and in synod, as it were, of select physicians" (5).
The actual functioning of an early medical team is

illustrated by the treatment given King Charles II in
1685:   "A pint of blood was extracted from his right
arm, and a half-pint from his left shoulder, followed
by an emetic, two physics, and an enema comprising
fifteen substances; the royal head was then shaved
and a blister raised; then a sneezing powder, more
emetics, and bleeding, soothing potions, a plaster of
pitch and pigeon dung on his feet, potions containing
ten different substances, chiefly herbs, finally for-
ty drops of extract of human skull, and the application of bezoar stone; after which his majesty died"
(49,88). It may be that each of the king's physicians
in turn applied his own favorite remedies.
   The need for controlled experiments was recognized
by some in the 18th century. A particularly interesting example is found in the writings of the British
philosopher George Berkeley, who was convinced of the
great curing powers of tar-water. The latter was prepared by mixing a gallon of water with a quart of tar
and after 3 days removing the supernatant. Tar-water
was used as a remedy by many, but considered quackery
by others. To settle the controversy, Berkeley proposed a controlled clinical trial as follows: Patients were to be "put into two hospitals at the same
time of the year, and provided with the same necessi-
ties of diet and lodging; and, for further care," he
said "let one have a tub of tar-water and an old woman; the other hospital, what attendance and drugs you
please" (6). If this trial had been carried out, the
results would have shown tar-water to be far more effective than the standard therapies of the day. There
is an obvious explanation. Humoral theories dominated
medical practice in those days and the treatments generally brought on dehydration. Berkeley's prescriptions, on the other hand, called for frequent drinking
of large glasses of tar-water (62,89). The remedy was
simply -- water.

THE NINETEENTH CENTURY

The modern, scientific attitude toward medicine
began emerging during the first decades of the 19th
century in France, made possible to a large extent by
the gradual development of a sound nosology. Examination of patients, classification of diseases, and
the observation of their natural course were assuming
increased importance. This approach reached its cul-
mination in the clinicopathologic investigations of
P. C. A. Louis, who was the first to make extensive
and systematic use of record keeping and data analysis, and to insist on their indispensability to medical methodology. He developed his procedure during a
period of 7 years that he spent full time studying
ward patients and their subsequent autopsies (91).
His "Numerical Method" consisted essentially of tabulating data for patients grouped according to various
characteristics, and comparing observed survival patterns and other parameters of prognosis. The most
famous application of his method was to the practice
of bleeding (65). He studied the effects of blood-
letting in series of patients with different diagnoses
and found essentially no difference in death rate or
duration and severity of symptoms between patients
bled or not bled and those bled at different stages
of their disease. His results, completely contradic-
ting the teachings of the day, caused a great uproar
in the medical community. But the ultimate outcome
was inevitable.

Louis' work on bleeding has been called "in some
ways the most significant study ever made in medical
method" (91), because of its far-reaching implications. He also developed guidelines to be followed
in designing prospective studies for evaluating different modes of treatment, in his Essay on Clinical
Instruction (64). The placing of Louis' Numerical
Method into a probabilistic framework was accomplished
by Jules Gavarret, a student of Poisson, in a work
that became the first textbook of medical statistics

(42). Louis had great influence on the development
of scientific medicine in the United States, since
many young Americans were then studying medicine in
Paris. Among them was Oliver Wendell Holmes.

The overwhelming problem with the subsequent rapid
evolution of this critical, objective approach to
medical practice was that it rejected existing treatments as worthless or even harmful, without being able
to provide anything to replace them. The result was
a long period of therapeutic nihilism in the orthodox
practice of medicine. To quote from the Medical Essays of Holmes: "Throw out opium, which the Creator
himself seems to prescribe, for we often see the scar-
let poppy growing in the cornfields, as if it were
foreseen that wherever there is hunger to be fed there
must also be pain to be soothed; throw out a few specifics which our art did not discover, and is hardly
needed to apply; throw out wine, which is a food, and
the vapors which produce the miracle of anesthesia,
and I firmly believe that if the whole materia medica,
as now used, could be sunk to the bottom of the sea,
it would be all the better for mankind, -- and all the
worse for the fishes" (58).

But people were suffering and they needed hope.
And they were willing to pay for it, in the form of
elixirs and nostrums and other promises of universal
cure. Thus, the 19th century became also the great
era of patent medicines, when quacks amassed large
fortunes at the expense of a helpless and gullible
public (53). One of the objects of great fear was the
disease called cancer. A popular remedy for it was
Swift's Specific, distributed by the Swift Specific
Company founded in 1879. It was a vegetable compound
based on a secret formula allegedly obtained from
Uanita, the daughter of a Creek Indian chieftain in
Georgia. Other newspaper ads included guarantees of
permanent cure at the Berkshire Hills Sanatorium in
Massachusetts, and a 40-year record of thousands cured
painlessly in two weeks in Rome, New York. Soothing,
balmy oils instead of surgery or plasters were offered

to cure all types of cancer at Dr. Bye's Sanatorium
in Indiana. And so the promises continued.

These two major movements -- quackery and therapeutic nihilism -- proceeded in parallel to the turn
of the century.

THE TWENTIETH CENTURY

We can consider the cancer problem today through
the eyes of some of its critics, saying how little has
really been accomplished, and that we have not found
a "cure." Or we can look back to see the enormous
progress that has been made, and that it has all been
made essentially in our century. The first few decades brought on results by developments in surgical
techniques and radiation therapy, followed since the
1950s by increasingly successful applications of
chemotherapy (32).

The discovery of antibiotics for the treatment of
infectious diseases and the development of antimalari-
al drugs, in a targeted program during World War II,
raised the possibility of a similar program to approach the problem of cancer. The first two drugs
found to have antitumor effect were nitrogen mustard,
developed originally for gas warfare, and the anti-
metabolite methotrexate. Because of the promising results obtained with these drugs, Congress in 1955
authorized the National Cancer Institute to establish
a Cancer Drug Development Program. The great surge of
research activity that this program precipitated continues to the present day (32).

In a recent paper, DeVita et al. (31) have outlined
the major developments leading to the effective cancer
therapy we have today. These include: (a) The development of en-bloc resection in surgery; (b) the discovery of X-rays by Roentgen, providing physicians
with an additional means of tumor treatment; (c) the
development of inbred systems of experimental animals
such as mice, and the successful transplantation of

tumors into these animals; the identification and
development of systemic modes of therapy have been
made possible because of the existence of these animal
systems; and (d) the development of the randomized
clinical trial. The first large-scale controlled
trial was designed by Sir Austin Bradford Hill and
implemented by the British Medical Research Council
in 1946 to evaluate the effect of streptomycin in the
treatment of pulmonary tuberculosis (56). Zubrod and
Schneiderman were instrumental in the introduction of
controlled trials into the U.S. cancer program. Among
the first trials were those reported by Frei et al.
in 1958 (39) for comparison of treatment regimens in
leukemia, and by Zubrod et al. in 1960 (103) for a
variety of solid tumors. These were collaborative
efforts of the NCI's National Cooperative Groups Program which, established in 1955, is still a major
mechanism for treatment evaluation.

The main events in the development of systemic
therapy, based on the syngeneic animal test systems,
have been suggested as the following (31): First,
demonstration that the fractional-kill hypothesis is
applicable to cancer, as it is to the action of anti-
septics on bacteria. This makes possible a quantification of the relationship of drug dose to tumor response and tumor volume. Second, much of the early
work in cancer chemotherapy research focused on testing the hypothesis that drugs alone can cure patients
with advanced cancer; this was first shown for choriocarcinoma. Finally, continued progress in studying
the pharmacology of antitumor drugs, their pharmaco-
kinetics and intermediary metabolism.

THE CANCER PROGRAM TODAY

The cancer drug development and clinical research
program is of very broad scope today, both here and
abroad. It is the inherent challenges posed by this
program that have given impetus to so much fruitful

research in statistical methodology. But it is important to keep in mind that the guiding thrust of successful advances in treatment has always been provided
by evolving concepts in biology as perceived by leading clinical investigators. A constant awareness of
this on the part of the biostatistician is absolutely
essential for productive interaction, because of the
sheer vastness of the overall effort.

There are a number of excellent reports on various
aspects of the NCI's drug development program (16,18-
20,30,32,46,80,99). The stages of development are:
acquisition of the substance, followed by screening
(4); then production and formulation, followed by preclinical toxicology, which involves testing in rodents
as well as larger mammals. Subsequent studies in humans are grouped into Phase I clinical trials, to establish tolerated dose levels and toxicity and observe
for any therapeutic effect; Phase II trials to measure
efficacy; and Phase III trials, controlled studies
aimed at showing effectiveness as compared with standard therapy. The final phase is the introduction of
the drug into general medical practice.

In 1975 the NCI's drug screening program tested
over 30,000 compounds. Of these, 36 made it to the
point of selection for toxicologic evaluation, and
just 8 were judged appropriate for clinical trial and
filed for Investigational New Drug approval with the
Food and Drug Administration (32,99). This largely
empirical, random process, which tested up to 40,000
compounds annually in rodents bearing L1210 leukemia
and other transplanted tumors, was supplanted in 1975
by a new, more directed approach based on chemical
and biological rationales. A reduced number of compounds, about 15,000 each year, is evaluated in a P388
murine leukemia system, which is more sensitive than
the L1210. The agents passing this prescreen are then
tested in 8 tumor systems: 3 matched pairs of tumors
of the same organ (lung, colon, breast), that is,
transplantable mouse tumors and human tumors growing
in nude mice, and in the two murine systems L1210

leukemia and B16 melanoma. The main issues of interest are the identification of new types of drugs, better prediction of specific tumor response by use of
the matched experimental tumors, and the question
whether human tumor xenografts are more useful for
predicting human response than transplanted mouse tumors. The full evaluation of this new approach will
require extensive data from clinical studies, but the
early results are promising (32).

A list of commercially available anticancer drugs
is shown in Figure 1 (32) by year of FDA approval.
The current system of drug approval is a complex procedure under the jurisdiction of the Food and Drug
Administration. It is based on a law passed by Congress in 1962, in the wake of the Thalidomide tragedy
(93). This law authorized the FDA to control the
clinical testing of new drugs, requiring manufacturers
to establish their safety and efficacy. Three phases
of testing were prescribed and informed consent was
to be obtained from each subject. (A further discussion of this is given in Chapter 5.)

Table 1 (16) shows a general overview of reported
drug activity for the major tumor types. The entry
for each cell is one of 4 categories: 0 to ++, ranging from inadequate evaluation to definite activity
against the tumor type in question; NE stands for "not
evaluated." The following observations are of interest: 57% of the 464 combinations are marked NE, that
is, they have not been evaluated. Of the remaining
201, 38% were either inadequate evaluations or drug
activity was not clearly established. Results were
definitely positive in 21% of combinations and negative in 41%. Given variations in drug regimen and
patient selection, the difficulties in combining results from different studies, and the perennial questions of sample size, one is struck by the enormity
of the inherent statistical problems.

A summary was also compiled for two-drug combinations considered most promising against the major tumors, based on those found most active as single

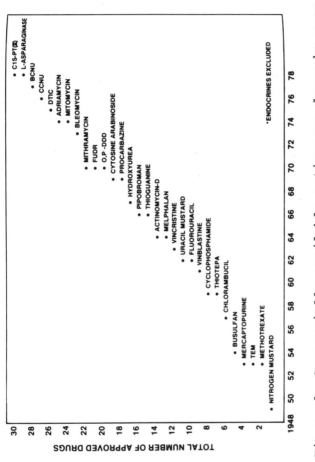

Figure 1. Commercially available anticancer drugs by year of approval. Reproduced from DeVita et al. (32), The drug development and clinical trials programs of the Division of Cancer Treatment, National Cancer Institute, Cancer Clinical Trials 2: 206 (1979), Masson Publishing USA, Inc., New York.

TABLE 1. Drug Activity by Tumor Type[a]

Drugs	Colon	Lung	Breast	Pancreas	Ovary	Prostate	Stomach
Alkylating agents							
Cytoxan	+	++	++	0	++	0	NE
Nitrogen mustard	–	++	+	NE	0	NE	NE
Chlorambucil	–	–	+	NE	+	NE	NE
Melphalan	–	–	++	NE	++	NE	NE
Busulfan	NE	–	NE	NE	NE	–	NE
Antimetabolites							
5-FU	++	–	++	++	++	+	++
Methotrexate	+	++	++	NE	NE	NE	NE
6-Mercaptopurine	–	–	–	NE	NE	NE	NE
6-Thioguanine	–	NE	NE	NE	NE	NE	NE
Ara-C	–	–	–	NE	NE	NE	NE
Mitotic inhibitors							
Vincristine	–	–	++	NE	–	0	NE
Vinblastine	–	–	++	NE	–	NE	NE
Antitumor antibiotics							
Dactinomycin	–	–	–	NE	NE	NE	NE
Mithramycin	–	0	–	NE	NE	0	NE
Daunorubicin	NE	NE	NE	NE	NE	NE	NE
Adriamycin	–	++	++	NE	+	+	NE
Bleomycin	–	–	–	NE	0	NE	NE
Mitomycin-C	++	+	+	–	NE	NE	++
Random synthetics and miscellaneous							
BCNU	++	+	+	–	0	NE	+
CCNU	++	+	+	NE	NE	NE	0
Methyl-CCNU	++	+	–	NE	NE	NE	0
Streptozotocin	–	–	–	–	NE	NE	NE
DTIC	–	–	–	NE	NE	NE	NE
Hexamethylmelamine	–	++	+	NE	+	0	0
Dibromodulcitol	–	–	+	NE	NE	NE	NE
Hydroxyurea	–	+	–	NE	NE	NE	NE
Procarbazine	–	+	–	NE	NE	NE	NE
L-Asparaginase	–	–	NE	NE	NE	NE	NE
Dibromomannitol	NE	NE	NE	NE	NE	NE	NE

TABLE 1. (continued)

Cervix	Head and neck	Bladder	Kidney	Esophagus	Brain	Testicle	Melanoma	Sarcoma
++	-	0	-	0	-	+	-	++
0	NE	NE	NE	0	-	+	-	NE
+	NE	0	0	NE	NE	+	-	+
-	NE	NE	NE	NE	NE	++	-	NE
NE	NE	NE	NE	NE	NE	NE	NE	NE
++	+	++	-	-	-	NE	-	NE
++	++	NE	NE	-	+	NE	-	NE
NE	NE	NE	NE	NE	NE	NE	-	NE
NE	NE	NE	NE	NE	NE	NE	NE	NE
NE	NE	NE	NE	NE	NE	NE	-	NE
+	NE	NE	NE	NE	-	0	-	++
NE	NE	NE	NE	NE	-	++	-	NE
NE	NE	NE	NE	NE	NE	++	+	++
NE	NE	NE	NE	NE	-	++	0	NE
NE	NE	NE	NE	NE	NE	NE	NE	NE
+	+	++	-	NE	NE	+	-	++
+	++	NE	0	-	0	++	-	NE
0	NE	NE	NE	0	NE	NE	0	NE
NE	0	NE	0	NE	++	NE	++	NE
NE	NE	NE	0	NE	++	NE	+	NE
NE	NE	NE	0	NE	+	NE	+	NE
NE	NE	NE	NE	NE	NE	NE	NE	NE
NE	NE	NE	NE	NE	0	NE	++	+
-	-	0	-	NE	NE	NE	-	NE
NE	0	NE	NE	NE	NE	NE	0	NE
0	0	0	-	NE	NE	NE	+	NE
NE	NE	NE	NE	NE	0	-	-	NE
NE	NE	NE	NE	NE	NE	NE	NE	NE
NE	NE	NE	NE	NE	NE	NE	NE	NE

[a] Adapted from Carter (16).

NE: not evaluated.

0: inadequate evaluation; a decision on drug activity is not possible.

-: adequate evaluation; drug inactive.

+: adequate evaluation; evidence of drug activity, but not clearly established.

++: adequate evaluation; drug definitely active.

agents (18). The percentage of combinations actually
tested ranges from 6 to 22%. Selection of drugs for
combination therapy is of course determined by additional criteria: The drugs should have minimal over-
lapping toxicity and different mechanisms of action,
and there may be other biochemical or pharmacologic
considerations. But the statistical questions just
raised remain.

Phase III clinical trials have proceeded from single agent or modality evaluations to multiagent regimen studies and those of combined modality treatment,
including surgery, radiation therapy, chemotherapy,
and immunotherapy. They have used both concurrent
randomized and historical controls. Recent developments include adjuvant therapy for minimal residual
disease (29). These studies have been carried out
over the years by individual institutions as well as
the cooperative group mechanism. About 20,000 new
patients are entered into cooperative group clinical
trials each year, submitted by some 760 participating
institutions (28). A book summarizing the work of
the cooperative groups has recently been published
(59). Another relevant recent publication is a review
by disease site of randomized trials in cancer (92),
part of the monograph series of the EORTC, the European Organization for Research on Treatment of Cancer.

A further indication of the scope of ongoing work
in clinical cancer research is given by the following:
The Proceedings of the 1981 annual meeting of the
American Society of Clinical Oncology and the American
Association for Cancer Research, each of which has a
membership of about 2700, included 781 abstracts dealing with clinical trials. The new edition of the Compilation of Experimental Cancer Therapy Protocol Summaries (25) lists 1574 ongoing Phase II and III studies, testing a total of 179 agents. Eighty-five percent of these trials are from the United States, but
there are others from around the world. The 1978 registry of controlled clinical trials of the UICC, the
International Union against Cancer, lists 945 cancer-

related trials conducted in 32 countries (36). A
search by MEDLARS, the computerized bibliography retrieval system of the National Library of Medicine,
produced a list of 351 journals publishing results of
clinical studies in human cancer.

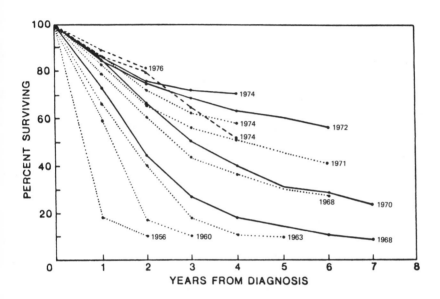

Figure 2. The improving survival of children with
acute lymphocytic and undifferentiated leukemia diagnosed between 1956 and 1976. Composite experience of
Cancer and Acute Leukemia Group B, the Children's Cancer Study Group and the Southwest Oncology Group. Reproduced by permission from Hammond, D. (50), Progress
in the study, treatment and cure of the cancers of
children, in: Burchenal, J. H., and Oettgen, H. F.,
eds., Cancer: Achievements, Challenges, and Prospects
for the 1980s, Vol. 2, Grune & Stratton (1981).

ACCOMPLISHMENTS AND FUTURE GOALS

A detailed overview of the major accomplishments
of the cancer program may be found in the proceedings
of a recent international symposium on cancer (12).
Enormous strides have been made in the control of
children's cancers. Figure 2 (50) shows survival
curves for leukemia, covering protocols begun by various cooperative groups over a 20-year period. The
progressive improvement in duration of survival from
diagnosis is dramatic. In Figure 3 (50) estimated
two-year survival rates are given for children with
solid tumors diagnosed over the last 40 years.
Hodgkin's disease and Wilms' tumor are now very close
to complete control. An example of successful treatment of an adult malignancy is that of Hodgkin's disease, with results shown in Figure 4 for successive
eras of treatment (61).

A summary of the estimated impact of therapy is
shown in Table 2, cited from the review paper by
DeVita et al. (32); it is based on 1977 incidence
data (15). The overall long-term survival rate is
now over 40% and about 60% if skin and in situ cervix
cancers are included. An update of this analysis,
with further details on the effect of different types
of chemotherapy, is given in a follow-up paper by
DeVita and associates (31).

Long-term cure of a proportion of patients with
advanced disease can now be achieved with chemotherapy
for 12 types of cancer. They include: acute lymphocytic leukemia in children, acute myelogenous leukemia
in adults, Hodgkin's disease, diffuse histiocytic
lymphoma, nodular mixed lymphomas, Burkitt's lymphoma,
Ewing's sarcoma, embryonal rhabdomyosarcoma, Wilms'
tumor, choriocarcinoma, testicular carcinoma, and
ovarian carcinoma. These are generally rare malignancies occurring in children and young adults and involve less than 10% of cases of cancer and of cancer
deaths each year. But for these age groups the successive decline in mortality in recent years is

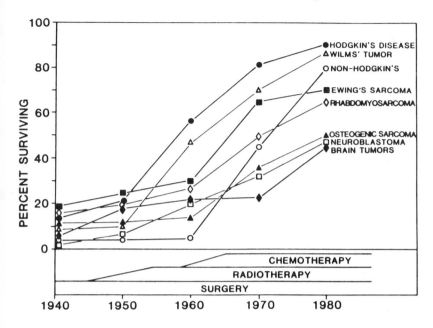

Figure 3. Progressive improvement in survival of children with solid tumors, 1940-1980. Proportion surviving two years from diagnosis. Data from multiple sources are shown relative to the chronology of the general application of the 3 principal therapeutic modalities to the tumors of children. Reproduced by permission from Hammond, D. (50), Progress in the study, treatment and cure of the cancers of children, in: Burchenal, J. H., and Oettgen, H. F., eds., Cancer: Achievements, Challenges, and Prospects for the 1980s, Vol. 2, Grune & Stratton (1981).

evident, as can be seen in Figure 5 (32). The decrease is more pronounced considering only the cohort of those under age 30, and is maintained even if one takes into consideration a possible decrease in the incidence of some cancers affecting this segment of the population. Cancer incidence is difficult to estimate and has been the subject of some controversy. (See Chapter 3 for further discussion.)

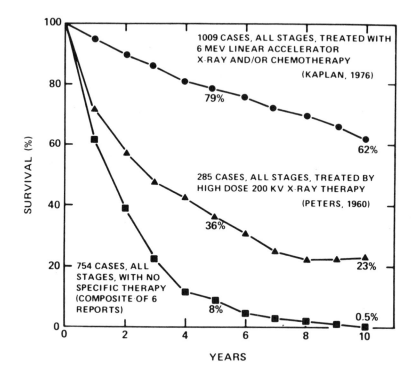

Figure 4. Survival of patients with Hodgkin's disease (all stages) in 3 therapeutic eras. Reproduced from Kaplan (61).

The need is urgent for new approaches for the 220,000 cancer patients each year who are expected to develop recurrent disease after treatment of their localized tumor. These patients are candidates for adjuvant chemotherapy, and numerous such studies are under way. Progress is already being made by reducing mortality due to recurrent breast cancer.

New areas of clinical investigation cover the full range of treatment modalities (31,32). In radiotherapy, they include study of high linear energy transfer (LET) radiation and of the interaction of drugs and radiation, and research in the use of agents

TABLE 2. Estimated Impact of Cancer Therapy, Based on 1977 Incidence Data[a,c]

Patient category	Number of cases	Percent
A. New cases, excluding skin and in situ cervix	700,000	100
B. Localized tumor	500,000	71
Remain free of tumor	280,000	40
Develop recurrent tumor[b]	220,000	31
C. Metastatic disease	200,000	29
"Effective" chemotherapy exists	92,000	
Possible to prolong life	60,000	
Treated for cure	32,000	
"Cured"	11,000	

[a]Total number of new cases: 1,000,000.
[b]Prime candidates for chemotherapy: 150,000.
[c]Table adapted from DeVita et al. (32).

functioning as radiosensitizers and radioprotectors. Studies are also being carried out on problems of toxicology related to these treatments, and on treatment interaction with alterations in temperature (hyperthermia).

Other treatment research areas include the development of modified surgical procedures and examination of the role of nutritional support. Research in pain control and antiemetic therapy is in progress, the latter to alleviate a serious side effect of both chemotherapy and radiation therapy. The development of new types of drugs is under study, and of biologic response modifiers such as immunoadjuvants and

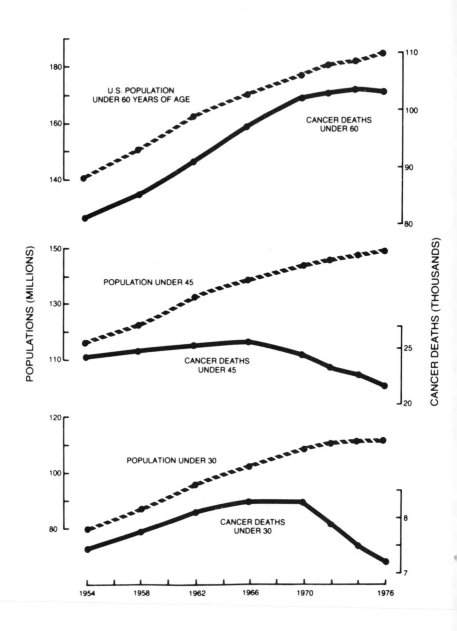

Figure 5. Cancer mortality and U.S. population trends, 1954-1976. Reproduced from DeVita et al. (32).

interferon. A relatively new area of investigation
is that of chemoprevention, aimed at controlling the
late effects of cancer therapy, which may include
treatment-induced second malignancies. Such agents
could also be of great importance for populations at
high risk for developing cancer.

Along the future path of new drugs for cancer and
the more efficient use of known ones is the challenge
of redefining histologic cancer categories in terms
of antigenic subsets. The study of surface antigens
of cancer cells has now been made possible through
the new techniques of hybridomas and their monoclonal
antibodies. And a more efficient screening procedure
for new drugs could ultimately be provided by homogeneous clones of human tumors, replacing the present
murine systems (102).

In all of these areas foreseen today as the approaches of tomorrow, there is seemingly endless potential for contributions by the statistician.

THE IMPACT OF STATISTICAL METHODOLOGY

This leads naturally to the question: How can we
assess the nature of the interface between biostatistics and clinical cancer research, and the impact of
statistical methodology?

The very high response rate to my letter reflects
a strong interest in this subject on the part of both
physicians and statisticians. There has been a great
deal of concern with methodology in clinical cancer
research, with several recent international symposia
devoted to this subject. The Committee on Controlled
Therapeutic Trials of the International Union against
Cancer has been engaged in a project to evaluate the
impact of controlled trials, using as their starting
point the studies registered with the UICC Information
Office (3,21,37). A major area of controversy has
been the use of concurrent randomized versus historical controls, and ethical considerations have figured

heavily in the arguments proposed in support of each
viewpoint.

There is an extensive literature dealing with principles and problems in the design of clinical trials
(104), and it is not my goal here to elaborate on
these. With the exception of Gehan (43), who has ad-
vocated the use of historical controls in some circumstances, statisticians stand firmly for the principles
of randomization and the randomized clinical trial.
But Gehan's position is by no means categorical;
throughout his career he has participated in the design and analysis of numerous randomized clinical trials. Among clinical investigators there is a much
broader scope of response, although the majority
strongly support the need for randomization. I am not
in a position to question the sincerity of medical
colleagues who argue against randomized trials on ethical grounds, which they see as deriving from the nature of the doctor-patient relationship (54). Very
interesting is the paper by Mathé (69) calling for
ecumenism in clinical trials, a free and open discussion of strengths and weaknesses of each approach.
He feels that the present controversy is healthy and
sums up his view by quoting Werner Heisenberg: "It
is probably true quite generally that in the history
of human thinking the most fruitful developments frequently take place at those points where two different
lines of thought meet."

Especially thought provoking are the comments by
clinical investigators suggesting that statisticians
develop new methods that are more appropriate for
clinical studies. To quote from just a few letters[*]:
"The biggest problem in clinical trial research is
the assumption that the perfect clinical trial

---

[*]The respondents to the survey are not identified by
name in this report. Selections of their relevant
published work are listed in the bibliography.

methodology is here .... We must continue to be open-
minded and to challenge our prejudices with new approaches ...." Another suggests "a continuing search,
and re-examination of the optimal experimental design
for studies. Biomedical therapeutic research is advancing very rapidly, and therefore there is a constant need to re-examine our biostatistical approaches." And from another letter: "I believe we should
pay more attention to developing methodology to replace randomized clinical trials, since most patients
don't care for them, and the essential ingredient in
these studies is still patients. If it is possible
to do proper studies some other way, we should attempt
to do so." Someone else writes: "As we move into the
area of prevention trials ... some variant of the randomized controlled trial will have to be utilized in
order that the costs of such trials do not exceed the
total budget of the NCI." Finally, from a statistician: "I would underline the unsatisfactory nature
of the classical Neyman-Pearson approach to clinical
trials. The more I think about this, the less happy
I am with the way of thinking which we have now suc-
ceeded in persuading clinicians to adopt."

The reaction to the question of impact of single
center versus cooperative group studies and the types
of controls used was surprising in that there was
virtually complete agreement among the respondents:
Nearly all significant discoveries in the treatment
of cancer have emerged from single center studies,
and have been based on historical controls.

The adjuvant studies in breast cancer were listed
as the single exception. Cooperative studies are essential, however, for the study of rare diseases. An
example given by several was the productive collaboration resulting in the development of successful treatment for Wilms' tumor.

In a more general way, the significant impact of
cooperative groups was recognized in several categories: Their main role is in confirmation and generalization of new findings, an indispensable part of

scientific discovery. Subjection of new claims to
systematic evaluation has also resulted in the disproving of numerous apparent advances reported by
smaller and uncontrolled studies. It would be difficult to overemphasize the importance of this contribution. The development of large-scale clinical trial
methodology has been another significant achievement.
This has included statistical design, protocol definitions of response and toxicity, uniform pathology review, and techniques of data management and analysis.
It is in this general area that the statistical approach has had its major impact.

By structuring the development of multidisciplinary
teams and enforcing the implementation of systematic
planning, data collection, and review, the cooperative
groups have brought a general awareness of principles
of scientific methodology to the clinical research
community. This has immense value independently of
the actual studies being carried out. One investigator said: "I don't believe methodology has much to do
with discovery." But another pointed out that while
new concepts may originate in the minds of single individuals, the frequent group discussions and systematic data analyses provide the best stimulus for the
germination of these insights.

The comments on statistical aspects of Phase I and
II trials were made generally by statisticians. The
need for good design is implicit but formal methodology is not required in the view of many clinical investigators. The problem of reproducibility of reported results is generally recognized, however. A
summary by Moertel of the wide range in response found
by a series of investigators studying the same agent
for treatment of the same disease is shown in Table 3
(74). Sample size is an extremely important issue.
It is interesting to note here that the higher response rates were all reported for studies with fewer
than 50 patients; the overall response rate for the
15 trials in this category was 37%. For the other 5
studies, which had sample sizes ranging from 87 to

TABLE 3. Results of Rapid Injection of 5-FU for Treatment of Advanced Carcinoma of the Large Bowel[a]

Reporting group	Number of patients treated	Objective regressions (%)
Sharp and Benefiel	13	85
Hall and Good	19	63
Rochlin et al.	47	55
Allaire et al.	17	47
Cornell et al.	13	46
Eyerly	12	42
Field	37	41
Bell	22	36
Weiss and Jackson	37	35
Ferguson and Humphrey	12	33
Hurley	150	31
Eastern Cooperative Group	48	27
Brennan et al.	183	23
Hyman et al.	30	20
Ansfield	141	17
Mayo Clinic	144	15
Ellison	87	12
Kennedy	22	9
Knoepp et al.	11	9
Olson and Greene	12	8

[a]Adapted from Moertel, C. G., and Reitemeier, R. J. (74), Advanced Gastrointestinal Cancer: Clinical Management and Chemotherapy, Harper and Row (1969).

183, the overall response rate was 20%.

What can one say about general impact? Several clinical investigators stated that the emergence of

the statistician as a full member of the research team
is in itself a significant achievement. In other
words, his presence is accepted as important, and the
approaches he represents are at least implicitly recognized as valid. "Statistical methodology has developed mechanisms of thinking which dominate clinical
science," someone wrote. And from a statistician:
"Clinical therapeutics has very high standards for
evidence, a sign that statistical principles have been
widely accepted."

MAJOR PROBLEMS

What is the main problem as recognized by statisticians and seen in the literature? Without question
this seems to be poor quality: small sample size and
inadequate design, preventing meaningful conclusions
in a disturbingly large proportion of published studies. References to several recent literature reviews
from this viewpoint are included in the bibliography
(35,40,85,90,101). Table 4 (77) illustrates a survey
of recent clinical trials in cancer; the median sample
size per treatment arm in these studies was about 50.
For the majority of these trials the sample size used
could provide reasonable power only for differences
so large as to be highly unlikely.

Another problem area is related to the function of
regulatory agencies. Some investigators feel that
present regulations impede progress and have an adverse impact on innovation. I am not qualified to
assess clinical aspects of the situation or the apparent problems of political pressure. I would, however,
like to share some of my own related experiences.

During the past 3 years I was a member of the Oncologic Drugs Advisory Committee of the Food and Drug
Administration, and also served on both of its subcom-
mittees: the subcommittee for preclinical toxicology,
and the subcommittee on clinical guidelines for the
evaluation of anticancer drugs. All committee

TABLE 4. Sample Sizes[a] for Comparative Studies of
Treatments in Cancer[b,f]

Size	M & L[c]	GI[d]	Breast cancer	Cancer[e]
0-9	4	3	10	
10-19	16	9	36	9
20-29	11	7	67	14
30-39	9	7	40	
40-49	5	4	25	
50-59	4	9	19	8
60-69	1	7	1	5
70-89	6	7	22	2
90-109	0	12	27	
110-129	0	2	10	
130-149	4	1	2	8
150-199	1	4	9	
200-299		5	3	4
300-499		4	12	4
500-799			2	
Total samples	61	81	285	54

[a]These sizes give the number of patients assigned to
one treatment. The sample sizes compared were usually approximately equal.
[b]The first 3 columns refer to studies reported in
Staquet (92); the last column pertains to clinical
trials published in Cancer and reviewed by Zelen et
al. (101).
[c]Multiple myeloma and chronic myelocytic leukemia.
[d]Gastrointestinal cancer.
[e]Approximate class intervals.
[f]Adapted by permission of the publisher from (77),
Reporting standards and research strategies for controlled trials, by Mosteller et al., Controlled Clinical Trials 1:45. Copyright 1980 by Elsevier Science
Publishing Co., Inc.

137

meetings are formal government hearings, open to the general public and the news media. The advisory committees are asked to make recommendations concerning action to be taken on new drugs, and in recent years the acceptance rate of their recommendations to the FDA has been over 98%. All voting is by show of hands. Held in hearing rooms crowded with spectators, and monitored by electronic recording devices, which on at least one occasion included network TV cameras, these meetings have provided by far the most dramatic encounters in my professional experience. With proponents of opposing views facing each other in an emotionally charged atmosphere, how does one discuss science? Arguments based on anecdotal evidence and uncontrolled studies are difficult to handle in a setting where the subtleties of the methodologic problems involved are beyond the technical expertise of the vast majority of those in attendance.

What concerned me most was the enormous amount of inconclusive and often worthless material presented to the committee for evaluation. Clinical trial methodology is now well developed; pharmaceutical companies are aware of it and they have adequate financial resources; the National Cancer Institute has in its turn provided abundant support. Patients have generally been available and time has not been a problem. Why then were in so many cases the proper studies not carried out? Why does the appeal so often have to be to "those poor suffering patients out there" who need new drugs, at a hearing of a regulatory agency concerned with scientific principles? In controversial reviews the committee vote usually fell along predictable lines, separating the clinically and the more research oriented members.

I personally believe that some form of regulation is necessary and that open hearings are an appropriate component of our system of government. But procedures can be modified to become more effective. An improvement in the FDA procedure as I observed it could be achieved by the appointment of a subcommittee

consisting of statisticians from the FDA, the NCI,
and the Oncologic Drugs Advisory Committee. This subcommittee would review the materials submitted in support of requests for action, and studies would not be
presented to the full advisory committee for discussion at an open hearing unless or until their conclusions met accepted standards of statistical evidence.
The long-term resolution of the problem clearly requires stronger input from the statistical profession
into the design and analysis of many of these clinical
studies.

Preclinical toxicology protocols are likewise the
subject of much controversy. I can only report on
statistical aspects of the problem, which again pertain to the poor quality of published studies. A case
in point is a 1979 review paper by Guarino et al.
(47). Striking discrepancies were revealed in estimated lethal dose levels even in tests repeated at
the same laboratories, under the same conditions, and
using the same mouse strains. In 9 of 16 studies reported, there was a lack of parallelism in pairs of
repeated experiments; in 12 of the studies the data
were insufficient for computer analysis and the probit
regression lines were obtained by visual inspection.
And yet, principles and methods of bioassay have been
well developed for many years.

To end this point on a positive note: The Oncologic Drugs Advisory Committee collaborated in the development of a basic set of guidelines for the clinical
evaluation of anticancer drugs, and these have just
been published by the Food and Drug Administration
(48).

Aside from the issue of regulation, there has been
the problem of delay in resolving major controversies
in treatment. An example sometimes mentioned is that
of breast cancer. Assessment of radical mastectomy
and the use of chemotherapeutic agents could have been
carried out much sooner (30). The scientific methodology, drugs, and related biological information have
been available. With 100,000 new cases of breast

cancer diagnosed each year and survival rates at a
plateau, why were these studies not done a long time
ago?

Another example, one in which I have been personally involved from the beginning, is the controversy
surrounding the treatment of osteogenic sarcoma. With
Marcove et al. (67-68,73) we published the first major
retrospective study of the disease, which was then
used by many investigators as historical control for
their own studies and subsequently confirmed by other
centers. Drastic recent improvements in survival experience have been attributed to the effect of adjuvant chemotherapy. But the Mayo Clinic has observed
greatly increased survival even in patients who received only the standard surgical treatment (95).
This problem, although under constant, wide-ranging
discussion for over 5 years, has still not been resolved (17,79; see also Chapter 6).

In order to present a balanced picture, let me also
cite an example illustrating just the reverse, namely,
excellent cooperation across disciplinary and institutional boundaries to address an important problem. I
was the statistician for a cooperative study planned
to investigate the late effects of cancer therapy in
long-term survivors of childhood cancers. Working
with D'Angio, Meadows, and associates, we began a pilot study with 3 institutions. Preliminary results
indicated an increased risk of a second cancer in the
field of irradiation for children who had received
antifolate drugs, and a slightly decreased risk for
those who had been given actinomycin D. Because of
the serious implications of the finding concerning
antifolate therapy, the decision was made to do a
larger study without delay, focusing on this issue.
A carefully planned case-control study was carried
out, based on 15,000 patient records from 10 cooperat-
ing institutions in the United States and Europe. The
required data were collected and analyzed in less than
one year. The early evidence for a harmful effect of
antifolates washed out in this larger study, whereas

the indicated protective effect of actinomycin D held
up and was now statistically significant. This result
was especially surprising because actinomycin D is
oncogenic in animals and a radiation enhancer (27).

CONCLUSION

Given this overview, the range of accomplishments
and problems we have been discussing, the question
arises: Can we reach a conclusion that is relevant to
the theme of this conference? In other words, are
there well-defined objectives that can be sought as
meaningful goals by today's biostatistician? I believe that the answer is yes, and that there are essentially two: initiative and scientific involvement.
    Exercising strong initiative, we should assume an
increasingly active role in implementing known methodology, to see to it that more of the clinical research
being carried out is scientifically informative. We
should be alert and exert influence when there is an
opportunity to settle an issue early by a properly
designed clinical trial. We should help to resolve
methodologic controversies, by engaging in continuous
dialogue with the medical community, including the
editors of medical journals. Reviewing the literature
and presenting the results of actual studies can be a
very persuasive argument, as has been shown in recent
papers by Mosteller and associates (45,75-77). This
report has addressed itself to clinical studies and
the evaluation of cancer treatment, but an equally
important and challenging field for the statistician
is that of cancer prevention (97; see also Chapter 2).
    As the second objective, we should be aware of the
state of scientific developments. A letter from a
clinical investigator states: "I am concerned, from
time to time, that left to their own devices, statisticians will often give short shrift to our ignorance
of biology." Close collaboration with good scientists
is probably the ideal way to overcome this problem.

These investigators are most likely to be following promising leads derived in the full context of our present knowledge. The suggestion in some of the letters that entirely new statistical approaches be developed for clinical trials needs to be examined carefully in the light of what is possible and in the long run desirable. In any case, increased professional interaction promoting a better understanding of scientific issues by the statistician is certain to be of benefit to all concerned.

Mathematics has traditionally been called either the queen or the handmaiden of science. Handmaiden or queen? But surely these are concepts of a bygone era. A modern woman does not wish to be either; what she seeks is partnership as an equal. It may be appropriate to set this as our goal, as we collaborate with biomedical scientists in the search for greater insight into life processes and the ultimate eradication of disease: equal partnership in sharing the responsibility and the challenge.

REFERENCES

1. Armitage, P. (1979), The analysis of data from clinical trials, The Statistician 28: 171-183.

2. Armitage, P. (1979), The design of clinical trials, Australian Journal of Statistics 21: 266-281.

3. Armitage, P., Bardelli, D., Galton, D. A. G., Gehan, E. A., Higgins, G. A., Magnus, K., Miller, A. B., Pocock, S. J., and Saracci, R. (1978), Methods and Impact of Controlled Therapeutic Trials in Cancer, Part I, UICC Technical Report Series, Vol. 36, Geneva.

4. Armitage, P., and Schneiderman, M. A. (1958), Statistical problems in a mass screening program,

Annals of New York Academy of Sciences 76: 896–908.

5. Bacon, F. (1623), De augmentis scientiarum, in: Robertson, J. M., ed., The Philosophical Works of Francis Bacon, Reprint, 1970, Books for Libraries Press, Freeport, New York.

6. Berkeley, G. (1752), Farther thoughts on tar-water, in: Fraser, A. C., ed., The Works of George Berkeley, Vol. 3, 1901, Clarendon Press, Oxford.

7. Box, J. F. (1978), R. A. Fisher, The Life of a Scientist, Wiley, New York.

8. Breslow, N. E. (1978), Perspectives on the statistician's role in cooperative clinical research, Cancer 41: 326–332.

9. Breslow, N. E. (1979), Clinical Trials, Technical Report No. 38, Department of Biostatistics, School of Public Health and Community Medicine, University of Washington, Seattle.

10. Brown, B. W. (1980), Statistical controversies in the design of clinical trials: Some personal views, Controlled Clinical Trials 1: 13–27.

11. Bull, J. P. (1959), The historical development of clinical therapeutic trials, Journal of Chronic Diseases 10: 218–248.

12. Burchenal, J. H., and Oettgen, H. F., eds. (1981), Cancer: Achievements, Challenges, and Prospects for the 1980s (2 Vols.), Grune & Stratton, New York.

13. Byar, D. P. (1979), The necessity and justification of randomized clinical trials, in:

Tagnon, H. J., and Staquet, M. J., eds., Controversies in Cancer: Design of Trials and Treatment, Masson, New York, pp. 75-82.

14. Byar, D. P., Simon, R. M., Friedewald, W. T., Schlesselman, J. J., DeMets, D. L., Ellenberg, J. H., Gail, M. H., and Ware, J. H. (1976), Randomized clinical trials: Perspectives on some recent ideas, The New England Journal of Medicine 295: 74-80.

15. Cancer Facts and Figures (1977), American Cancer Society, New York.

16. Carter, S. K. (1977), Phase III studies and the strategy for integrating chemotherapy into a combined modality approach, in: Methods of Development of New Anticancer Drugs, U.S.A.-U.S.S.R. Monograph, National Cancer Institute, Bethesda, Maryland, pp. 93-100.

17. Carter, S. K. (1980), The dilemma of adjuvant chemotherapy for osteogenic sarcoma, Cancer Clinical Trials 3: 29-36.

18. Carter, S. K., and Goldin, A. (1977), Experimental models and their clinical correlations, in: Methods of Development of New Anticancer Drugs, U.S.A.-U.S.S.R. Monograph, National Cancer Institute, Bethesda, Maryland, pp. 63-74.

19. Carter, S. K., and Selawry, O. (1977), Phase II clinical trials, in: Methods of Development of New Anticancer Drugs, U.S.A.-U.S.S.R. Monograph, National Cancer Institute, Bethesda, Maryland, pp. 81-92.

20. Carter, S. K., Selawry, O., and Slavik, M. (1977), Phase I clinical trials, in: Methods of Development of New Anticancer Drugs, U.S.A.-

U.S.S.R. Monograph, National Cancer Institute,
Bethesda, Maryland, pp. 75-80.

21. Cascinelli, N., Davis, H. L., Flamant, R.,
    Kennio, Y., Lalanne, C. M., Muggia, F. M.,
    Rozencweig, M., Staquet, M. J., and Veronesi, U.
    (1981), Methods and Impact of Controlled Thera-
    peutic Trials in Cancer, Part II, UICC Technical
    Report Series, Vol. 59, Geneva.

22. Chalmers, T. (1975), Randomization of the first
    patient, Medical Clinics of North America 59:
    1035-1038.

23. Chalmers, T. C., Block, J. B., and Lee, S.
    (1972), Controlled studies in clinical cancer re-
    search, The New England Journal of Medicine 287:
    75-77.

24. Cochrane, A. L. (1972), Effectiveness and Effi-
    ciency, Nuffield Provincial Hospitals Trust,
    London.

25. Compilation of Experimental Cancer Therapy Proto-
    col Summaries (1981), International Cancer Re-
    search Data Bank, National Cancer Institute,
    Bethesda, Maryland.

26. Cox, D. (1980), Summary views: A statistician's
    perspective. Cancer Treatment Reports 64: 533-
    535. (Proceedings of Symposium on Designs for
    Clinical Cancer Research, April 13-15, 1978,
    New Orleans, Louisiana.)

27. D'Angio, G. J., Meadows, A., Miké, V., Harris, C.,
    Evans, A., Jaffe, N., Newton, W., Schweisguth, O.,
    Sutow, W., and Morris-Jones, P. (1976), Decreased
    risk of radiation-associated second malignant neo-
    plasms in actinomycin-D-treated patients, Cancer
    37: 1177-1185.

28. Davis, H. L., Durant, J. R., and Holland, J. F.
    (1980), Interrelationships: The groups, the NCI
    and other governmental agencies, in:
    Hoogstraten, B., ed., Cancer Research: Impact of
    the Cooperative Groups, Masson, New York,
    pp. 371-390.

29. DeVita, V. T. (1977), Adjuvant therapy: An over-
    view, in: Salmon, S. E., and Jones, S. E., eds.,
    Adjuvant Therapy of Cancer, Elsevier/North-
    Holland Biomedical Press, Amsterdam, pp. 613-645.

30. DeVita, V. T. (1978), The evolution of therapeu-
    tic research in cancer, The New England Journal
    of Medicine 298: 907-910.

31. DeVita, V. T., Henney, J. E., and Hubbard, S. M.
    (1981), Estimation of the numerical and economic
    impact of chemotherapy in the treatment of can-
    cer, in: Burchenal, J. H., and Oettgen, H. F.,
    eds., Cancer: Achievements, Challenges, and
    Prospects for the 1980s, Vol. 2, Grune &
    Stratton, New York, pp. 859-880.

32. DeVita, V. T., Oliverio, V. T., Muggia, F. M.,
    Wiernik, P. W., Ziegler, J., Goldin, A.,
    Rubin, D., Henney, J., and Schepartz, S. (1979),
    The drug development and clinical trials programs
    of the Division of Cancer Treatment, National
    Cancer Institute, Cancer Clinical Trials 2: 195-
    216.

33. Editorial, Protracted war on cancer, The New York
    Times, June 12, 1981.

34. Farewell, V. T., and D'Angio, G. J. (1981), A
    simulated study of historical controls using real
    data, Biometrics 31: 1-8.

35. Feinstein, A. R. (1974), A survey of statistical

procedures in general medical journals, Clinical
Pharmacology and Therapeutics 15: 97-107.

36. Flamant, R., and Fohanno, C. (1978), Controlled
Therapeutic Trials in Cancer, UICC Technical Report Series, Vol. 32, Geneva.

37. Flamant, R., and Sancho-Garnier, H. (1980),
Knowledge acquisition in oncology from randomized
therapeutic trials, Bulletin of Cancer 67: 446-
449.

38. Forrest, D. W. (1974), Francis Galton: The Life
and Work of a Victorian Genius, Paul Elek,
London.

39. Frei, E., Holland, J. F., Schneiderman, M. A.,
Pinkel, D., Selkirk, G., Freireich, E. J,
Silver, R. T., Gold, G. L., and Regelson, W.
(1958), A comparative study of two regimens of
combination chemotherapy in acute leukemia, Blood
13: 1126-1148.

40. Freiman, J. A., Thomas, A. B., Smith, H.,
Kuebler, R. R. (1978), The importance of beta,
the type II error and sample size in the design
and interpretation of the randomized control trial, The New England Journal of Medicine 299: 690-
694.

41. Freireich, E. J, and Gehan, E. A. (1979), The
limitations of the randomized clinical trial, in:
DeVita, V. T., and Busch, H., eds., Methods in
Cancer Research, Vol. 17, Academic Press, New
York, pp. 277-309.

42. Gavarret, J. (1840), Principes Generaux de
Statistique Medicale, Paris.

43. Gehan, E. A., and Freireich, E. J, (1974),

Non-randomized controls in cancer clinical trials, The New England Journal of Medicine 290: 198–203.

44. George, S. L. (1980), Statistical design for pediatrics: Past, present, and future, in: VanEys, J., and Sullivan, M. P., eds., Status of the Curability of Childhood Cancers, Raven Press, New York, pp. 47–59.

45. Gilbert, J. P., McPeek, B., and Mosteller, F. (1977), Statistics and ethics in surgery and anesthesia, Science 198: 684–689.

46. Guarino, A. M. (1979), Pharmacologic and toxicologic studies of anticancer drugs: Of sharks, mice and men (and dogs and monkeys), in: DeVita, V. T., and Busch, H., eds., Methods in Cancer Research, Vol. 17, Academic Press, New York, pp. 91–174.

47. Guarino, A. M., Rozencweig, M., Kline, I., Penta, J. S., Venditti, J. M., Lloyd, H. H., Holzworth, D. A., and Muggia, F. M. (1979), Adequacies and inadequacies in assessing murine toxicity data with antineoplastic agents, Cancer Research 39: 2204–2210.

48. Guidelines for the Clinical Evaluation of Antineoplastic Drugs (1981), Food and Drug Administration, U.S. Department of Health and Human Services, Rockville, Maryland.

49. Haggard, H. W. (1929), Devils, Drugs, and Doctors, Harper and Brothers, New York.

50. Hammond, D. (1981), Progress in the study, treatment and cure of the cancers of children, in: Burchenal, J. H., and Oettgen, H. F., eds., Cancer: Achievements, Challenges, and Prospects for

the 1980s, Vol. 2, Grune & Stratton, New York, pp. 171-190.

51. Healy, M. J. R. (1979), Does medical statistics exist? Bias 6: 137-182.

52. Healy, M. J. R. (1981), 'Null' results in clinical trials. (Unpublished manuscript.)

53. Hechtlinger, A. (1970), The Great Patent Medicine Era, Or Without Benefit of Doctor, Grosset and Dunlap, New York.

54. Hellman, S. (1979), Randomized clinical trials and the doctor-patient relationship, Cancer Clinical Trials 2: 189-193.

55. Herson, J. (1979), Predictive probability early termination plans for Phase II clinical trials. Biometrics 35: 775-783.

56. Hill, A. B. (1962), Statistical Methods in Clinical and Preventive Medicine, Oxford University Press, New York.

57. Hippocrates (1962), Jones, W. H. S., trans., Vol. 1, Heinemann, London.

58. Holmes, O. W. (1891), Medical Essays, Houghton, Mifflin and Company, Boston.

59. Hoogstraten, B., ed. (1980), Cancer Research: Impact of the Cooperative Groups, Masson, New York.

60. Jones, S. E. (1978), How to evaluate improvements in cancer treatment: The debate continues, Biomedicine 28: 55-57.

61. Kaplan, H. S. (1976), Hodgkin's disease and other

human malignant lymphomas: Advances and prospects, Cancer Research 36: 3863-3878.

62. King, L. S. (1958), The Medical World of the
    Eighteenth Century, University of Chicago Press,
    Chicago.

63. Lee, Y. J., Staquet, M., Simon, R., Catane, R.,
    and Muggia, F. (1979), Two-stage plans for pa-
    tient accrual in Phase II cancer clinical trials,
    Cancer Treatment Reports 63: 1721-1726.

64. Louis, P. C. A. (1834), Essay on Clinical In-
    struction (trans.), P. Martin, London.

65. Louis, P. C. A. (1836), Researches on the Effects
    of Blood-Letting (trans.), C. G. Putnam, Boston.

66. Mantel, N. (1980), A miscellany of statistical
    and other considerations for clinical trials,
    Controlled Clinical Trials 1: 3-11.

67. Marcove, R. C., Miké, V., Hajek, J. V.,
    Levin, A. G., and Hutter, V. P. (1970), Osteogen-
    ic sarcoma under the age of 21:   A review of 145
    operative cases, Journal of Bone and Joint Sur-
    gery 52A: 411-423.

68. Marcove, R. C., Miké, V., Hajek, J. V.,
    Levin, A. G., and Hutter, V. P. (1971), Osteogen-
    ic sarcoma in childhood, New York State Journal
    of Medicine 71: 855-859.

69. Mathé, G. (1978), Towards ecumenism for compara-
    tive trials, Biomedicine 28: 2-6.

70. Meier, P. (1975), Statistics and medical experi-
    mentation, Biometrics 31: 511-529.

71. Meier, P. (1979), Terminating a trial: The

ethical problem, Clinical Pharmacology and Therapeutics 25: 633-640.

72. Miké, V., and Good, R. A. (1977), Old problems,
new challenges. Introduction to Birnbaum Memorial Symposium "Medical Research: Statistics and
Ethics." Science 198: 677-678.

73. Miké, V., and Marcove, R. C. (1978), Osteogenic
sarcoma under the age of 21: Experience at Memorial Sloan-Kettering Cancer Center, in:
Terry, W. D., and Windhorst, D., eds., Immunotherapy of Cancer: Present Status of Trials in
Man, Raven Press, New York.

74. Moertel, C. G., and Reitemeier, R. J. (1969), Advanced Gastrointestinal Cancer: Clinical Management and Chemotherapy, Harper and Row, New York.

75. Mosteller, F. (1979), Problems of omission in
communications, Clinical Pharmacology and Therapeutics 25: 761-764.

76. Mosteller, F. (1981), Innovation and evaluation,
Science 211: 881-886.

77. Mosteller, F., Gilbert, J. P., and McPeek, B.
(1980), Reporting standards and research strategies for controlled trials, Controlled Clinical
Trials 1: 37-58.

78. Mosteller, F., Gilbert, J. P., and McPeek, B.
(1982), Controversies in design and analysis of
clinical trials, in: Shapiro, S., and
Louis, T. A., eds., Clinical Trials: Issues and
Approaches, Marcel Dekker, New York.

79. Muggia, F. M., and Louie, A. C. (1978), Five
years of adjuvant treatment of osteosarcoma:

More questions than answers, Cancer Treatment
Reports 62: 301-305.

80. Muggia, F. M., Rozencweig, M., Chiuten, D. F.,
Jensen-Akula, M. S., Charles, L. M.,
Kubota, T. T., and Bono, V. H. (1980), Phase II
trials: Use of a clinical tumor panel and over-
view of current resources and studies, Cancer
Treatment Reports 64: 1-9.

81. Peto, R. (1978), Clinical trial methodology, Biomedicine 28: 24-36.

82. Peto, R. (1982), Statistical aspects of cancer
trials, in: Halnan, K. E., Boak, J. L.,
Crowther, D., von Essen, C. S., Orr, J. S., and
Peckham, M. J., eds., Treatment of Cancer,
Chapman & Hall, London.

83. Peto, R., Pike, M. C., Armitage, P.,
Breslow, N. E., Cox, D., Howard, S. V.,
Mantel, N., McPherson, K., Peto, J., and
Smith, P. G. (1976), Design and analysis of randomized clinical trials requiring prolonged observation of each patient, Part I, British Journal of Cancer 34: 585-612.

84. Peto, R., Pike, M. C., Armitage, P.,
Breslow, N. E., Cox, D. R., Howard, S. V.,
Mantel, N., McPherson, K., Peto, J., and
Smith, P. G. (1977), Design and analysis of randomized clinical trials requiring prolonged observation of each patient, Part II, British Journal of Cancer 35: 1-39.

85. Pocock, S. J., Armitage, P., and Galton, D. G.
(1978), The size of cancer clinical trials: An
international survey, in: Methods and Impact of
Controlled Therapeutic Trials in Cancer, Part I,
UICC Technical Report Series, Vol. 36, pp. 5-32.

86. Rosenberg, S. A. (1977), Personal comments on problems of interpretation of clinical trials presented at the Conference on the Adjuvant Therapy of Cancer, in: Salmon, S. E., and Jones, S. E., eds., Adjuvant Therapy of Cancer, Elsevier/North-Holland Biomedical Press, Amsterdam, pp. 609-611.

87. Schneiderman, M. (1977), The numerate sciences: Epidemiology and biometry, Journal of the National Cancer Institute 59: 633-644.

88. Shapiro, A. K. (1960), A contribution to a history of the placebo effect, Behavioral Science 5: 109-135.

89. Shapiro, A. K. (1966), The curative waters and warm poultices of psychotherapy, Psychosomatics 7: 21-23.

90. Shor, S., and Karten, L. (1966), Statistical evaluation of medical manuscripts, Journal of the American Medical Association 195: 1123-1128.

91. Shryock, R. H. (1969), The Development of Modern Medicine, Hafner Publishing Company, New York.

92. Staquet, M., ed. (1978), Randomized Trials in Cancer: A Critical Review by Sites, Monograph Series of the European Organization for Research on Treatment of Cancer, Vol. 4, Raven Press, New York.

93. Swazey, J. P. (1978), Protecting the "animal of necessity": Limits to inquiry in clinical investtigation, Daedalus 20: 129-145.

94. Sylvester, R. J., and Staquet, M. J. (1980), Design of Phase II clinical trials in cancer using

decision theory, Cancer Treatment Reports 64: 519-524.

95. Taylor, W. F., Ivins, J. C., Dahlin, D. C., Edmonson, J. H., and Pritchard, D. J. (1978), Trends and variability in survival from osteosarcoma, Mayo Clinic Proceedings 53: 695-700.

96. Tukey, J. W. (1977), Some thoughts on clinical trials, especially problems of multiplicity, Science 198: 679-684.

97. Upton, A. C. (1978), Progress in the prevention of cancer, Preventive Medicine 7: 476-478.

98. Walker, H. (1931), Studies in the History of Statistical Method, Williams Wilkins, Baltimore.

99. Wood, H. B. (1977), Selection of agents for the tumor screen of potential new antineoplastic drugs, in: Methods of Development of New Anticancer Drugs, U.S.A.-U.S.S.R. Monograph, National Cancer Institute, Bethesda, Maryland, pp. 15-35.

100. Zelen, M. (1979), A new design for randomized clinical trials, The New England Journal of Medicine 300: 1242-1245.

101. Zelen, M., Gehan, E., and Glidewell, O. (1980), Biostatistics, in: Hoogstraten, B., ed., Cancer Research: Impact of the Cooperative Groups, Masson, New York, pp. 291-312.

102. Zubrod, C. G. (1981), Development of anti-cancer therapy, in: Burchenal, J. H., and Oettgen, H. F., eds., Cancer: Achievements, Challenges, and Prospects for the 1980s, Vol. 2, Grune & Stratton, New York, pp. 1-10.

103. Zubrod, C. G., Schneiderman, M. A., Frei, E.,

et al. (1960), Appraisal of methods for the study
of chemotherapy of cancer in man: Comparative
therapeutic trial of nitrogen mustard and tri-
ethylene thiophosphoramide, Journal of Chronic
Diseases 11: 7-33.

104. A selection of references concerning the design
of clinical trials is listed in the bibliography
above: 1-2, 8-10, 13-14, 22-24, 26, 34, 41,
43-44, 51-52, 55, 60, 63, 66, 70-72, 78, 81-84,
86, 94, 96, 100. Additional references may be
found in chapters throughout this volume.

CHAPTER 5

Clinical Trials: Exploring Ethical, Legal, and Psychological Issues

Panel Discussion
VALERIE MIKÉ, *Chairman*
GEORGE J. ANNAS
ERIC J. CASSELL
JIMMIE C.B. HOLLAND
ROBERT J. LEVINE

V. Miké: In the book review section of yesterday's edition of The New York Times (27) there was a review of a newly published book entitled Bad Blood: The Tuskegee Syphilis Experiment (14). It is the story of a medical experiment started in 1932 and sponsored by the U.S. Government, in which 400 black sharecroppers afflicted with syphilis were kept under observation without being given any treatment. They were never told that they had syphilis, and were not told that effective treatment was being withheld, even after penicillin became widely available. The experiment continued for an unbelievable 40 years and was stopped only in 1972 when the Associated Press broke the story. Although perhaps the most horrible, this is by no means an isolated incident in the recent history of medical practice. Henry Beecher, in his paper "Ethics and Clinical Research," published in 1966 in The New England Journal of Medicine (2), and M. H. Pappworth, in his book Human Guinea Pigs, published in 1967 (20), called attention to a long series of highly unethical practices in experimentation on human subjects.

Today, barely a decade later, the new field of bioethics has come into its own as a major discipline. There are institutes and scholarly journals devoted to its study (3,13), and a 4-volume encyclopedia of bioethics has been published (8). Experimentation on humans is now closely regulated by the Federal Government.* There is also a great deal of interest in these matters on the part of the general public, paralleling the rise of what is called consumerism in medicine. A modern theory of medical ethics is under development (28).

At today's panel discussion we plan to concentrate on specific issues related to clinical trials, especially those affecting the cancer patient. We are not doing this merely as a cultural exercise, but because the statistician cannot contribute to the development of a meaningful design if he is not aware of other aspects of what is a rather complex situation. The multidisciplinary approach is a characteristic of medical research at its best in the 1980s. Our panelists will make opening statements, addressing legal, psychological, and ethical aspects of clinical trials and the nature of the physician-patient relationship.

LEGAL ASPECTS OF CLINICAL TRIALS

G. J. Annas: I am a lawyer, and for the next few minutes I will talk about the law, to give you a perspective on what the legal issues are concerning human experimentation and the rights of subjects. I think almost any lawyer giving this presentation would

---

*The first code of ethics for human experimentation concerned with the rights of the subject was developed at the trial of war criminals by the Nuremberg Military Tribunal in 1947 (26). The most current general document is the Declaration of Helsinki of the World Medical Association, as revised in 1975. The texts of the Nuremberg Code and the Declaration of Helsinki are reproduced at the end of this chapter. Further material on codes of medical ethics may be found in (8), (17), and (23).

identify the same issues.

I will introduce the topic by discussing a case that did not involve human experimentation. It concerned a physician, Dr. Fleming, who was flying back to Rochester, New York, from Kansas City and he was, as is not terribly uncommon, afraid of flying. During the flight, the plane encountered very heavy weather. Dr. Fleming, although his seatbelt was fastened, was thrown against the window next to which he was sitting, his glasses were smashed, his face was bruised, and he claimed to have suffered a mild heart attack. He sued the airline. What did he sue for? He sued for failure to inform. He said that the airline had a duty to warn him before he got on that plane concerning what it knew about the weather conditions. It turns out that the following was known before takeoff: Heavy thunderstorms were predicted, with surface wind gusts of 50-70 miles per hour, cloud tops to 45,000 feet, and isolated tornadoes and hailstorms, which could cause moderate to severe turbulence. Dr. Fleming said that if he had known about those weather reports, he would not have flown and thus would not have been injured. The airline said that it could not possibly tell everyone about everything, that this would upset the passengers and cause turmoil at the airport. It was simply not feasible from a business perspective to inform passengers about the conditions.

A New York court disagreed, ruling in favor of the physician. It stated in part: "Such conditions aloft, although possibly not extreme enough to prevent takeoff, are sufficiently serious to be a matter of significant concern to prospective travelers. Although an airline must bear the ultimate responsibility for deciding whether conditions permit a safe flight, it must not arrogate to itself a decision which rightly belongs to each passenger, namely, whether to fly under conditions which, although not hazardous, might prove to be emotionally or physically traumatizing" (1).

We can use this analogy to say that this is

essentially the law with regard to human experimentation. An investigator may believe that his protocol is ethically, medically, and scientifically acceptable, but in the end it has to be up to each individual potential subject whether or not to enroll in the clinical trial. The law seeks to protect the self-determination, or autonomy, of individual subjects by requiring physicians and other researchers to disclose to those potential subjects certain information before they are asked to enroll in the study.

Henry Beecher described a number of unethical trials in his important 1966 paper that was mentioned in the introduction (2). He reviewed several randomized clinical trials that involved withholding a known effective treatment and randomizing patients between a placebo and an effective treatment. Robert Veatch in 1973 updated that study (29), and noted, with regard to randomized clinical trials: "Shocking as it may seem, no established principle of medical ethics requires that subjects be informed that one of the risks of an experimental procedure is that there is a control group included in the research design." And he states why he thinks that this is essentially wrong and that the subjects have a right to know that there are other people in the study and that they may be in a control group, receiving a placebo, or in some other group. More recently, there has been a rise in at least the basic view among researchers that something needs to be done with informed consent, and if you read the medical literature now you will see in most reports of randomized clinical trials some statement about informed consent.

I would like to cite from two articles published in the April 16 issue of The New England Journal of Medicine. One study involved routine early endoscopy in upper-gastrointestinal-tract bleeding (22). The authors state: "The patients agreed to undergo endoscopy if they were randomly assigned to that group. Approval was obtained from our Human Subjects Review Committee." That is all they say about informed

consent. The other study involved randomizing between
a placebo and doxycycline treatment for college women
who had urinary infections (25); the authors say that
the women provided informed consent. I am not arguing
that informed consent was not provided in either of
these studies. I am simply stating that we do not
know from reading these reports how informed consent
was obtained, how much information was given to patients, and whether the patients had an opportunity
to say no. In the endoscopy study it is indicated
that 8 patients refused. In the study involving the
young college women the refusal figure is not given.
Only the statement is made that the patients were eligible to be entered into the study if, as one of the
conditions, they provided informed consent. Of 87
women randomized in this double-blind study, 6 did not
complete all follow-up visits. No further information
on them is supplied in the paper.

The primary point I would like to make is that
there seems to be a confusion in medical centers between the consent form and the consent process. Tre-
mendous emphasis is put on the consent form, and you
will see very often in these studies the phrase that
the patient signed the consent form. Now, that is
probably the lawyers' fault as much as anything, because lawyers always emphasize the signing of documents. But we need to be very clear that the issue
in consent is not the signature on the form. Forms
are not designed to protect patients; they are designed to protect hospitals and doctors. But one can
make them protect patients, and two steps are required
to do this. First, the consent form should be written
in language the average patient can understand, and
second, the patient should receive a copy of it some
time before being asked to sign it, so that he can
read it and think about it and ask more questions.
If the side effects of one of the arms of a randomized
clinical trial are expected to be much worse, if patients are told, "We don't know which treatment is
better, we really don't know," then they will take the

treatment with the fewer side effects. That would be the logical thing to do, and if the majority do not do that, then you have to wonder whether they were treated honestly, fairly, and noncoercively in the consent process.

The main legal issue concerning informed consent is to protect the subject's autonomy, to let him make up his own mind whether to be part of the trial. This is a process of information exchange and the consent form is not proof that the process actually took place, but only a device used to document it in a hospital chart.

PSYCHOLOGICAL ASPECTS OF CLINICAL TRIALS

J. C. B. Holland: One of the most important, least studied and controlled variables in clinical trials is the psychologic variable. The attitude of physician-investigator and patient and their interaction in regard to the patient's accepting and complying with treatment have been little explored. There have been clinical trials in cancer for over 25 years in the United States. Notable by its absence, however, has been a measurement of patients' quality of life while they were receiving a particular treatment regimen, or why patients chose to accept and adhere to treatment by randomized protocol. Patients have been carefully monitored for drug effects and drug toxicities, with each quantified for level. No data were collected, nevertheless, on how they felt or how they were observed by others to be functioning while treated on a specific treatment arm. The first systematic observations of this type were begun in 1976 in the Cancer and Leukemia Group B (CALGB) clinical trials group.

The National Cancer Institute recommended that the cooperative clinical trials groups become multimodal, providing the opportunity through CALGB for the beginning participation of psychiatry as one of the modalities, joining at that time with surgery and pathology. Beginning then we developed a simple observer and

self-report that has been included in CALGB protocols
(11). The patient is requested by the nurse to indicate how he feels, using a list of adjectives. An observer, the research nurse, also rates the patient in
a similar manner. This provides an assessment of how
the patient is feeling, what his mood is, and his
total function, both physical and social. We have
now studied approximately 1000 patients with this simple measurement. Data from a protocol just completed
on small cell lung carcinoma are of interest. The
survival rate was approximately 25% at 36 months for
the two treatment arms; toxicity was also similar. On
the psychosocial data, however, one treatment arm was
found to be associated with significantly greater fa-
tigue and dysphoria (24). When treatment is aimed at
palliation, then quality of life during the treatment
chosen becomes important. The psychosocial data provided in this protocol led to the information that
allowed one to identify the treatment associated with
better quality of life.

We now are able to ask more sophisticated questions
in the CALGB protocols. Depression, pain, and nausea
and vomiting are all being studied, to develop ways
to quantify the subjective components.

Another very important variable in a clinical trial
is the physician-patient relationship, the interaction
between the physician-investigator and the patient.
The major question in this regard has related to the
interaction of doctor and patient around the signing
of the informed consent document. While it serves to
protect doctor and hospital, the question has been increasingly raised as to the possibly deleterious effects it may have as currently practiced. The Psychosocial Collaborative Oncology Group, a cooperative
group of 3 centers funded by the National Cancer
Institute, has carried out a formal study of this
problem (21). One hundred fifty patients have been
interviewed 1-3 weeks and 3 months after accepting
treatment and signing consent for investigational
chemotherapy at one of the 3 institutions. They were

asked in the first structured interview about their
recall of the consent procedure and what they felt
about the interview with the doctor and about the consent form. Over 80% of patients stated that it was
the discussion with the doctor which led them to accept treatment. The primary reasons given were that
they trusted the doctor, they hoped that the treatment
would help them, and they feared the consequences of
the disease if they did not accept it. Less than 1%
of these patients indicated that the informed consent
form itself had been instrumental in their decision.
Most patients could not remember more than 2 or 3 of
the side effects listed on the form, which were as
many as 18 in some cases.

Given the high anxiety level, the information over-
load given, and the clear indication that the interaction with the physician is the key part of the procedure for informed consent, should we not be thinking
about how to make the consent form more helpful to the
patient? When standard readability tests were applied
to several cooperative group protocol consent forms,
the latter fell between the reading level of a professional required for The New England Journal of Medicine and that of a college graduate (19). The consent
form should be written to be understandable to patients; they should be allowed to take it home and
discuss treatment with their family. The physician
interview should take two sessions, if necessary, to
allow "hearing" the information with lessened anxiety.
Taking a tape recording of the session home to listen
to it again is also helpful.

Compliance is another aspect of this problem. Taking the full dose of prescribed treatment is clearly
important; the ambiance of the clinic provided by physician and staff can be a key factor. Patients should
feel that "somebody gives a damn" about their discom-
forts and troublesome side effects. Even if these can
only be diminished to a minor extent, the fact that
staff are trying to help is important.

Why do people who are facing disease that is

advancing and has not responded to the usual treatments seek out unproved remedies, such as laetrile? The most common reason patients have given in one study for asking for laetrile was because "the doctor told me there was nothing else he could do for me." Clearly, curative treatment must give way to supportive treatment at times, but there is never a time that the physician has a right to say nothing more can be done. Patients hear this as abandonment. Patients may experience a better sense of care by the physician who honestly offers continued care and investigational protocols. It is better to have patients and their families know about clinical trials, what they are, how they are designed, recognizing that they have a basis for potential efficacy, such as trials based on another tumor and animal studies. The unproved remedies have no such solid basis for trial, while promising cure at no risk.

The psychologic variable in clinical trials must be studied in the patient, in the physician, and in the staff. Only by recognizing and gaining understanding of this "uncontrolled" variable can the quality of our studies be improved (12).

ETHICAL ASPECTS OF CLINICAL TRIALS

R. J. Levine: My first official trip to this medical center was in 1957 when I spent the summer here as a visiting medical student. At our very first orientation meeting the director of the medical student program told us that the sign over the door read "Memorial Hosptial for Cancer and Allied Diseases." He said that it was our obligation to persuade each and every patient that he had one of the allied diseases, because no patient could tolerate being informed that he had cancer. We have come a long way since then.

The range of ethical problems encountered in the course of planning or conducting a clinical trial is very large, and I shall focus on just a few. I have selected some that are especially vexing from the

perspective of those with an interest in the statistics of clinical trials.

First, there is a consensus that the ethical justification for beginning a controlled clinical trial requires, at a minimum, that the investigators be able
to state an honest null hypothesis. We have problems
with the fact that the introduction of new therapies
in the United States is commonly done in an uncontrolled fashion. Biases and prejudices based on early
uncontrolled experiences often create serious debates
as to whether one can justify a controlled clinical
trial. There is an even more serious problem with the
null hypothesis, which generally consists of a statement that certain gross measures of outcome are equal,
for example, that 5 years after the initiation of either therapy A or therapy B, the probability that the
patient will still be alive is the same. But this may
be very different from the perspective of the patient,
who may find the quality of life offered by one or the
other of the treatments to be as important as the
eventual outcome. A dramatic illustration of this was
provided by a randomized clinical trial performed to
compare the results of radical mastectomy with wide
excision in the treatment of early breast cancer. The
two treatments were judged to be potentially equivalent in terms of life expectancy and probability of
local recurrence. However, one of the alternatives
was, to quote the surgeons who did the study, "of a
mutilating character." For this reason, from the perspective of the patients the two approaches to therapy
should not have been presumed equivalent.

The second problem I will state is the subject of
current spirited controversy. As one proceeds with a
clinical trial, one begins to develop preliminary data
that may suggest a trend toward disproving the null
hypothesis. Thus, at some point it may appear that
therapy A is either more beneficial or less harmful
than therapy B. At this point the question arises:
Do the investigators have an obligation to disclose
preliminary trends? Must they inform subjects who are

already enrolled in the protocol that, although the
results are not yet statistically significant, therapy
A is beginning to seem to be better than therapy B?
If patients who are already enrolled are so informed,
how many of them might drop out and secure therapy A
outside the protocol? If you are obliged to inform
new prospective subjects of the preliminary trends,
how many may refuse to enroll because they want what
seems to be the superior therapy? I am willing to argue that the withholding of preliminary data can be
justified ethically (17).

A third problem is the following: All of our ethical codes and all regulations require that research
subjects must be promised absolute freedom to withdraw
from the protocol at any time. Statisticians are familiar with the problems that are presented by high
withdrawal or high dropout rates. Karen Lebacqz and
I have proposed that limits can be imposed on the absolute liberty granted research subjects by our ethical codes and regulations. Some of our arguments are
grounded in the ethical obligation to keep promises
or to maintain commitments (18). Other arguments may
be grounded in patient benefits. For example, in trials of certain antiarrythmic drugs, abrupt withdrawal
without consultation with the physician-investigator
may result in serious arrythmias and in some cases
death.

Another problem concerns compliance. It is essential that those who have the obligation to analyze and
interpret the data know how many patients are actually
taking all of the drug that has been prescribed for
them. In many clinical trials substantial numbers of
patients take no therapy whatever, and an even larger
number of subjects miss occasional doses of the drug.
What we commonly do is to monitor for compliance.
This presents several problems. The most effective
approaches to compliance monitoring require that we
use techniques to measure drug-taking behavior without
letting the subjects know exactly what we are doing or
why. Such activities are at least potentially

deceptive, and deception is generally incompatible with the ethical norms calling for informed consent. Now, if all we want to know is the general level of compliance within a population, for example, and we have several hundred or several thousand subjects in a randomized clinical trial, we can resolve this problem simply. We can tell them that we are going to do certain maneuvers without letting them know the purpose of the maneuvers. We can have the subjects agree to remain unaware of the purpose of these maneuvers until the clinical trial has ended. This type of interaction is called research with consent to having the purpose undisclosed, and within certain limits of risk and inconvenience it can be justified ethically (17).

However, if what we plan to do through our compliance monitoring is to identify specific individuals who are poor compliers, then we have a problem. We may then find it necessary to say to some of these individuals that without their knowledge we have been monitoring their drug-taking behavior and we have found that they are not taking their drugs. Formally, confrontations of this sort are called inflicted insights. Protocols presenting the possibility that it will be necessary to inflict on research subjects insights that they might consider unwelcome or offensive are very difficult to justify, and I believe that they should be very difficult if not impossible to justify. It is possible to inform subjects that covert means will be used to observe their compliance behavior. It is also possible to tell them that in the event poor compliers are identified they will be offered special assistance in enhancing their compliance. However, many subjects who would rather not be spied on will then refuse to enroll in the protocol. For this reason, the general data on compliance within the protocol will be neither representative nor comprehensive. It will be generally very difficult, if not impossible, to achieve simultaneously the goal of identifying individual poor compliers for purposes of

improving compliance, and the goal of developing general information on compliance within representative
populations.

THE PHYSICIAN-PATIENT RELATIONSHIP

E. J. Cassell: I think that one of the important advances in medicine during this past decade has been
the increased acceptance of the controlled clinical
trial. This has introduced into the practice of medicine some of the science that the laboratory promised
in the care of patients but which has not, until now,
made it to the bedside. We talk about the ethical
aspects of research not as a nuisance that has been
imposed on research. Ethics are the rules that guide
the interactions of human beings. Clinical research
is done by people on other people, and these are
merely rules that guide that interaction, relatively
complicated rules because human interaction is complicated. Thus, we are not talking about some new requirement. We are talking about something that makes
clinical research fit the world for which it was designed, the world of people taking care of other people.
    The relationship between physician and patient is
something that has not been given enough attention in
American medicine. We generally act as though when
people get better from a disease, it is because something was done to them to make them better. That is
not quite true even in brief illness and it certainly
is not the case in a long illness such as malignant
disease. Malignant disease has reintroduced to the
world, certainly to the United States, a situation
that has not been around for decades, the long-term,
chronically ill person who ultimately dies. It is
the tuberculosis, or osteomyelitis of our era. In
such patients there is no way of even pretending that
it is the drugs or technology that make the sick better. We must recognize that, in fact, doctors take
care of patients. It is the relation between the two

which is the vehicle of care. The patient who takes
medication has to believe that it has been given in
good faith; that it is not poison meant to kill. It
is like crossing the street. There is a car coming
just as the light turns green and I walk across, believing that the driver of that ton-and-a-half vehicle
is going to stop for me. I believe that because we
have relationships; we are partners in the social contract, even though strangers. The contract that makes
medical care possible is the doctor-patient relationship; and that relationship is fundamental (4,6).

Clinical research offers a special problem. The
researcher, although a physician, and although caring
for those patients, has an obligation to his research
which overrides the obligation to a particular patient, if the two come in conflict. Knowledge is the
goal. The primary care physician, on the other hand,
has a basic commitment to the patient, whose welfare
is the primary goal.

We are talking here about a basic aspect of medicine, the doctor-patient relationship, a relationship
we understand very poorly at best. There are new conflicts arising that must be resolved to achieve a kind
of clinical research that can best enhance medical
care. Dr. Holland pointed out that patients go after
things like laetrile often when they have been told
that there is nothing more we can do. Such a statement reflects the belief that a treatment is the drug
and not what people do for other people. As a prac-
ticing physician, I say that there is never nothing
more that we can do. We can always do something. The
something, however, may be simply to take care of people while they die, and that is a very potent thing
to do.

SIDE EFFECTS VERSUS BENEFITS OF CHEMOTHERAPY

V. Miké: Cancer chemotherapy is highly toxic and not
yet generally effective. Since the vast majority of
patients on chemotherapy experience only the side

effects and none of the benefits, what are the ethical
and legal implications of the situation? It has been
estimated by DeVita et al. in a recent publication (7)
that of the 200,000 or so patients receiving chemotherapy today we can show significant benefit for approximately 38,000 or 19%. In other words, over 80%
derive only side effects and no benefit.

G. J. Annas: From the legal point of view it would
seem to me to be an important part of informed consent
to give patients some idea of what you expect to be
the risks and benefits. If only 20% of the 200,000
patients across the nation receiving chemotherapy have
benefitted, then patients should have that baseline
information. You have a right to tell them that your
study is different and you think the results are going
to be better, if you have reason to believe that.

E. J. Cassell: This has always been a very troubling
question to me. We do not have this treatment versus
another that is 90% effective, with no side effects.
We are talking about generally fatal diseases. When
children were dying of leukemia, when the remission
rate was 10%, we might have said that we were killing
9 children for every child that we put into remission.
In fact, we never stated it that way, although that
was what we were doing. Instead of dying of bleeding,
which they would have, they died of infection. But
now, 10 years later, we are no longer killing 9 children to put one into remission; we are putting most of
the children into remission and for prolonged remissions. We could not be here without having been
there. I resolve the issue for myself by discussing
with my patient what our problems are, what is offered
to us, with the side effects, and where we would like
to go (5). But then, when I see someone with overwhelming side effects, it is hard to remember that we
have another goal. But the goal itself becomes part
of the treatment. Most people, certainly in our
world, do not just wait for things to happen to them.

The alternatives are worse, we say, and so we proceed.

R. J. Levine: I agree mostly with what Dr. Cassell said.   I think though that it is more constructive not to speak in terms of killing 90% of the children.   It is true that a little more than 10 years ago about 90% of the children treated for leukemia died while they were being treated with therapy that seemed to produce no remission.   But we did not kill them.   What we did instead was perhaps to change the nature of their terminal illness.   If we had found that we shortened the lives of 90% of all people, of all children, that were being treated with investigational chemotherapies for leukemia, we would certainly have discontinued that work.   In all of medicine it is quite impossible to deliver the one to one: "I will do this thing to you and this will be the consequence."   In all of our therapy we say, "I will do this thing to you and, given 100 people like you with the same disease, increase by a certain percentage the likelihood of a cure.   If we take out your stomach because you have a peptic ulcer, we will vastly increase the likelihood that you will never bleed from a peptic ulcer.   On the other hand, there is one chance in 200 that you will die."   Or it could be one chance in 400; it depends on who is doing it and where.   What we expect the patient to do then is to consider this, to consider various alternatives.   Does he want to go all the way and take the risk of death, or does he want to go on for years with medical therapy, perhaps bleeding from time to time and, perhaps, having to have an emergency gastrectomy sometime?   I would not like to see this too oversimplified.

J. C. B. Holland: The issue of hope is important in this discussion.   Not many people can live feeling totally hopeless.   Most cancer patients today are well informed that they have a serious disease for which treatments are uncertain, and they have a fair knowledge of what the treatments are.   Even if the

percentage to benefit is low, there is still the opportunity to say: "Well, I may be in that percentage;
I would rather do that than nothing."

PHASE I TRIALS AND THE TERMINAL PATIENT

V. Miké: A related problem is that of Phase I clinical
trials, which are mostly concerned with establishing
the tolerated dose of a new agent. In these studies
the drugs are given to patients in the terminal stages
of disease who are no longer responding to established
forms of therapy, and drug efficacy is not a primary
goal. Is some form of subtle pressure exerted on
these patients so that they remain as subjects of
study for the greater good of future generations, and
are we then depriving them of time to face death, "a
peaceful death?" What is the role of the hospice
movement, which seems to be very successful in England
but is not growing very fast in this country?

J. C. B. Holland: By and large, patients sort themselves out by seeking out hospice, if that is what
they choose, or a research institution like Memorial
Sloan-Kettering if they want to "fight to the end."
Someone who comes here to Memorial Sloan-Kettering,
who is very ill, is often the patient who will want to
participate in Phase I trials, wanting the "newest
treatments that are around." The person who feels,
"Don't hassle me, I just want to die quietly," will
usually find his way to hospice or home care. The
hospice movement in this country is becoming better
organized, with better collaboration with primary care
facilities to enhance continuity of care. Continuity
seems important, particularly in cases of terminal
illness, when a sense of abandonment by primary physicians can occur with transfer to a free-standing hospice unit. Surely the hospice philosophy, with maximal time at home and maximal shared time with family,
is a goal to be pursued by both the hospital-based
care and hospice care.

R. J. Levine: There are scientific problems involved
in Phase I drug testing using a terminally ill population (17). But the probability of benefit, although
extremely small, is not zero, so that the risk-benefit
ratio is not infinity. If a patient, given the full
information, still agrees to enter the trial, then I
would show respect for that person's choice of how to
spend the last days of his life.

G. J. Annas: The main issue we have to be concerned
about with this population is coercion and the question of whether they are really consenting to this.
There is no problem if they are consenting to be volunteers.

E. J. Cassell: There is a kind of coercion involved
here that is very subtle and that perhaps cannot be
avoided. Sick people are not the same as healthy people; they are very different. Patients are afraid to
change; they are afraid to move or go. It is a kind
of coercion which is almost not coercion, it is almost
part of the relationship. And that is why the trust
that is inherent in that must not be breached easily.
Patients do not want to leave this hospital to go to
another place, so that we have to be careful that the
consent we are getting is not one that says, "Don't
abandon me. I will do whatever you want because otherwise it looks like you are going to abandon me."

SOCIAL CLASSES AND CLINICAL RESEARCH

V. Miké: It has been said that the outrageous practices of even the recent past were generally inflicted
on the poor and ignorant, the lower socioeconomic
classes, such as the sharecroppers in Tuskegee. What
is the situation in terms of socioeconomic status of
the patients who go on Phase I trials? Is there an
association?

J. C. B. Holland: I do not think so. We have looked

briefly at socioeconomic background of patients participating in CALGB protocols. There is a wide spectrum of ethnic, economic, and educational backgrounds.

V. Miké: It is estimated that less than 5% of the cancer patients in this country are on formal scientific
protocols. Which 5% of the social stratum is that?

R. J. Levine: Don't you think they are mostly people
who live in cities where the protocols are being carried out?

J. C. B. Holland: Protocols are changing; there are
now more and more participating community hospitals.
It also depends on where the academic center is; some
are in relatively rural areas, drawing on rural patients.

R. J. Levine: Most of the patients on our research
unit live within the county and seem to be a cross
section of the community.

PERSONAL SAVINGS FOR EXPERIMENTAL TREATMENT

V. Miké: I would like to turn to a financial aspect
of clinical research procedures. Unless the protocol
is on full grant support, the patient's life savings
may be wiped out by some of these extremely expensive
regimens, although he may receive no personal benefit.
What are the legal and ethical aspects of the situation?

G. J. Annas: We may begin to see some law suits for
deceit. I doubt that many people would spend their
life savings in pursuit of something that the physicians told them had not much chance of being effective. If the patient is fully informed and still
agrees to participate, then we have a general doctor-
patient contract and there is no legal problem.

E. J. Cassell: This is a very sad situation and the solution is not immediately apparent. The cost of the therapy should be part of the consent form. It should be clear to a patient when he enters the protocol that he may be paying for the tests and for at least some of the drugs and what the extent of the costs will be. But we still have the problem I mentioned earlier of the patient being in a coercive setting.

J. C. B. Holland: In the study I discussed earlier, in which we studied the informed consent procedure, we had the documents the patients signed and their perceptions of benefit were vastly different. Their expectation of benefit was nearly always above what they had actually been told by the physician and what was stated in the consent form. It was not a question of deceit or misrepresentation, but perhaps a basic human need to see greater potential benefit than had been presented. There is essentially nothing we can do about this, and all treatments cannot be free under our present system.

FEDERAL REGULATIONS: LEGAL AND ETHICAL?

V. Miké: It is less than 10 years since the Tuskegee scandal, but the pendulum seems to have swung to the other extreme. Many clinical investigators feel that the current degree of Federal regulation is excessive and that it actually hinders progress in clinical research. Although the regulations are legal, can it be that they are unethical? The point has been made that not doing experimentation when there is so little hope with existing therapy is unethical.

G. J. Annas: Of course there can be unethical laws by some criteria, because there are different systems of ethics. Are human experimentation regulations as currently formulated by the Federal Government unethical and do they hinder cancer research? This statement cannot be justified, given the amount of funding

the National Cancer Institute has provided and the
number of trials carried out in the last decade. We
are always trying to balance the interests of society
with the interests of the subject. Given the issues
discussed earlier, we cannot say that at this time
the balance weighs with the subject.

RANDOMIZED TRIALS AND THE NEW FEDERAL GUIDELINES

K. E. Stanley: I would like clarification on a point
in the new guidelines for human research. Do the
guidelines require that the patient be informed if
there is a randomized basis for his assigned treatment? The regulations speak of the patient understanding the objective of the study, but specifically,
is it required that the patient know that his therapy
was chosen by a chance mechanism?

R. J. Levine: New guidelines for human research have
been issued by both HHS and FDA (9,10); neither set
of regulations requires stating that the therapy will
be assigned at random. What they do though is perhaps
implicitly require this. In the optional elements of
informed consent in both sets of regulations, it is
suggested that patients be told how many other patients there are in the clinical trial, but this is
left to the discretion of the Institutional Review
Board.

CONCLUDING REMARKS

V. Miké: I would like to ask for a brief concluding
statement from each panelist.

J. C. B. Holland: An important aspect of clinical
trials that we have not touched on is the statistician's responsibility. You are the keepers of the
morals of the clinical trial. It is up to you to interpret what is going on, to point out the biases to
clinicians and those who are not as knowledgeable

about design principles as you are. We all carry biases and prejudices into the conduct of clinical trials, but within the framework of trying to do what is right. We make many mistakes; informed consent is far short of the mark, but the efforts for change are in the right direction.

G. J. Annas: I would like to second that. I think that the current state of the art in human experimentation is the Institutional Review Board. Very often, however, IRBs either have one biostatistician or none and the statistical issues are not addressed or addressed only improperly, because the issues are not understood. It is your responsibility to make certain that the investigator has a good chance of entering a sufficient number of patients to make the study statistically meaningful, and that patient selection and randomization are carried out in an objective manner. Just from a statistical point of view alone you can make that point to the investigator better than anyone else.

R. J. Levine: I would like to make a final comment on informed consent. The IRB has the general assignment from the Federal Government and within its own institution to monitor all ethical aspects of research. The consent form is something that the IRB seems greatly preoccupied with; not informed consent, but the consent form. Informed consent is the discussion between an investigator, commonly a doctor, and a subject who is also commonly a patient. It is difficult to write scripts for dialogues between two people one has never met. The consent form should be looked on as an indication of the minimal amount of information that the IRB considers necessary to be conveyed to the subject. It is expected that the subject will ask questions and have elaborations, so that technical concepts can be adequately communicated. The key factor is the interaction between the physician and the patient (15-17).

E. J. Cassell: I spent the first half of my professional life as an epidemiologist, and I have a strong
desire for an increased statistical power to solve the
problems that were discussed here today. One of the
exciting areas where the statistical approach is least
developed is the subjective aspect of the care of patients. It would be desirable to have a method for
knowing whether something is reproducibly true without
what we presently call objective measures, numbers,
and scales that do not represent what we are seeking.
This is an area where ultimately statistics will be
just as important as it is in the more established
fields of research. We have only taken a step along
a road. A recent introduction into this road has been
the understanding that ethics are a fundamental part
of all clinical research. The road is going toward
the resolution of the problem: "What is the best
thing I can do for my patient?"

REFERENCES

1. Annas, G. J., Glantz, L. H., and Katz, B. F.
   (1977), Informed Consent to Human Experimentation:
   The Subject's Dilemma, Ballinger, Cambridge,
   Massachusetts.

2. Beecher, H. K. (1966), Ethics and clinical research, The New England Journal of Medicine 274:
   1354-1360.

3. Bibliography of Society, Ethics and the Life Sciences (1979-1980), The Hastings Center, Institute
   of Society, Ethics and the Life Sciences,
   Hastings-on-Hudson, New York.

4. Cassell, E. (1976), The Healer's Art: A New Approach to the Doctor-Patient Relationship,
   Lippincott, Philadelphia.

5. Cassell, E. (1978), Informed consent in the therapeutic relationship: Clinical aspects, in: Encyclopedia of Bioethics, Macmillan and Free Press,
New York.

6. Cassell, E. (1978), Therapeutic relationship:
Contemporary medical perspective, in: Encyclopedia
of Bioethics, Macmillan and Free Press, New York.

7. DeVita, V. T., Henney, J. E., and Hubbard, S. M.
(1981), Estimation of the numerical and economic
impact of chemotherapy in the treatment of cancer,
in: Burchenal, J. H., and Oettgen, H. F., eds.,
Cancer: Achievements, Challenges, and Prospects
for the 1980s, Vol. 2, Grune & Stratton, New York,
pp. 859-880.

8. Encyclopedia of Bioethics (1978), Macmillan and
Free Press, New York.

9. FDA: Rules and regulations: Protection of human
subjects (1981), Federal Register 46: 8942-8980.

10. Final regulations amending basic HHS policy for
the protection of human research subjects (1981),
Federal Register 46: 8366-8391.

11. Holland, J. C., Bahna, G., McKegney, P.,
Silberfarb, P., Tross, S., and Glidewell, O.
(1980), Psychiatric research in multi-modal cancer
clinical trials in CALGB (Abstract), Proceedings
of the American Society of Clinical Oncology 21:
354.

12. Holland, J. C., and Rowland, J. H. (1981), Psychiatric, psychosocial, and behavioral interven-
tions in the treatment of cancer: An historical
review, in: Weiss, S., Hurd, A., and Fox, B.,
eds., Perspectives on Behavioral Medicine,
Academic Press, New York, pp. 235-260.

13. IRB: A Review of Human Subjects Research (1979-), published 10 times a year by The Hastings Center, Institute of Society, Ethics and the Life Sciences, Hastings-on-Hudson, New York.

14. Jones, J. H. (1981), Bad Blood: The Tuskegee Syphilis Experiment, The Free Press, New York.

15. Lebacqz, K., and Levine, R. J. (1978), Informed consent in human research: Ethical and legal aspects, Encyclopedia of Bioethics, Macmillan and Free Press, New York.

16. Levine, R. J. (1978), Research, Biomedical. Encyclopedia of Bioethics, Macmillan and Free Press, New York.

17. Levine, R. J. (1981), Ethics and Regulation of Clinical Research, Urban and Schwarzenberg, Baltimore.

18. Levine, R. J., and Lebacqz, K. (1979), Ethical considerations in clinical trials, Clinical Pharmacology and Therapeutics 25: 728-749.

19. Morrow, G. (1980), How readable are subject consent forms? Journal of the American Medical Association 244: 56-58.

20. Pappworth, M. H. (1967), Human Guinea Pigs, Beacon Press, Boston.

21. Penman, D., Bahna, G., Holland, J. C., Morrow, G., Morse, I., Schmale, A., and Derogatis, L. (1980), Patients' perception of giving informed consent for investigational chemotherapy (Abstract), Proceedings of the American Association for Cancer Research 21: 188.

22. Peterson, W. L., Barnett, C. C., Smith, H. J.,

Allen, M. H., and Corbett, D. B. (1981), Routine early endoscopy in upper-gastrointestinal-tract bleeding: A randomized, controlled trial. The New England Journal of Medicine 304: 925-929.

23. Reiser, S. J., Dyck, A. J., and Curran, W. J., eds. (1977), Ethics in Medicine, MIT Press, Cambridge, Massachusetts.

24. Silberfarb, P., Holland, J. C., Bahna, G. F., Anbar, D., Maurer, H., and Comis, R. (1981), Differences in psychologic response on two treatment regimens for localized small cell lung carcinoma (SCLC) (Abstract), Proceedings of the American Association for Cancer Research 22: 158.

25. Stamm, W. E., Running, K., McKevitt, M., Counts, G. W., Turck, M., and Holmes, K. K. (1981), Treatment of the acute urethral syndrome, The New England Journal of Medicine 304: 956-958.

26. Swazey, J. P. (1978), Protecting the "animal of necessity": Limits to inquiry in clinical investigation, Daedalus 20: 129-145.

27. The New York Times (1981), Book Review, June 21, p. 9.

28. Veatch, R. M. (1982), A Theory of Medical Ethics, Basic Books, New York.

29. Veatch, R. M., and Sollitto, S. (1973), Human experimentation: The ethical questions persist. The Hastings Center Report 3(3): 1-3.

NUREMBERG CODE*

1. The voluntary consent of the human subject is absolutely essential.

This means that the person involved should have legal capacity to give consent; should be so situated as to be able to exercise free power of choice, without the intervention of any element of force, fraud, deceit, duress, over-reaching, or other ulterior form of constraint or coercion; and should have sufficient knowledge and comprehension of the elements of the subject matter involved as to enable him to make an understanding and enlightened decision. This latter element requires that before the acceptance of an affirmative decision by the experimental subject there should be made known to him the nature, duration, and purpose of the experiment; the method and means by which it is to be conducted; all inconveniences and hazards reasonably to be expected; and the effects upon his health or person which may possibly come from his participation in the experiment.

The duty and responsibility for ascertaining the quality of the consent rests upon each individual who initiates, directs or engages in the experiment. It is a personal duty and responsibility which may not be delegated to another with impunity.

2. The experiment should be such as to yield fruitful results for the good of society, unprocurable by other methods or means of study, and not random and unnecessary in nature.

3. The experiment should be so designed and based on the results of animal experimentation and a knowledge of the natural history of the disease or

---

*Reprinted from Trials of War Criminals before the Nuernberg Military Tribunals under Control Council Law No. 10, Vol. 2, U.S. Government Printing Office, Washington, D.C. (1949), pp. 181-182.

other problem under study that the anticipated results will justify the performance of the experiment.

4. The experiment should be so conducted as to avoid all unnecessary physical and mental suffering and injury.

5. No experiment should be conducted where there is an a priori reason to believe that death or disabling injury will occur; except, perhaps, in those experiments where the experimental physicians also serve as subjects.

6. The degree of risk to be taken should never exceed that determined by the humanitarian importance of the problem to be solved by the experiment.

7. Proper preparations should be made and adequate facilities provided to protect the experimental subject against even remote possibilities of injury, disability, or death.

8. The experiment should be conducted only by scientifically qualified persons. The highest degree of skill and care should be required through all stages of the experiment of those who conduct or engage in the experiment.

9. During the course of the experiment the human subject should be at liberty to bring the experiment to an end if he has reached the physical or mental state where continuation of the experiment seems to him to be impossible.

10. During the course of the experiment the scientist in charge must be prepared to terminate the experiment at any stage, if he has probable cause to believe, in the exercise of the good faith, superior skill and careful judgment required of him that a continuation of the experiment is likely to result in injury, disability, or death to the experimental subject.

DECLARATION OF HELSINKI[*]
Recommendations Guiding Medical Doctors
in Biomedical Research Involving Human Subjects

Introduction

It is the mission of the medical doctor to safeguard the health of the people. His or her knowledge and conscience are dedicated to the fulfillment of this mission.

The Declaration of Geneva of The World Medical Association binds the doctor with the words "The health of my patient will be my first consideration," and the International Code of Medical Ethics declares that "Any act or advice which could weaken physical or mental resistance of a human being may be used only in his interest."

The purpose of biomedical research involving human subjects must be to improve diagnostic, therapeutic and prophylactic procedures and the understanding of the aetiology and pathogenesis of disease.

In current medical practice most diagnostic, therapeutic or prophylactic procedures involve hazards. This applies a fortiori to biomedical research.

Medical progress is based on research which ultimately must rest in part on experimentation involving human subjects.

In the field of biomedical research a fundamental distinction must be recognized between medical research in which the aim is essentially diagnostic or therapeutic for a patient, and medical research, the essential object of which is purely scientific and without direct diagnostic or therapeutic value to the

---

[*]Adopted by the 18th World Medical Assembly, Helsinki, Finland, 1964 and as revised by the 29th World Medical Assembly, Tokyo, Japan, 1975. Reprinted with permission of The World Medical Association.

person subjected to the research.

Special caution must be exercised in the conduct of research which may affect the environment, and the welfare of animals used for research must be respected.

Because it is essential that the results of laboratory experiments be applied to human beings to further scientific knowledge and to help suffering humanity, The World Medical Association has prepared the following recommendations as a guide to every doctor in biomedical research involving human subjects. They should be kept under review in the future. It must be stressed that the standards as drafted are only a guide to physicians all over the world. Doctors are not relieved from criminal, civil and ethical responsibilities under the laws of their own countries.

I. Basic Principles

1. Biomedical research involving human subjects must conform to generally accepted scientific principles and should be based on adequately performed laboratory and animal experimentation and on a thorough knowledge of the scientific literature.

2. The design and performance of each experimental procedure involving human subjects should be clearly formulated in an experimental protocol which should be transmitted to a specially appointed independent committee for consideration, comment and guidance.

3. Biomedical research involving human subjects should be conducted only by scientifically qualified persons and under the supervision of a clinically competent medical person. The responsibility for the human subject must always rest with a medically qualified person and never rest on the subject of the research, even though the subject has given his or her consent.

4. Biomedical research involving human subjects cannot legitimately be carried out unless the importance of the objective is in proportion to the

inherent risk to the subject.

5. Every biomedical research project involving human subjects should be preceded by careful assessment of predictable risks in comparison with foreseeable benefits to the subject or to others. Concern for the interests of the subject must always prevail over the interests of science and society.

6. The right of the research subject to safeguard his or her integrity must always be respected. Every precaution should be taken to respect the privacy of the subject and to minimize the impact of the study on the subject's physical and mental integrity and on the personality of the subject.

7. Doctors should abstain from engaging in research projects involving human subjects unless they are satisfied that the hazards involved are believed to be predictable. Doctors should cease any investigation if the hazards are found to outweigh the potential benefits.

8. In publication of the results of his or her research, the doctor is obliged to preserve the accuracy of the results. Reports of experimentation not in accordance with the principles laid down in this Declaration should not be accepted for publication.

9. In any research on human beings, each potential subject must be adequately informed of the aims, methods, anticipated benefits and potential hazards of the study and the discomfort it may entail. He or she should be informed that he or she is at liberty to abstain from participation in the study and that he or she is free to withdraw his or her consent to participation at any time. The doctor should then obtain the subject's freely given informed consent, preferably in writing.

10. When obtaining informed consent for the research project the doctor should be particularly cautious if the subject is in a dependent relationship to him or her or may consent under duress. In that case the informed consent should be obtained by a doctor who is not engaged in the investigation and who

is completely independent of this official relationship.

11. In the case of legal incompetence, informed
consent should be obtained from the legal guardian in
accordance with national legislation. Where physical
or mental incapacity makes it impossible to obtain informed consent, or when the subject is a minor, permission from the responsible relative replaces that of
the subject in accordance with national legislation.

12. The research protocol should always contain a
statement of the ethical considerations involved and
should indicate that the principles enunciated in the
present Declaration are complied with.

II. Medical Research Combined with Professional Care
(Clinical Research)

1. In the treatment of the sick person, the doctor
must be free to use a new diagnostic or therapeutic
measure, if in his or her judgment it offers hope of
saving life, reestablishing health or alleviating suffering.

2. The potential benefits, hazards and discomfort
of a new method should be weighed against the advantages of the best current diagnostic and therapeutic
methods.

3. In any medical study, every patient -- including
those of a control group, if any -- should be assured
of the best proven diagnostic and therapeutic method.

4. The refusal of the patient to participate in a
study must never interfere with the doctor-patient
relationship.

5. If the doctor considers it essential not to obtain informed consent, the specific reasons for this
proposal should be stated in the experimental protocol
for transmission to the independent committee (I, 2).

6. The doctor can combine medical research with
professional care, the objective being the acquisition
of new medical knowledge, only to the extent that

medical research is justified by its potential diagnostic or therapeutic value for the patient.

III. Non-therapeutic Biomedical Research Involving Human Subjects (Non-Clinical Biomedical Research)

1. In the purely scientific application of medical research carried out on a human being, it is the duty of the doctor to remain the protector of the life and health of that person on whom biomedical research is being carried out.

2. The subjects should be volunteers -- either healthy persons or patients for whom the experimental design is not related to the patient's illness.

3. The investigator or the investigating team should discontinue the research if in his, her or their judgment it may, if continued, be harmful to the individual.

4. In research on man, the interest of science and society should never take precedence over considerations related to the well-being of the subject.

CHAPTER 6

Issues in the Design of Clinical Trials

Panel Discussion
JOHN C. BAILAR, III, *Chairman*
BYRON W. BROWN, JR.
JEROME J. DeCOSSE
EDMUND A. GEHAN
JAMES F. HOLLAND

J. C. Bailar: The subject of clinical trials is one of great interest to both medical and biostatistical professionals. Some of the issues in study design have been the center of much controversy in recent years. I know that the members of our panel, each of whom has had considerable experience in conducting clinical trials, will provide us with a very stimulating discussion.

VIEWS OF A MEDICAL ONCOLOGIST

J. F. Holland: I have divided cancers into 3 kinds without reference to their histology or their location: curable cancers, subcurable cancers, and pre- curable cancers. Curable cancers are those in which more than half of the patients can be cured by chemo- therapy. Subcurable cancers are those in which more than half of the patients can be cured, but it takes

This work was supported in part by the Mobil Corpora- tion, the Rockefeller Foundation, and National Cancer Institute Grants CA-12014 and CA-30138.

both chemotherapy and a local or regional approach, such as surgery or radiotherapy, to accomplish the cure. And it may well be that surgery alone could cure a portion and chemotherapy alone could not cure any, but together they cure more than 50%. Precurable cancers are some 80% of neoplasms. Surgery with its ancient traditions and radiotherapy in its middle age await the youthful expression of chemotherapy and of future disciplines to elevate these to be curable or subcurable.

I introduce these categories in order to make a point about discoveries in cancer research: Namely, the discovery of cures in most of the curable cancers was so dramatic, so miraculous that it seems to have occurred by revelation. Choriocarcinoma was first cured when patients at the National Cancer Institute with "incurable" choriocarcinoma participated in a clinical pharmacology experiment of methotrexate dose schedules. M. C. Li recognized that there was a change in the titer of their chorionic gonadotropin and thus quickly converted a new finding into something that made sense. The lead was rapidly exploited by Hertz and Li (15). Other curable cancers have had similar quantum leap discoveries. I do not think controlled trials will make major discoveries of curable cancers.

In the curable cancers, once the revelation has been found, controlled trials make sense. In the subcurable cancers it is necessary to identify some lead of importance and then controlled trials are essential. Curable types of kidney, liver, and lung tumors are known among the precurable cancers. Ordinarily what we see are minor deviations from expectancy as a lead, and then controlled trials establish these small step-by-step advances. The series of successive controlled trials in acute lymphocytic leukemia of children provides an enlightening example. Although it might have been possible successively to pick the best regimen of the prior study for the next comparison, that is not what happened. Several studies introduced

innovations. The largest step was due to the use of
a whole new principle, the concept of induction and
bulk reduction of the tumor by vincristine and prednisone, and then the application of more intensive
treatment. As we get farther and farther toward cure,
the increments in percentage survival are smaller,
and the numbers required to demonstrate statistical
significance are greater. In the most recent 3 studies of the Cancer and Leukemia Group B 500-600 children were entered per study. It is difficult to provide conclusive evidence in the final curative steps,
since luekemia is a rare disease, afflicting about
4000 children in the country each year. Also, as the
treatment becomes more successful, fewer doctors refer
their patients elsewhere for study. We need new statistical techniques, other than randomized trials, to
establish that a disease is cured. Progress in mark-
ing the tumor by immunologic means should make it
easier to know when the patient is cured.

There is a controversy concerning osteogenic sarcoma treatment. One group, Edmonson et al. (8), has
not found a difference between adjuvant chemotherapy
and surgery only in a preliminary report of a controlled trial from the Mayo Clinic. Miké (17,18),
Gehan (12), and others have reported a 20% survival
at best for osteogenic sarcoma with surgery alone,
whereas recent survival results have been much better
at the Mayo Clinic for this group of patients (20).
We have studied patients with osteogenic sarcoma using
the drug adriamycin, and analyzed those who did and
did not adhere to the protocol (6). Adherence was
more often a physician's characteristic than a patient's, since thresholds for dose adjustments of
parenteral drugs were clearly stipulated. The behavior of some physicians in altering dose at less rigorous thresholds because of concern for drug toxicity
led to greater danger from the tumor. Those who received the appropriate protocol dose (with the dose
adjustments as called for) had superior disease-free
survival. In my opinion, a controlled trial that

commits a group of patients with osteogenic sarcoma
at random to no treatment other than surgery is an
unethical relegation of patients to a highly mortal
regimen. It has been said to me, "If you had randomized at the beginning it would not be necessary now."
However, we deliberately did not randomize in the beginning. When a disease kills 80% of the children
that it affects, and a treatment is in hand that has
made significant impact on the advanced metastatic
disease, sequential trial appears the most ethical.
Rosen at Memorial Sloan-Kettering has subsequently
done even better than our early trial. His recent
findings with multiple combination chemotherapy indicate a disease-free survival of about 75% (19). A
controlled study between two treatments is reasonable
and desirable but certainly not one involving a treatment consisting of surgery alone.*

When Richard Cooper entered the practice of medical
oncology, he no longer encountered patients with acute
leukemia, but was confronted with women with breast
cancer. He devised a multicombination drug regimen
for breast cancer that had convergent toxicity on the
tumor and divergent toxicity on the host. He put together 5 drugs: vincristine, prednisone, cyclophosphamide, methotrexate, and fluorouracil. He treated
women with metastatic breast cancer and observed better results than any theretofore reported. Because
women who had 4 or more metastatic axillary nodes at
the time of operation had an 85% probability of relapse from their surgery within 10 years, he began
treating them early after surgery. The trial was conducted sequentially without controls. Its effects,
if not the study itself, have revolutionized the practice of breast cancer surgery in this country. The
first 73 patients he treated with chemotherapy are

---

*This topic is further discussed by Dr. O'Fallon be-
low; see also Chapter 4. Ed.

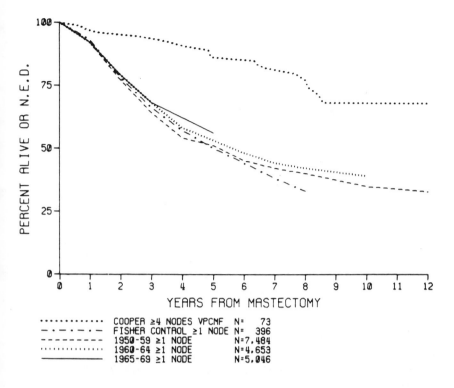

COOPER ≥4 NODES VPCMF   N=   73
FISHER CONTROL ≥1 NODE   N=   396
1950-59 ≥1 NODE   N=7,484
1960-64 ≥1 NODE   N=4,653
1965-69 ≥1 NODE   N=5,046

Figure 1. Comparison of survival experience of breast
cancer patients on Cooper regimen (5) with that of
the Fisher control group (9) and 3 groups from the
National Cancer Institute End Results Section (2).
The Cooper curve represents disease-free survival.
The last 3 curves show relative survival rates, which
are lower than the corresponding observed survival
rates, so that the comparison is still appropriate.

compared with 17,183 American women from the End Results Section of the National Cancer Institute (2) in
Figure 1, which is an updated version of results reported in (5). One of my statistical colleagues says
there are some data that do not need statistics, and
these are some of them. The universe of 17,183 women
had one node or more containing cancer in the axilla,

and their relative survival rates are shown for 3 consecutive time periods. Cooper's patients had 4 metastatic nodes or more, which is much more adverse prog-
nostically, and the curve shows disease-free survival
which appears to plateau at 67% at 9 years. The
Cooper regimen minus vincristine, CMFP, was used at
the National Cancer Institute and found to be a highly
active combination of drugs in metastatic breast cancer. Subsequently the NCI group studied CMF alone
versus melphalan (L-PAM) in metastatic cancer and then
in the adjuvant circumstance, the latter by contract
to Bonadonna and colleagues in Milan. Bonadonna et
al. (3) reported an extraordinarily important study
of CMF versus no treatment after surgery, demonstrat-
ing in a controlled comparative fashion that the
chemotherapy was effective. I made reference to
Cooper's data in an editorial I wrote at the time
about Bonadonna's study (13). The absence of controls
in Cooper's work precluded assertion of statistical
significance, but clearly the study was of great biologic and heuristic significance.

　　We analyzed 100 patients, of whom the 73 who received chemotherapy only are shown in Figure 1 (5).
The other 27 women received radiotherapy, the classic
treatment, after their surgery but before the chemotherapy. Twenty-two of the 27 are dead. In a
matched-pair analysis accounting for age, tumor diam-
eter, node number, and pathologic type, the patients
who received chemotherapy only do significantly better, as can be seen in Figure 2, which is an update
of results reported in (14). This finding has been
rejected by many radiotherapists because it was not
done as a prospectively controlled comparison. It is
a lead indicating the possibility that major unantici-
pated interactions between treatments may occur, however.

　　I am disturbed about some of today's problems, not
the least of which are that physicians are reluctant
to randomize patients because sometimes patients are
reluctant to be randomized. A patient goes to a

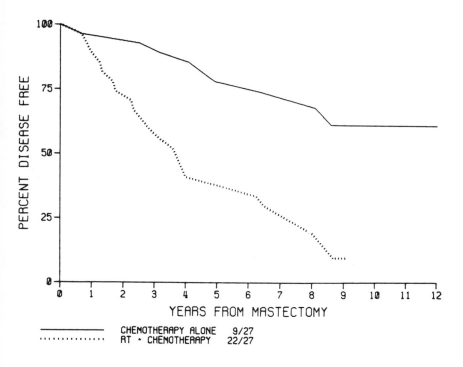

Figure 2. Disease-free survival curves for 27 matched pairs of breast cancer patients who received chemotherapy only or radiotherapy plus chemotherapy.

physician and says, "Do what's best for me." If a doctor says, "I don't know what's best," patients often seek another doctor for a second opinion. It is difficult to tell someone whose life is at stake, "Medicine doesn't really know what's best for you, therefore we'll randomize you." It may sound easy in the lecture hall but it is not so easy at the bedside. Furthermore, the vast majority of cancer patients are not referred to the major centers for treatment. Patients are being cared for in their doctor's office, where they would rather be, particularly if the doctor tells them: "There is no real basis for you to go to New York, I can do everything they would do for you

here." That is very reassuring to patients. There
is a decrease in patient referral for the very problems that we need to investigate. The same number of
patients fill the beds in the centers, but they are
often patients with rarer diseases, or patients at
the end stages of their diseases, rather than early
where the major advances can be made.

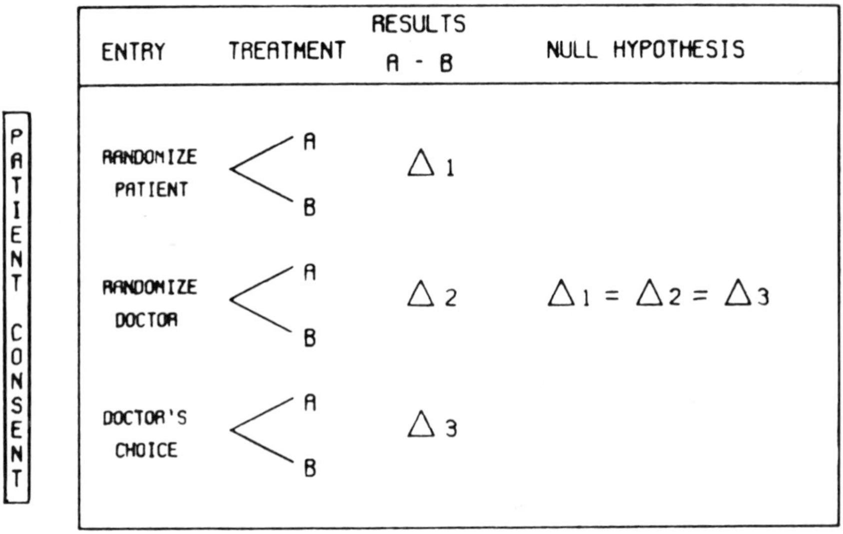

Figure 3. Proposed randomization design.

Oliver Glidewell and I designed a test of the process of randomization, which I outline in Figure 3.
In one arm we would randomize patients as usual. Another group of physicians (or possibly institutions)
would be randomized to give all patients treatment A
or all treatment B. In the third category some physicians could administer the treatment they are sure is
better. This, after all, is how most cancer treatments have been found that are successful and curative. In this design, "doctors at random" become the
controls for "doctors by choice." One would look at
the 3 arms with the same analytic dispassion and the

same criteria for assessment, comparing the difference
of treatments A and B when given by doctor's choice,
when the doctors are randomized, or when the patients
are randomized.

The controlled randomized study is now held in the
highest esteem, but it has many drawbacks. It is not
a way to get large patient volumes, for example.
What is gained in volume using our methodology may
make up in reliability for what is lost in the smaller
numbers of a randomized study.

It is not easy to get people to stay in academic
medicine. Many good oncologists are in urban and suburban communities, extraordinarily busy, and they may
have a major role to play in clinical investigation.
The difference between treatments A and B could be
constant over the arms of this design, even though
each type of investigator got different values for A
and for B, and one might find alternative ways to
reach the same answer with confidence.

THE ISSUES AS SEEN BY A STATISTICIAN

E. A. Gehan: I recently gave a talk on what every
clinician needs to know about the design of clinical
trials.   I later realized, however, that it is really
what statisticians need to know also.   That is, statisticians need to know the statistical aspects of
these very same issues.   There are 3 types of clinical
trials: Phase I, Phase II, and Phase III, and we are
talking about Phase III trials in the present context.

In designing Phase III trials, we first need to
know about writing protocols and the things to look
for in reviewing protocols.   In my experience, a main
point is the feasibility of the study and, in particular, the number of patients needed.   Many studies
are started and never completed, or not completed
adequately enough to answer the main question of interest, simply because the patient accrual was too
low.   This is an important area that needs the attention of statisticians.   Second, we need to know about

issues relating to stratification and other techniques of adjusting for prognostic factors. Third, we need to know the arguments for and against randomization and the types of clinical trial that have proved useful, such as factorial and other special designs. Fourth, a statistician should be an expert in techniques for analysis of data and should be able to teach a physician an understanding of the concepts used in analysis.

There are further considerations in planning controlled clinical trials. The objectives are very important. In some cases, statisticians have taken as the objective to select the better of the two treatments under study. I believe, however, that what is really wanted is selection and estimation. Given that a drug has gone through Phase I and Phase II studies, it is only ethical to be doing a randomized Phase III trial if it is known that the treatments are not different in effectiveness by an order of magnitude. Thus, the major objective should be to select the better of the two treatments and to say something about how effective each one is. Also, patients should be comparable not only at entry into study but while they are managed on study, and with respect to the criteria for their evaluation at the conclusion of study.

I have always been surprised that whereas statisticians acknowledge that historical controls can be of value in clinical studies, not more of them have actually planned historical control studies in some circumstances. Let me review briefly some of the arguments for historical controls. First, all knowledge is historical. Even those using randomized trials have to believe this, or otherwise they could not believe their own results. Second, in cancer we do have definitions of response and toxicity that are objective and, therefore, comparable over time. Third, we can assure comparability of groups of patients when we have information concerning the major prognostic factors. Fourth, recruitment of patients is much easier for nonrandomized studies. A person may not be willing to travel far if there is a chance he will not receive the new treatment. Fifth, it is clear that studies with historical controls need fewer patients than randomized studies designed to meet equivalent objectives (11,16). Sixth, there is no ethical dilemma either prior to or during the conduct of the study in a historically controlled study.

People have argued that the most convincing evidence is from the randomized trial. I do not believe that. There are some very controversial randomized and nonrandomized studies. The most convincing evidence is from confirmatory studies. If we stratify patients and/or use methods of adjustment for prognostic factors, we can estimate the difference in effectiveness between treatments adjusting for elements of noncomparability between the historical control series and the concurrent series. Note that it is an assumption here that to use historical controls we have to know something about prognostic factors. The record of accomplishment of nonrandomized studies in cancer has already been mentioned. In essence, the major advances in treatment have come from the nonrandomized studies.

I would like also to present some of the arguments for the use of randomized studies. These arguments appeared in the paper by Byar et al. in The New England Journal of Medicine (4). I think some of the force of that article arises from the fact that many different institutes from NIH were represented among the coauthors on the paper.

The first argument in favor of randomization is that there is an unbiased allocation of patients to treatments. I have always thought that I worked with reputable investigators who know something about patient features related to prognosis and would not deliberately bias studies to give misleading results. Thus, I do not think this first point is always a strong argument for randomization. Second, there is comparability of patients on each treatment on the average in the randomized study. However, this cannot be guaranteed in any particular study. Third, inferences can be based on randomization models. This is an argument that does not carry much weight with clinicians. It is basically a theoretical argument. Fourth, there is unbiased estimation of treatment effects.

When historical data are fairly old and one cannot rely on them to predict results for the current study, then a randomized study is appropriate. For example, when there have been substantial improvements in diagnosis and in staging of patients, this makes it very difficult to construct comparable groups of patients for use in a historically controlled study.

Freireich, Keating, and I have incorporated the clinician's and patient's preferences for treatment, as well as the option for randomization, into a new design for comparative clinical trials. We think that our design will remedy some of the problems that occur in controversial studies when patient accrual may be very low, when some doctors may prefer one treatment over another, and when the study may otherwise go nowhere. For the design to be useful, we must know something about the patient characteristics related to prognosis. Figure 4 outlines our proposal for an informed consent design. Let me note that our proposal is related to Dr. Holland's in that a clinician may prefer one treatment or have no preference. Also, some of the nomenclature used is because of the relation to Zelen's paper on prerandomization and randomized designs (21). Here, the doctor seeks consent for whichever treatment he prefers. For those who prefer the randomized design, if a doctor gets consent for the patient to enter the randomized trial, the patient is simply randomized to the new or standard treatment. If the patient refuses and prefers, for example, the new treatment, he receives the new treatment. If the patient prefers the standard, he gets the standard.

We let the doctor treat according to his particular preference. If the doctor prefers the new treatment,

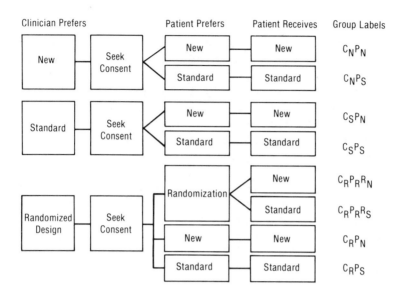

Figure 4. Alternative design for comparative clinical trials. C = Clinician, P = Patient, R = Randomized patient. Subscripts: N = New, S = Standard, R = Randomization. For example, C_N = Clinician prefers New Treatment.

he seeks the patient's consent to give that treatment. If the consent is received, he administers the new treatment. I expect that most of the patients would prefer the new treatment in this situation. Similarly, if the doctor prefers the standard and tries to persuade the patient of that, I would expect that most of the patients would choose the standard treatment. But if the patient's preference is opposite that of the doctor's, the doctor should be willing to administer the other treatment.

Some of the standard types of design are subcategories of our proposal. For example, if all patients receive the new treatment in this design, then we can compare the new versus standard in historical control patients. If all patients are randomized, then we

have the usual randomized trial. If all patients receive the standard treatment, however, then one should
reexamine the basis for studying the new treatment.

We think that patient accrual will be stimulated
by this design, especially in controversial studies.
The patient will be fully informed and will have the
option to pick the new treatment or the standard
treatment or to be randomized. We will be able to
study the effect of a physician's preference on the
outcome of treatment. Some have argued that if a doctor prefers a new treatment he might obtain better
results than a doctor who administers a new treatment
when he has no preference for one of the two treatments. There are many implications of this design.
However, the main implication for this discussion is
that our design is an attempt to provide an alternative to the strictly randomized study.

VIEWS OF A SURGICAL ONCOLOGIST

J. J. DeCosse: My comments will represent some of my
thinking about interactions between clinicians and
biostatisticians. They will not address some of the
specifics of the proposed designs just presented,
which to me appear to be more a study of randomization
than a study of cancer.

I am a user of biostatistical support. I am deeply
grateful for the help biostatisticians have provided
my clinical colleagues and me. But I worry, and I
worry because I am not at all sure that we understand
one another fully. We clinicians are guilty of a bad
habit of congenitally overestimating available, eligible patients. The biostatistician ought to regularly
discount our optimism. We do not know as much as we
think we do about the natural history of human cancers. With rare exceptions, prognostic factors are
not well understood. I believe the nature of some
human cancers changes over periods of time for reasons
we do not understand. Certainly this is true of stomach cancer and, as has come up twice already, it is

intriguing that the results of surgical treatment of osteogenic sarcoma have changed over time at the Mayo Clinic, with neither a change in treatment nor a change in the microscopic criteria for diagnosis. Hence, I find retrospective comparisons exceedingly worrisome.

Let me pose a dilemma. When we engage in a randomized trial the basic ethical setting is that we do not know which of the two treatments is better. Since they are considered to be essentially the same, it is ethically permissible to compare these two treatments. We have a degree of belief in both the conventional and the new treatment that we propose to test. Yet there is information we have acquired that expresses a certain degree of belief that the new treatment may be better. It seems that the trial in which we are about to engage ought to incorporate some of that prior information, and the results of the trial ought to either add or subtract from that degree of belief.

I am an ardent advocate of the randomized trial but I worry that we clinicians have forced too much complexity on trial design. Too often we have sold a bill of goods to the biostatistician about prospective stratifications. Too often there have been inappropriate and unnecessary add-ons that have unduly increased complexity and obscured the important questions.

Another problem that concerns me is the complex web of referral patterns and how the population sample in a tertiary care center such as here may not be representative of the total population with that tumor. For example, among all patients with large bowel cancer one expects about two patients with colon cancer for every patient with rectal cancer. At Memorial Sloan-Kettering, that ratio is reversed because of a particular interest in rectal cancer and rectal preservation. We have very good results in our treatment of large bowel cancer but it may be that some patients are too sick to travel here and those patients make results in the community hospital look worse. Also,

it does not help to compare institutions by stage because I believe there may be shifts to the right or
to the left in an institution within any given stage.
All this may be an argument for multiple institutional
trials of cancer treatment where a broader and more
representative population base can be scrutinized.
On the other hand, it would seem that confounding variables such as the extent of operation, the precision
of radiation therapy, and uniformity of pathology are
better controlled in a single center trial.

Another point of difficulty is that in cancer
treatment research small differences may be important.
If one compares the results of no treatment in breast
cancer with results of various treatments, perhaps 2
or 3 of every 10 patients are helped, and even that
difference is disputable. Then, if one compares the
results of different kinds of treatment among these
20-30%, differences at best are small. However, if
you are a patient with breast cancer looking at treatment options, even one additional chance in 100 is important. I do not know how to address this worry
short of enormous sample size.

This leads to two other thoughts. I worry that
clinicians have not always given the facts to the biostatistician about what they do. In the case of
breast cancer there is so much variability in the
thoroughness of what we label mastectomy and in the
completeness of prosection of the specimen by pathologists that this heterogeneity ought to dilute or ob-
scure true differences that may exist among treatments
(7). I suspect that radiation therapy may be equally
variable but on paper it looks better. The other
thought is that survival is not the only thing patients are concerned about these days. I do not know
how to do it, but we have to learn how to express the
quality of life in some semiquantitative way for appropriate consideration in treatment planning. There
needs to be a dialogue among biostatisticians and clinicians to develop and validate more precise considerations of the quality of life.

The whole idea is to end up with a "yes" or "no" answer to the question being asked. I worry that even the biostatistician cannot make a silk purse out of a sow's ear when the question is either poorly phrased or when the state of the art does not permit an unambiguous answer.

This leads to two conclusions. First, there is an ellipsis in the conclusions of a manuscript, which goes something like, "Under the conditions of the study we found such and such." Perhaps that ellipsis ought to be explicit in publications about cancer treatment. Second, the study of human cancer is exceedingly complex. There are many traps. They are not always initially apparent. Dr. Miké may not care for the appellation of biostatistics as handmaiden or queen,* but how about mountain climbing guide leading the clinician out of the traps? We have no choice except to perfect our science and ourselves and we have to do it together.

A STATISTICIAN RESPONDS

<u>B. W. Brown</u>: I am very pleased about the idea of scientifically examining the question of making scientific progress. This is the thrust of both Dr. Holland's and Dr. Gehan's proposals. The question of making scientific progress is worth examining especially when you see the strong feelings and the difficulties of doing scientific work when the experimental object is a patient.

The question of historical studies and methods is an interesting one. Although some prefer historical studies while others prefer randomized trials, everyone agrees that if you want to do a valid study of a scientific question there is some advantage in randomly allocating the experimental objects to the

---

*See conclusion of Chapter 4. Ed.

treatments. A major advantage of randomization is to
eliminate one source of bias in the allocation of
treatments to experimental units by not allowing the
physician to decide which patient gets which treatment. A second advantage, which in fact is the reason
for randomization as first introduced by Fisher, is
to provide a foundation for statistical inference,
for P-values, standard errors, and other measures of
the reliability of an inference. The price paid for
these advantages is inefficiency, as Dr. Holland and
Dr. Gehan have observed. By using historical controls, for example, you can achieve the same power
with one-fourth as many patients as would be required
by the randomized study.

Nobody disagrees with these things. Every experimental situation has to be solved by itself in view
of the situation, in discussion with the physicians,
statisticians, and other people involved in the study,
and in consideration of where the study will be reported and who will be persuaded by the results.

I would like to make a comment on Dr. Holland's
proposal. There are problems with randomly assigning
the physician to the use of one treatment or another,
in that you still allow the doctor, in a sense, to
select his patients for the study. You have not
eliminated bias in quite the effective way you do by
randomizing patients to the treatments. The physician, knowing that he is always going to use treatment
A, can withhold certain patients from treatment A, or
from entry into the study, and the problem such selection bias can create will have to be examined in any
statistical analysis of the results. Of course, this
problem can be even more acute among the physicians
who are allowed to elect the treatment they will use.

I would like to comment on some points raised by
Dr. DeCosse. The first is the question of referral
and the bias that comes from referral patterns in a
standard randomized clinical trial. Generally, when
you randomize patients to treatment A or B in a study,
the statistical inferences, the P-values, the standard

errors, and so on, refer only to those patients and
what might have been if the assignments had been different. You are left to wonder whether in fact you
can generalize from the result in the patients studied
to patients at another institution or to patients followed in the general practice of the community. On
the other hand, the experiment itself, with the randomization, should provide a valid inference to the
question of whether it is better to treat patients one
way or another within the institution of study, or
within the cluster of institutions from which the patients were referred. And that is the most we can
hope for. A second point concerns balancing. You
worry about placing too much burden on the statistician to balance the study on 5 prognostic factors,
some of which you may not even be sure are important.
Do not worry about it. We have simple methods for
achieving balance on many prognostic factors, and I
feel that we should use them, even though one or another factor may not be as predictive as we think.

A physician-scientist should worry, however, about
trying to draw many inferences from the same slim set
of data. Statisticians know something about how to
measure the reliability of inferences when you put a
large burden on a small set of data by attempting to
draw a number of different conclusions. Perhaps we
should try to put the brakes on your enthusiasm for
asking questions, by explaining more clearly how reliability is attenuated by asking too many questions
of the same study.

THE OSTEOGENIC SARCOMA CONTROVERSY[*]

J. R. O'Fallon: The Mayo Clinic osteogenic sarcoma
study has been mentioned several times during this

---

[*]This is in response to comments made by Dr. Holland.
See also discussion of this issue in Chapter 4. Ed.

meeting. I did not foresee that it was going to figure so prominently, so I did not come prepared to discuss it. However, I would like to make a few comments
about this controversial study because it illustrates
a couple of ethical issues.

Osteogenic sarcoma is a malignant bone tumor encountered primarily among young people. It has a
rather large literature, including some important papers in which Dr. Miké was a coauthor and statistician. Immediate amputation has been the treatment of
choice for many decades and still is used frequently
at the Mayo Clinic. Within the past 10 years, several
adjuvant chemotherapeutic regimens have been developed, which are currently believed to be effective.
One of them is high-dose methotrexate given with cit-
rovorum rescue. This particular regimen must be used
very carefully. It frequently involves repeated hos-
pitalizations for several days over the course of a
year; and its side effects are sometimes very serious
and occasionally fatal. It is very expensive, costing
upward of $1000 per month. Furthermore, its long-term
effects are not completely known, even now. Certainly
it is not a treatment that should be used without substantial evidence of effectiveness.

The problem with the adjuvant chemotherapy used today and with methotrexate in particular is that its
efficacy has been established by comparison with historical controls from earlier years (going back generally to the early 1960s) and sometimes even from
other institutions. In 1976, the Mayo Clinic reviewed
its historical data and discovered to its surprise
that osteogenic sarcoma patients treated with surgery
alone appeared to be getting better, that is, appeared
to be surviving longer as a trend in time without
change in treatment. In fact, the Mayo Clinic's most
recent surgery-only patients have survival and
disease-free interval distributions quite similar to
those of patients treated with methotrexate during the
same years, both at Mayo and elsewhere (20).

Supported by this evidence, in 1976 investigators

at Mayo proposed that a randomized study be done to
compare the efficacy of adjuvant high-dose methotrexate with that of surgical treatment alone. There was
a problem with this, however, because in 1975 the NCI
had sent a memorandum informing physicians throughout
the country of the apparent value of adjuvant treatment with either high-dose methotrexate or doxorubic-
in. When Mayo attempted to do its randomized controlled clinical trial, it was very difficult to get
patients to accept it, and many physicians were reluctant to refer patients to the Clinic. The clinical
trial limped along for about 3 years with patient accrual being very slow, but the study was continued
until nearly 40 patients were collected. The result
of this rather limited trial has been the same from
the earliest examination of the data to the latest:
There is no great difference observed between the two
treatment arms. There certainly is no significant
difference (8). Now, people around the world who have
heard the preliminary reports have begun to say, "Maybe we do need a clinical trial with some kind of concurrent comparison group untreated with chemotherapy
but receiving amputation."

This controversy involves ethical considerations
on many levels. One of them is the ethics of using an
unproved, highly toxic, and expensive treatment in the
presence of information that suggests that it may not
be effective after all. Another is the ethics of pub-
licly declaring a regimen to be the treatment of
choice without adequate evidence of its worth in controlled trials, thereby making the performance of de-
finitive clinical comparisons virtually impossible.*

---

*A randomized clinical trial in osteogenic sarcoma, of
surgery plus chemotherapy versus surgery only (with
chemotherapy after progression of disease), is now being undertaken by a 6-institution consortium sponsored
by the National Cancer Institute. Ed.

THE CASE FOR RANDOMIZATION IN CLINICAL TRIALS

M. H. Gail: I would like to consider a hypothetical
example of a comparative study to illustrate why many
authors favor randomization. Suppose you wanted to
find out whether the polio vaccine was useful. In an
extreme case let us suppose that we would allow the
parents to decide whether the child gets the vaccine
or not, and then we would follow each of the children.
So we would have a follow-up on one set of children
who got the vaccine and on another set who did not get
the vaccine but were followed. And if we followed
these children carefully we might be able to determine
that there appeared to be a treatment difference. But
at the end of the study we would have to begin to ask
a whole series of questions. Were the people who
chose to get the polio vaccine, were those children
who actually received the vaccine, different in some
fundamental way from those who did not receive the
vaccine? Do we know what those fundamental ways are?
We would hope that we had measured some of those
things so that we could invoke adjustment procedures,
but we would ultimately be left still wondering whether we had adjusted for all the appropriate factors.
     The contrasting situation was the situation that
actually evolved in that setting. There were so many
people involved in these trials that we probably measured very few covariates. But the conclusion that
there was a real difference was based on the randomization itself. One wonders what the conclusion would
have been in the absence of randomization.

J. F. Holland: Could I ask a question of Dr. Gail?
What do you think is the solution to the problem of
patient numbers, if indeed someone persuaded you that
there were problems in recruiting patients to studies?

M. H. Gail: If it became impossible to conduct randomized studies because the numbers were not there
then I would try to do the best I could with observa-

tional studies. I would see what happened to patients
who actually got one treatment and see what happened
to patients who actually got another treatment. I
would do the best I could to try to find the adjustment variables. I would have to confront many of the
uncertainties that an epidemiologist confronts.

PATIENT ACCEPTANCE OF RANDOMIZATION

J. J. DeCosse: Dr. Holland stated the concept that
patients do not like to be randomized. I would argue
that the worst opponents of randomization are the physicians themselves. If you have a good doctor-patient
relationship, if you have confidence in yourself and
your ability to say you do not know to the patient,
and if the patient is at all reasonable, he will accept your judgment and on the whole opt for randomization. The thought that patients just do not want to
know that there are two treatments that may be equal
is not true.

J. F. Holland: I have conducted a great many randomized trials, as you know. I believe that your perspective, Dr. DeCosse, as the Chairman of Surgery at
Memorial Sloan-Kettering is not that of the surgeon in
general practice. If this surgeon tells a patient
that he does not really know the best treatment, he
is likely to lose his practice. Therefore, self-
preservation is a factor and, I believe, we are deny-
ing ourselves access to some 80% of the cancer patients. It may turn out that our hypothesis is wrong.
It may turn out that you cannot conduct trials the way
I have proposed to do, but at least we should test the
design and that to me is the beauty of it. I am not
advocating nonrandom studies.

J. J. DeCosse: No, the evidence for my view is not so
much from here because we have our problems. The evidence comes from engaging in a couple of trials in the
United Kingdom where the willingness of patients to

enter trials is greater. I do not believe it is the
patient population in this country which is at fault.
I think it is very often the insecurity of the physician.

J. C. Bailar: I think part of this may be a matter of
language. As physicians, we should not be saying to
our patients in these circumstances, "I do not know."
It is much better to say, "It is not known," and to
make it clear to the patient that there is a general
question, not just a matter of one's own confidence.
I am concerned also that we are skipping around part
of the question. If we think there may be fewer than,
say, 40 patients available, the limitation on case
material may prohibit a good randomized trial. Are
we then to believe that we can learn more from a nonrandomized trial with that same number of patients?
If we are primarily concerned about random error the
answer is clearly "no," whereas I think those who disagree with this argument are more concerned about nonrandom error. Is that a fair statement?

DIFFERENCES IN QUALITY OF HISTORICAL CONTROLS

B. W. Brown: Yes. It is a question of balancing more
bias against less bias and the other advantages that
come with randomization. There is one other point to
be made about historical controls. We talk as if we
know what we mean when we say historical controls and,
to be fair to Dr. Gehan's side of this argument, there
is a wide spectrum of kinds of historical control data, ranging from dim personal remembrances of what
might have gone on in the clinic 3 years ago, to looking at detailed reports of investigators who have
gathered data carefully. As Gehan and Freireich (11)
mention in their paper, data collected in the same way
by the same definitions, by the same physicians, in
the same hospital over the last two years may be a
fairly good historical control for a study now to be
embarked on. I think the design decision can depend

heavily on which of these situations prevails. However, though Dr. Gehan has a point, I wish that I had
been one of the authors of the Byar et al. paper (4)
because I argue as strongly as I can in most instances
for randomization. It is one of the basic blocks of
good science.

THE NEED FOR A BALANCED VIEW

E. A. Gehan: I would like to reply first to Dr.
Brown's comment about trying some of the new designs.
I think the value of such studies can only be proved
by their actual conduct. One of the examples that
comes to mind is a study in the Southwest Oncology
Group that proposed to study surgery alone versus surgery plus FAM treatment for stomach cancer patients
which continues to go along at a snail's pace. I
think it is basically because many physicians participating in the study believe that since FAM has been
shown to be effective in the patient with advanced
stomach cancer, it would tend to be effective in the
adjuvant setting and, therefore, that one should not
randomize. But our study is a randomized one, and a
problem we will have to face is what to do with the
patients who were randomized to surgery plus no further treatment but who have received FAM because they
heard about the treatment and sought it elsewhere, or
for some other reason received the treatment. This
has happened to at least 10% of the patients in the
surgery alone group. So, the conduct of the study and
accrual of patients is a problem that arises even in
the randomized studies.
   In reply to Dr. Gail's comments, I would prefer to
analyze the data from a randomized study. There are
certainly fewer problems. But I think the basic problem is the ethical aspect of the study. I think that
one should not design a study for others that one
would not be willing to participate in, if one happened to be a patient. I have known many statisticians, and some that have had cancer. I have never

heard of one that has been a participant as patient
in a randomized study. It is sometimes difficult to
weigh the evidence from various studies, but I think
we do have to consider the ethical aspects of clinical
trials. Although there are problems with historically
controlled studies, the ethical side of such studies
should persuade us to be willing to try and analyze
them using all the techniques that we have and to try
to convince others of their effectiveness.

SEQUENTIAL DESIGNS

V. Miké: The area of sequential trials is one that is
discussed a great deal in statistical circles. Sequential designs have not really taken hold in the
medical setting and they may be impossible to use in
cancer clinical trials because of the essentially
multivariate nature of the situation, and also because
the outcome is generally not known for some time. But
clinical investigators often ask us about these methods.

E. A. Gehan: I think that sequential designs with the
objective only of selecting the better of two treatments should generally not be used. The sequential
trial is a carryover of a mathematical probability
problem, which has an apparent relation to cancer
clinical trials, but which I do not believe has real
application in the field of cancer research. As I
stated in my opening presentation, I think the objective in most Phase III trials is to select the better
treatment and estimate the effectiveness of each; the
latter requirement is usually not sufficiently well
met in sequential trials.

If I may continue by commenting on the sequential
aspects of studies, I would like to relate a brief experience which occurred in the early days of Cancer
and Leukemia Group B that has influenced my attitude
toward sequential trials. The clinical trial was a
randomized study of 6MP versus placebo in the

maintenance of remissions in acute leukemia (10).
Dr. Holland was a participant in this study. The
trial was designed according to one of the Armitage
sequential schemes (1) for comparing pairs of patients
with respect to length of remission. One patient got
6MP, and one got placebo; after 18 pairs of patients
we were able to stop the study deciding that 6MP was
the better treatment. It worked out that 6MP had a
27-week median length of remission and placebo had a
9-week median length of remission.

In talking about the results of that trial, the
physicians would say that an "estimate" of the difference in median lengths of remission was 18 weeks.
Clearly, a good estimate of this difference could not
be based on only 18 patients in each group. We could
conclude that 6MP was better than placebo in this
case, but we could not give a precise estimate of how
much better it was.

While that was a reasonable study to do at the
time, I think that at present we also want to be able
to estimate the differences between the treatments
and to say something about the effectiveness of each
treatment. I think we need sequential trials where
we put enough patients on study to meet the estimation
requirement. If, at that point, we still cannot decide which is the better of the two treatments, then
we might consider a sequential study beginning at that
point to determine which treatment is better. But it
would be a different form of sequential trial than
has been proposed in the past.

CONCLUDING REMARKS

J. C. Bailar: I would like to summarize some of what
I hear as the major points of disagreement. They seem
to focus on the nature and the use of controls, which
is a matter of much wider interest in biostatistics,
clinical science, and even science in general.

In the evaluation of treatment of human beings for
medical conditions there are really 4 general kinds

of approaches, not all of which are equally applicable
to matters of cancer. One is the crossover design in
which each patient gets, in succession, two or more
treatments that are considered candidates for evaluation. There are many variations on crossovers: They
may be randomized, there may be certain sequences that
are chosen in preference to others, and so forth. A
second approach is what some of my colleagues have
begun calling parallel designs. These are the ordinary kinds of clinical trials in which one group of
patients gets treatment A, another group gets treatment B, and there is no crossover feature, although
these different treatment groups are developed and
followed by the same group of investigators during
the same period of time. A third general approach
which, like the crossover designs, has more limited
applicability to questions of cancer comprises the
self-controlled designs in which one compares the status of the patient before treatment with the status
after treatment, sometimes long after treatment, when
one thinks that perhaps the treatment effects have
disappeared. The fourth is that group of approaches
that we call external controls. These are the studies
in which the controls are developed outside the study
proper, generally by other people in other settings,
perhaps within the same institution, but at a prior
time. Historical controls are one form of external
control. Much of the discussion here has been around
the appropriate nature and use of these external controls. We all do externally controlled or historically controlled studies. Phase I trials are examples. There are no internal controls in Phase I
studies.

It seems to me that we should not come down hard
for one or the other approach, but that we should
rather try to develop an understanding, perhaps a set
of questions that we should ask about each situation
for evaluation and each set of data for analysis, that
will help us to determine the strengths of one or the
other kind of approach. I do not think this is

entirely unreasonable. One might ask, for example, about historically controlled studies in general or about externally controlled studies of all types, whether the hypothesis being examined was in fact developed prior to the generation of the data. If it was not, one is likely to have some serious troubles in inference. One might ask if the results would be of equal medical or scientific interest if somehow they had been turned around. If you find in your historically controlled study that treatment A looks better than treatment B, you might learn something, but I think you would learn a bit more if you could assure yourself that you would be at least as much interested if it turned out in the end that treatment B was better than treatment A. This is again a way of avoiding some of the biases that people fear creep into this kind of approach. A third question might be whether the data are really symmetric. Do you know the same kinds of things about one group as you do about the other? I think there are a number of other such questions that might be asked about the use of external controls and that careful attention to these matters might improve their use.

We cannot do randomized clinical trials on everything that is of interest. These trials are too expensive in all resources. They are time consuming, ponderous, and have to be pointed toward the questions that really require that sort of apparatus. So we have the prior step, as I see it, of trying to screen out the situations where we can either develop a reasonably satisfactory answer in some other way, such as by the use of historical controls, or where we find that we do not really need an answer.

The whole problem, in a sense, comes down to the nature of what we would regard as a satisfactory degree of proof, that is, an adequate demonstration that one treatment is or is not better than another. Now the nature of proof is a matter that has concerned mathematicians for centuries, and scientists in other fields for decades at least. I regard a proof, and I

think many scientists also regard a proof, as a means
to convince oneself that something is true. And if
we adopt this definition in our work it is going to
mean that my standards of proof may not entirely match
yours. I am not sure that this is inappropriate. I
think that this entire matter of the nature and the
use of controls in developing an understanding of what
is going on with one or another treatment still needs
a lot more careful attention.

REFERENCES

1. Armitage, P. (1975), Sequential Clinical Trials
   (2nd ed.), Wiley, New York.

2. Axtell, L. M., Asire, A. J., and Myers, M. H.,
   eds. (1976), Cancer Patient Survival, Report No.
   5, [DHEW Pub. No. (NIH) 77-992], U.S. Government
   Printing Office, Washington, D.C.

3. Bonadonna, G., Brusamolino, E., Valagussa, P.,
   Rossi, A., Brugnatelli, L., Brambilla, C.,
   De Lena, M., Tancini, G., Bajetta, E.,
   Musumeci, R., and Veronesi, U. (1976), Combination
   chemotherapy as an adjuvant treatment in operable
   breast cancer, The New England Journal of Medicine
   294: 405-410.

4. Byar, D., Simon, R., Friedewald, W.,
   Schlesselman, J., DeMets, D., Ellenberg, J.,
   Gail, M., and Ware, J. (1976), Randomized clinical
   trials, The New England Journal of Medicine
   295: 74-80.

5. Cooper, R. G., Holland, J. F., and Glidewell, O.
   (1979), Adjuvant chemotherapy of breast cancer,
   Cancer 44: 793-798.

6. Cortes, E. P., Holland, J. F., Wang, J. J., and

Glidewell, O. (1975), Adriamycin (NSC-123127) in 85 patients with osteosarcoma, Cancer Chemotherapy Reports 6: 305-313.

7. DeCosse, J. J., Donegan, W. J., Sedransk, N., Jones, N. F., and Claudon, D. B. (1980), Operative procedures: Is standardization feasible or necessary? Cancer Treatment Reports 64: 419-423.

8. Edmonson, J. H., Green, S. J., Ivins, J. C., Gilchrist, G. S., Cregan, E. T., Pritchard, D. J., Smithson, W. A., Dahlin, D. C., and Taylor, W. F. (1980), Methotrexate as adjuvant treatment for primary osteosarcoma, Letter to the Editor, The New England Journal of Medicine 303: 642-643.

9. Fisher, B., Slack, N., Katrych, D., and Wolmark, N. (1975), Ten year follow-up results: Patients with carcinoma of the breast in a cooperative clinical trial evaluating surgical adjuvant chemotherapy, Surgery, Gynecology & Obstetrics 140: 528-534.

10. Freireich, E. J, Gehan, E., Frei, E., Schroeder, L., Wolman, I., Anbari, R., Burgert, O., Mills, S., Pinkel, D., Selawig, O., Moon, J., Gendal, B., Spurr, C., Storrs, R., Haurani, F., Hoogstraten, B., and Lee, S. (1963), The effect of 6-mercaptopurine on the duration of steroid-induced remission in acute leukemia: A model for evaluation of other potentially useful therapy, Blood 21: 699-716.

11. Gehan, E. A., and Freireich, E. J (1974), Nonrandomized controls in cancer clinical trials, The New England Journal of Medicine 290: 198-203.

12. Gehan, E. A., Sutow, W. W., Uribe-Botera, G., Romsdahl, M., and Smith, T. L. (1978), Osteosarcoma: The M. D. Anderson Experience, in: Terry, W. D., and Windhorst, D., eds., Immunother-

apy of Cancer: Present Status of Trials in Man, Raven Press, New York, pp. 271-282.

13. Holland, J. F. (1976), Breast cancer and chemo-therapy, Science 192: 1062-1063.

14. Holland, J. F., Glidewell, O., and Cooper, R. G. (1980), Adverse effect of radiotherapy on adjuvant chemotherapy for carcinoma of the breast, Surgery, Gynecology & Obstetrics 150: 817-821.

15. Holland, J. F., and Hreshchyshyn, M. M., eds. (1967), Choriocarcinoma, Vol. 3, UICC Monograph Series, Springer-Verlag, Berlin.

16. Makuch, R., and Simon, R. (1979), Sample size considerations for non-randomized comparative studies, Journal of Chronic Diseases 33: 175-181.

17. Marcove, R. C., Miké, V., Hajek, J. V., Levin, A. G., and Hutter, R. V. (1970), Osteo-genic sarcoma under the age of 21. A review of 145 operative cases, Journal of Bone and Joint Surgery 52-A: 411-423.

18. Miké, V., and Marcove, R. C. (1978), Osteogenic sarcoma under the age of 21: Experience at Memorial Sloan-Kettering Cancer Center, in: Terry, W. D., and Windhorst, D., eds., Immunother-apy of Cancer: Present Status of Trials in Man, Raven Press, New York, pp. 283-292.

19. Rosen, G., Caparros, B., Huvos, A. G., Kosloff, C., Nirenberg, A., Cacavio, A., Marcove, R. C., Lane, J. M., Mehta, B., and Urban, C. (1982), Pre-operative chemotherapy for osteogenic sarcoma: Selection of postoperative adjuvant chemotherapy based on the response of the primary tumor to pre-operative chemotherapy, Cancer 49: 1221-1230.

20. Taylor, W. F., Ivins, J. C., Dahlin, D. C.,
    Edmonson, J. H., and Pritchard, D. J. (1978),
    Trends and variability in survival from osteosar-
    coma, Mayo Clinic Proceedings 53: 695-700.

21. Zelen, M. (1979), A new design for randomized
    clinical trials, The New England Journal of Medi-
    cine 300: 1242-1275.

Part IV
Practical Considerations

CHAPTER 7
Design and Implementation of Clinical Trials

MARTIN L. LESSER

The purposes of this chapter on the design and implementation of clinical trials are threefold: (a) to discuss the basic principles and types of study designs, including what are frequently referred to as Phase I, Phase II, and Phase III clinical trials in cancer research; (b) to present various methods of sample size calculation in fixed-sample trials; (c) to discuss techniques of implementing a clinical trial, with particular emphasis on the randomization process.

Closely related issues pertaining to the design of clinical trials are discussed elsewhere in this volume. Specifically, the use of randomized or historical controls is considered in Chapter 6; sequential designs are considered in Chapter 14.

TYPES OF CLINICAL TRIALS AND THEIR STRUCTURE

A clinical trial is a prospective study that is designed to investigate the effect of a therapeutic

This work was supported by National Cancer Institute Grant CA-08748.

regimen on a given disease. In cancer clinical trials, the therapy under investigation might typically
be surgery, chemotherapy, radiotherapy, immunotherapy,
or some combination of these modalities.

Phase I Trials

A Phase I trial is an exploratory trial, the purpose of which is to assess the frequency and degree
of harmful side effects (i.e., toxicity) of the proposed therapy. Although the assessment of therapeutic
effect may not be conclusive, such studies should allow for early observation of therapeutic activity.
When feasible, pharmacology studies (e.g., absorption
and bioavailability) should be performed (11). In
cancer research, the Phase I trial usually involves
the investigation of a new drug or combination of
drugs on patients who have failed or are not candidates for conventional therapy. After a drug dose
level has been found with the highest acceptable level
of toxicity, the therapy can be evaluated for efficacy. Phase I trials are, of course, not limited to
drugs. In immunotherapy trials, interest might center
on finding an acceptable dosage of a biologic response
modifier; in studies of hyperthermia, it is important
to determine what temperature levels can be applied
to a tumor with minimal damage to surrounding normal
tissue.

Phase I studies should be designed so that initial
drug doses are well below the level at which toxic effects might be expected. Generally, a schedule of escalating doses is followed. Initial doses and subsequent escalations should be justified by preclinical
data or other relevant considerations (11).

Since toxicity resulting from treatment will be
reported in these studies (as well as in Phase II and
III described below), standardized grading of toxicity, for reporting purposes, is encouraged. Miller et
al. (14) recommend a specific grading scheme.

Formal statistical procedures may not be essential at this stage. However, the analysis of Phase I data presents a unique challenge to the statistician, since these studies often result in unstructured data sets which may be difficult to interpret.

Phase II Trials

The objective of the Phase II trial is to determine the level of effectiveness of a particular therapeutic regimen (e.g., antitumor activity) and to further define the nontherapeutic effects (e.g., toxicity) of such therapy.

A Phase II trial initially consists of a preliminary study to determine whether there is a sufficient level of therapeutic activity to warrant the further investigation of the treatment.

To this end, a sample size should be established which specifies the number of treatment failures that must be observed before the treatment can be rejected with a certain probability of error (11). The section entitled "Sample Size and Power Determination" provides information on such sample size calculations. If there is evidence of therapeutic potential, then the trial is continued and additional patients are entered in order to precisely estimate a parameter that is a measure of efficacy.

Since the main goal of this type of trial is to estimate a measure of "success," it is essential that such a measure be defined precisely; this is one aspect of the design of a Phase II trial about which the statistician should be particularly concerned.

The therapeutic effect of a treatment regimen is usually measured by a "response rate." In most cancer clinical trials the term "response" refers to disappearance of all measurable disease or to some specified decrease in tumor size (e.g., 50% decrease), although the response need not always be thought of in this sense. For example, response could be defined as the relief of pain or nausea or the attainment of a specified change in a biochemical parameter. Obviously, the definition of response depends on the objective of the clinical trial.

In any case it is important to enumerate all characteristics that must be present in order that a patient be classified as a responder, as well as the time interval in which these characteristics must be observed. Thus, for example, in a drug trial, a "complete response" might be defined as the disappearance of all measurable disease for at least 30 days. (Note that in this definition, a patient's disease must be measurable in order to be evaluated in the trial.)

Finally, response to treatment is not always dichotomous; many trials classify patients as either complete, partial, or nonresponders. The important point is that the categories be mutually exclusive and exhaustive.

Phase III Trials

Once a treatment has been tested in a Phase II trial, it is usually subjected to another test in order to determine its efficacy relative to one or more other therapeutic regimens. Such a comparative trial is known as a Phase III trial.

Generally, the Phase III study is designed to compare definitively a new treatment with the existing established standard. In addition, the nontherapeutic effects are further evaluated, especially in the context of determining the risks and benefits of the new treatment relative to the standard.

It should be pointed out that a drug that has passed through Phase II testing may be compared directly with a standard therapy or may be incorporated into an established regimen of treatment, resulting in a "drug combination." This drug combination may then be compared with the standard therapy.

The process of designing a Phase III trial requires that attention be given to several important issues.

Purpose of the Trial. In order to properly design
a trial, the objective of the trial must be clearly
stated. The purpose of the Phase III trial is to compare response rates, disease-free intervals, or survival times, although other outcomes might be investigated. In specifying the purpose of the trial, one
should make reference to the group of patients and to
the modes of therapy to be studied.

Generally speaking, it is wise to focus on only
one or two (well-formulated) questions when defining
the objective of the study. Such a study is usually
of greater value than one that is designed to address
numerous questions, since the latter type of study
often results in complex designs, large required sample sizes, inference problems, and dilution of effort
of the participating investigators.

Number of Treatment Arms. Since sample size is
critical in the conduct of a Phase III trial, it is
important to keep to a minimum the number of treatment
groups (arms) to be studied in order to assure a reasonable number of patients per arm. Frequently, a
trial will be composed of just two arms (e.g., new vs.
standard treatment); however, situations do arise
where more than two therapies are compared simultaneously.

The statistician should also keep in mind that, in
most cases, multiple arm trials may have to be analyzed using methods of multiple comparisons and that
such methods should be available for the types of
variables being studied. Furthermore, inferences
from multiple comparisons procedures can sometimes be
difficult to interpret.

Nature of the Control Group. When comparing a new
treatment with standard or placebo (control group) it
must be decided how the controls are to be selected.
This group could be comprised of patients who were
treated in the past by the standard treatment (historical controls) or they could be a concurrent group of

patients (concurrent controls). In most cases, concurrent controls are selected by randomization, whereby a patient is assigned to the control or treatment group at random (randomized controls).

There has been considerable discussion in recent years as to the appropriateness of historical controls in clinical trials. Those who favor only randomized trials claim that bias in treatment assignment is eliminated and that patients in all treatment groups are comparable, whereas historical controls may not be comparable with, and the procedures and evaluation criteria used may not be the same as for the group currently under study.

The opposing view is that there exist situations in which the use of historical controls presents little or no problem and that any differences in prognostic factors between groups can be handled using specialized statistical methods including covariate adjustment or matching. Furthermore, proponents argue that in such trials the ethical questions surrounding randomization are not present and that the costs of investigation are much lower. These issues are discussed further in Chapters 4, 5, and 6.

In any case, the study design should explicitly state from what population and by what method the controls are to be selected.

Patient Selection. When designing a clinical study, careful attention should be given to defining the patient population to be studied. A list of criteria for patient eligibility and ineligibility should be drawn up which clearly specifies which patients are to be selected for study. Such criteria should be as objective as possible and should be subject to verification for each patient.

Comparability of Patients. Patients in each treatment arm should be comparable with respect to prognostic factors in order to avoid confounding. Confounding occurs when the observed difference between treatment groups cannot be attributed solely to the differing treatments. For example, suppose that the patients receiving treatment A are observed to perform better than those receiving treatment B and that the treatment B group consisted mostly of patients with advanced disease, while treatment A was administered primarily to patients with early stages of disease. Then it is possible that the observed difference is due, in whole or in part, to the differing types of patients in the groups and not entirely to the treatments.

When employing historical controls, this situation can be problematic, although the use of randomization does not assure comparability of patients either. In the section entitled "Implementation of Clinical Trials", a method for achieving a considerable degree of comparability in randomized trials (stratification) is given.

The following fictitious example illustrates how differences in therapeutic modalities may "naturally" induce lack of comparability of patients in a trial: Suppose that patients with biopsy-proved carcinoma of the prostate are randomized to either surgery alone (prostatectomy) or radiation therapy (RT) alone and that an eligibility requirement is that patients have stage $T_1 N_0 M_0$ disease (i.e., tumor is within the capsule, surrounded by normal glandular tissue, no evidence of nodal involvement or distant metastasis); this is an early stage of disease. Although all patients would be clinically staged, only those assigned to surgery would have the opportunity to be surgically staged. Thus, for instance, a surgeon operating on a patient declared clinically stage $T_1 N_0 M_0$ may (in conjunction with the pathologist) find that the tumor has, in fact, invaded the capsule, resulting in a reclassification to $T_2 N_0 M_0$. Consequently, this patient is ineligible for the trial. The RT patients are only clinically staged and, hence, cannot be reclassified by the more accurate surgical procedure.

It is clear that if surgical patients are excluded

on the basis of surgical staging, then this group will consist of "true" $T_1N_0M_0$ patients while the RT group will always have some patients who have a more advanced stage of disease due to clinical staging error. Thus, the two groups will not be comparable from the start; the surgical group starts out with patients who on the whole will have a better prognosis.

One solution to this problem is that the eligibility criterion state that patients must be clinical stage $T_1N_0M_0$ and that exclusion is not permitted based on surgical staging. Of course, this solution may violate ethical principles, since a patient with known T_2 disease may necessarily require treatment that he does not receive in the trial. Nevertheless, this example shows how different treatment arms may be associated with different "baseline" characteristics of patients.

End Point Variables. In addition to rates of response, several other measures of treatment efficacy may be compared. The two most common end points are disease-free interval and survival.

a. Disease-Free Interval (Remission Duration). If, after therapy, a patient is judged as being free of disease, one may wish to measure the length of time that the patient remains in that state. This period of time is known as the disease-free interval, remission duration, or time to recurrence of disease.

The point at which a patient is classified as disease free, as well as the criteria used to make such a classification, should be well defined. Furthermore, the methods of follow-up should be the same for all patients and clearly set forth in the protocol (more on protocol-writing in the last section).

b. Survival Time. In cancer clinical trials, a patient's survival time is, perhaps, the most frequently studied end point variable. The determination of survival time is made by measuring length of life from

a certain time of reference, such as time of diagnosis, time of initiation of therapy, or time of completion of therapy. Furthermore, when analyzing survival
time data it is important to distinguish between a
patient who dies with disease present and one who dies
with no evidence of disease, since these two types of
deaths are often treated differently.

Criteria for Evaluation. The criteria used for
evaluating a patient's performance on therapy, whether
it be response, survival time, or any other end point,
should be the same for each treatment group. Patients
should have the same scheduling of follow-up examinations and diagnostic procedures, although this may not
always be the case. For example, in a trial of surgery versus chemotherapy, patients in each treatment
group may be scheduled for, say, a physical examination, blood counts, and biochemistries every 3 months,
a chest X-ray every 6 months, and a bone scan every
year. However, the patients receiving chemotherapy
may, in addition, require a hospitalization every
month (for administration of chemotherapy) during
which time the patient is monitored very closely and
has more contact with his physician. Thus, it is possible that recurrences or progression of disease may
tend to be detected earlier in the latter group as
compared with the former, thus resulting in possible
bias.

Also, when measuring a time variable (e.g., survival time), time should be measured from the same reference point in all treatment groups. Frequently,
time is measured from diagnosis of disease, initiation
of therapy, completion of therapy, or some other
point. Whatever the reference point, it should be
well defined and the same for each group.

Blinding. A method of reducing bias in a trial is
to introduce "blinding." In a double-blind trial
neither the patient nor his physician knows which
treatment is being given, permitting the physician to

evaluate his patient more objectively; furthermore, it decreases the chance that the patient will respond differently just because he knows which therapy he is receiving. Obviously it is not always feasible to run a double-blind study; if the treatments are "surgery" and "no surgery" then both the patient and physician will know the treatment identity; in a trial of "chemotherapy" versus "no chemotherapy," the chemotherapy group might exhibit symptoms of toxicity, while the other group would not, thus enabling the physician to guess which patients are receiving drug therapy.

A less stringent type of blind study is the single-blind trial, where either the patient or the physician (but only one of them) does not know the nature of the treatment.

Although a blind study is highly desirable as a means of reducing bias, it does require more logistical planning and bookkeeping and it is often not as readily understood or accepted by patients.

Sample Size. In order that reliable results may be obtained, a sufficient number of patients must be entered into a clinical trial. The maximum possible number of patients that can participate in a trial is determined, in part, by "usual" patient accrual for the type of disease being studied, duration of the trial, restrictions on patient eligibility, and limitations of facilities and personnel.

The required number of patients for a Phase II or III trial can be computed in several different ways based on different criteria. A detailed discussion of sample size determination is given in the next section.

Ethics. Ethical problems are intrinsic to the conduct of studies involving human subjects. Some of the more important ethical issues relate to (a) randomization, (b) informed consent, (c) withdrawal of a patient from study, and (d) termination of the study.

It is not infrequent that one is faced with the situation where ethical concern conflicts with the need for adherence to study design. A discussion of some of these issues can be found in Chapter 5 of this volume.

SAMPLE SIZE AND POWER DETERMINATION

This section deals with the calculation of sample size and power for clinical trials and provides examples of such calculations. Some tables for sample size/power calculations are given and references are made to publications in which others can be found. For a further discussion of clinical trials design, see references 2, 7, 12, 16, 18, and Chapter 4 of this volume. Reference 1 is a computer program for calculating sample size and power in clinical studies.

Phase I Trials

Since the goal of the Phase I study is primarily to establish dose-related toxicities and since formal statistical analysis may not be required, sample size and power calculations are usually not given. However, Schoenfeld (17) provides some sample size guidelines for pilot studies which might be applied to Phase I studies. In any event, some estimate of expected patient accrual should be provided.

If the Phase I trial is to include a pharmacology study, the statistician might want to provide some sample size requirements in order that the study be appropriately analyzed by regression analysis or analysis of variance, for example.

Phase II Trials

In the early stages of a Phase II trial, one would like to reject a treatment as soon as there is evidence that the response rate is <u>less</u> than some

specified proportion r, where r is a minimum clinically acceptable success rate. Thus, in a drug trial
one might not be interested in a drug that has less
than, say, a 15% response rate.

Table 1 shows the number of consecutive failures
that must be observed in order to reject the hypothesis that the therapeutic response (i.e., success) rate
is at least r, with a Type I error probability P.

Example 1. A Phase II trial is to be carried out to
determine if a new drug has any therapeutic activity.
If the drug's success rate is less than 15% then we
would like to discontinue testing of the drug as soon
as possible. According to Table 1, with P = .05 and
r = 15%, one would reject r ≥ 15% if 19 consecutive
failures are observed. If at least one success out
of 19 trials is observed then the drug is subjected to
further testing with the accrual of more patients.

The number of patients required in a Phase II trial
to estimate a response rate with given precision (d)
is given in Table 2, assuming 95% confidence.

Example 2. If the response rate to therapy is expected
to be approximately 30% and we wish to estimate that
rate to within d = ±10% (using a 95% confidence interval) then 81 patients are required.

Due to limited expected patient accrual over the
proposed duration of a trial, one may not always be
able to accession the number of patients indicated in
Table 2. Instead, one may wish to ask: Given that n
patients can be expected to enter the trial, with what
precision can a response rate (r) be estimated? Using
a 95% confidence interval and the normal approximation

TABLE 1. Number of Consecutive Failures Required to Ensure That a Treatment Having Response Rate r Will Be Rejected with Probability at Most P[a]

			Response rate in % (100r)							
P	5	10	15	20	25	30	35	40	45	50
.05	59	29	19	14	11	9	7	6	6	5
.10	45	22	15	11	9	7	6	5	4	4

[a]The number n of consecutive failures required is given by the expression $n \geq \ln P / \ln(1-r)$.

TABLE 2. Number of Observations Required to Estimate the Response Rate r with Desired Precision (i.e., 95% Confidence Interval of Length 2d)[b]

			Response rate (%)			
d (%)	5	10	20	30	40	50
1	1825	3457	6147	8067	9220	9604
5	73	139	246	323	369	385
10	–	35	62	81	93	97
15	–	–	28	35	41	43
20	–	–	16	21	24	25
25	–	–	–	13	15	16

[b]The sample size n required is given by the expression $n = r(1-r)(1.96/d)^2$.

TABLE 3A. Number of Patients Needed in an Experimental and a Control Group for a Given Probability of Obtaining a Significant Result (One-Sided Test)[a]

Smaller proportion of success (P_1)	Larger minus smaller proportion of success $(P_2 - P_1)$													
	.05	.10	.15	.20	.25	.30	.35	.40	.45	.50	.55	.60	.65	.70
.05	330	105	55	40	33	24	20	17	13	12	10	9	9	8
	460	145	76	48	39	31	25	20	19	15	13	11	10	9
	850	270	140	89	63	37	41	34	21	25	22	18	16	14
.10	540	155	76	47	37	30	23	19	16	13	11	11	9	8
	740	210	105	64	41	38	30	24	20	17	15	12	11	10
	1370	390	195	120	81	60	46	41	35	28	24	20	17	16
.15	710	200	94	56	43	32	26	22	17	15	11	10	9	8
	990	270	130	77	52	43	34	26	23	19	16	12	11	10
	1820	500	240	145	96	69	52	41	37	30	24	22	18	16
.20	860	230	110	63	42	36	27	23	17	15	12	10	9	8
	1190	320	150	88	58	46	36	29	23	18	16	12	11	10
	2190	590	280	160	105	76	57	44	39	30	27	22	18	16
.25	980	260	120	69	45	37	31	23	17	15	12	10	9	..
	1360	360	165	96	63	46	38	30	23	18	16	12	11	..
	2510	660	300	175	115	81	60	46	40	33	27	22	17	..
.30	1080	280	130	73	47	37	31	23	17	15	11	10	..	..
	1500	390	175	100	65	46	38	30	23	18	16	12	..	..
	2760	720	330	185	120	85	61	47	39	32	24	20	..	..
.35	1160	300	135	75	48	37	31	23	17	15	11	..	..	..
	1600	410	185	105	67	46	38	30	23	18	15	..	..	..
	2960	750	340	190	125	85	61	46	39	30	24	..	..	..
.40	1210	310	135	76	48	37	30	23	17	13	..	..	..	..
	1670	420	190	105	67	46	38	30	23	17	..	..	..	..
	3080	780	350	195	125	84	60	44	37	28	..	..	..	..
.45	1230	310	135	75	47	36	26	22	16	..	..	..	..	..
	1710	430	190	105	65	44	36	26	20	..	..	..	..	..
	3140	790	350	190	120	81	57	41	34	.	..	..	..	..
.50	1230	310	135	73	45	36	26	19	..	..	..	..	..	..
	1710	420	185	100	63	41	35	24	..	..	..	..	..	..
	3140	780	340	185	115	76	52	39	..	..	..	..	..	..

Upper figure: $\alpha = .05$, $1-\beta = .80$
Middle figure: $\alpha = .05$, $1-\beta = .90$
Lower figure: $\alpha = .01$, $1-\beta = .95$
[a] Modified from Cochran and Cox (3).
Reproduced from Gehan and Schneiderman (8).

TABLE 3B. Number of Patients Needed in an Experimental and a Control Group for a Given Probability of Obtaining a Significant Result (Two-Sided Test)[a]

Smaller proportion of success (P_1)	Larger minus smaller proportion of success ($P_2 - P_1$)													
	.05	.10	.15	.20	.25	.30	.35	.40	.45	.50	.55	.60	.65	.70
.05	420	130	69	44	36	31	23	20	17	14	13	11	10	8
	570	175	93	59	42	37	31	24	21	18	16	13	12	11
	960	300	155	100	72	54	42	38	33	27	24	20	18	16
.10	680	195	96	59	41	35	29	23	19	17	13	12	11	8
	910	260	130	79	54	40	36	29	24	20	17	16	13	11
	1550	440	220	135	92	68	52	41	38	32	26	23	19	17
.15	910	250	120	71	48	39	31	25	20	17	15	12	11	9
	1220	330	160	95	64	46	40	31	26	22	18	16	13	11
	2060	560	270	160	110	78	59	47	41	35	29	24	21	18
.20	1090	290	135	80	53	42	33	26	22	18	16	12	11	9
	1460	390	185	105	71	51	43	33	28	23	18	16	13	11
	2470	660	310	180	120	86	64	50	44	36	27	24	21	17
.25	1250	330	150	88	57	44	35	28	22	18	16	12	11	..
	1680	440	200	115	77	56	45	36	29	23	18	16	12	..
	2840	740	340	200	130	95	68	52	45	36	29	24	19	..
.30	1380	360	160	93	60	44	36	29	22	18	15	12	..	..
	1840	480	220	125	80	56	46	36	29	23	18	16	..	..
	3120	810	370	210	135	95	69	53	45	36	29	23	..	..
.35	1470	380	170	96	61	44	36	28	22	17	13	..	..	..
	1970	500	225	130	82	57	46	36	28	22	17	..	..	..
	3340	850	380	215	140	96	69	52	44	35	26	..	..	..
.40	1530	390	175	97	61	44	35	26	20	17	..	..	..	..
	2050	520	230	130	82	56	45	32	26	20	..	..	..	..
	3480	880	390	220	140	95	68	50	41	32	..	..	..	..
.45	1560	390	175	96	60	42	33	25	19	..	..	..	..	..
	2100	520	230	130	80	54	43	32	24	..	..	..	..	..
	3550	890	390	215	135	92	64	47	38	..	..	..	..	..
.50	1560	390	170	93	57	40	31	23	..	..	..	..	..	..
	2100	520	225	125	77	51	40	29	..	..	..	..	..	..
	3550	880	380	210	130	86	59	45	..	..	..	..	..	..

Upper figure: $\alpha = .05$, $1-\beta = .80$
Middle figure: $\alpha = .05$, $1-\beta = .90$
Lower figure: $\alpha = .01$, $1-\beta = .95$
[a]Modified from Cochran and Cox (3).
Reproduced from Gehan and Schneiderman (8).

239

to the binomial distribution, the half-width of the
interval can be computed as

$$d = 1.96 \sqrt{\frac{r(1-r)}{n}} .$$

Although most Phase II trials in oncology deal with
the estimation of some proportion (usually a response
rate) this may not always be so. One could also be
interested in estimating some biochemical parameter
or, perhaps, median survival time. Tables of sample
size for estimating the mean of a normal distribution
can be found in Cohen (4); refer to Gross (10) for
sample size calculations related to estimating parameters associated with survival distributions.

Phase III Trials

Statistical power is a critical factor in the Phase
III trial since this type of trial is expected to be
greatly informative with respect to assessing the usefulness of the proposed new therapy. Given below are
methods of sample size calculation for two-arm trials
where the variables may be proportions, means, or median survival times.

Comparing Two Proportions. Tables 3A and 3B (8)
give the number of patients needed in each arm for a
given probability of obtaining a significant result,
as a function of the true proportions in each arm.
These tables were modified from Cochran and Cox (3).

Example 3. If the response rate for treatment A is expected to be about 25% and the rate for treatment B
might be as high as 60%, then with 45 patients per
arm, such a difference can be detected with probability 0.90 (P=.05, two-sided test).

If one wishes to compute power as a function of

sample size (rather than sample size as a function of power) formulas and tables for power can be used (3,6).

Comparing Two Means. If the comparison of treatments is to be based on the difference between two means, then Table 4 (5) can be used, provided the t-test applies. In this situation, the null hypothesis is $H_0:\mu_1=\mu_2$. Let $D=\delta/\sigma$, where $\delta=|\mu_1-\mu_2|$, the true absolute difference between means, and σ denotes the common population standard deviation. In practice, σ is not known and one must choose a value for D. Cohen (4) provides some guidelines for estimating D when previous data are not available. Table 4 gives the number of observations required to carry out a two-sample t-test of level α, power $1-\beta$, with standardized difference D.

Example 4. Patients with cancer of the esophagus are randomized to either oral nutrition or total parenteral nutrition and the mean changes in body weights in each group are to be compared at 6 weeks after start of treatment. A two-sided 5% level t-test is to be used with power 0.90. Based on previous studies, a standardized difference between the means of magnitude D = 0.8 is of clinical importance. Table 4 shows that 34 patients are needed in each arm of the trial.

Multisample Comparisons. Calculation of sample size for the comparison of more than two treatments can often be complicated. Cohen (4) provides tables for the comparison of more than two proportions or more than two means. A "shortcut" method for determining sample size or power in such situations is as follows: If there are k>2 treatments, choose two treatments whose comparison is of the most interest and specify the difference worth detecting. Then, compute sample size or power for this two-sample problem. The computed

TABLE 4. Number of Observations for t-Test of Difference Between Two Means[a]

	Level of *t*-test																			
	0.01					0.02					0.05					0.1				
Single-sided test	α = 0.005					α = 0.01					α = 0.025					α = 0.05				
Double-sided test	α = 0.01					α = 0.02					α = 0.05					α = 0.1				
β =	0.01	0.05	0.1	0.2	0.5	0.01	0.05	0.1	0.2	0.5	0.01	0.05	0.1	0.2	0.5	0.01	0.05	0.1	0.2	0.5
Value of $D=\dfrac{\delta}{\sigma}$																				
0.05																				
0.10																				
0.15																				
0.20																				137
0.25															124					88
0.30										123					87					61
0.35					110					90					64				102	45
0.40					85					70				100	50			108	78	35
0.45				118	68				101	55			105	79	39		108	86	62	28
0.50				96	55			106	82	45		106	86	64	32		88	70	51	23
0.55			101	79	46		106	88	68	38		87	71	53	27	112	73	58	42	19
0.60		101	85	67	39		90	74	58	32	104	74	60	45	23	89	61	49	36	16
0.65		87	73	57	34	104	77	64	49	27	88	63	51	39	20	76	52	42	30	14
0.70	100	75	63	50	29	90	66	55	43	24	76	55	44	34	17	66	45	36	26	12
0.75	88	66	55	44	26	79	58	48	38	21	67	48	39	29	15	57	40	32	23	11
0.80	77	58	49	39	23	70	51	43	33	19	59	42	34	26	14	50	35	28	21	10
0.85	69	51	43	35	21	62	46	38	30	17	52	37	31	23	12	45	31	25	18	9
0.90	62	46	39	31	19	55	41	34	27	15	47	34	27	21	11	40	28	22	16	8
0.95	55	42	35	28	17	50	37	31	24	14	42	30	25	19	10	36	25	20	15	7
1.00	50	38	32	26	15	45	33	28	22	13	38	27	23	17	9	33	23	18	14	7

242

TABLE 4. (continued)

Value of $D = \dfrac{\delta}{\sigma}$																					Value of $D = \dfrac{\delta}{\sigma}$
1·1	42	32	27	22	13	38	28	23	19	11	32	23	19	14	8	27	19	15	12	6	1·1
1·2	36	27	23	18	11	32	24	20	16	9	27	20	16	12	7	23	16	13	10	5	1·2
1·3	31	23	20	16	10	28	21	17	14	8	23	17	14	11	6	20	14	11	9	5	1·3
1·4	27	20	17	14	9	24	18	15	12	8	20	15	12	10	6	17	12	10	8	4	1·4
1·5	24	18	15	13	8	21	16	14	11	7	18	13	11	9	5	15	11	9	7	4	1·5
1·6	21	16	14	11	7	19	14	12	10	6	16	12	10	8	5	14	10	8	6	4	1·6
1·7	19	15	13	10	7	17	13	11	9	6	14	11	9	7	4	12	9	7	6	3	1·7
1·8	17	13	11	10	6	15	12	10	8	5	13	10	8	6	4	11	8	7	5		1·8
1·9	16	12	11	9	6	14	11	9	8	5	12	9	7	6	4	10	7	6	5		1·9
2·0	14	11	10	8	6	13	10	9	7	5	11	8	7	6	4	9	7	6	4		2·0
2·1	13	10	9	8	5	12	9	8	6	5	10	8	6	5	3	8	6	5	4		2·1
2·2	12	10	8	7	5	11	9	7	6	4	9	7	6	5		8	6	5	4		2·2
2·3	11	9	8	7	5	10	8	7	6	4	9	7	6	5		7	5	5	4		2·3
2·4	11	9	8	6	5	10	8	7	6	4	8	6	5	4		7	5	4	4		2·4
2·5	10	8	7	6	4	9	7	6	5	4	8	6	5	4		6	5	4	3		2·5
3·0	8	6	6	5	4	7	6	5	4	3	6	5	4	4		5	4	3			3·0
3·5	6	5	5	4	3	6	5	4	4		5	4	4	3		4	3				3·5
4·0	6	5	4	4		5	4	4	3		4	4	3			4					4·0

[a]Reproduced from Davies, O. L., ed. (5), The Design and Analysis of Industrial Experiments (2nd ed.), Hafner Publishing Company (Longman Group Limited), New York, (1967).

243

sample size per arm can then be used as a guide for
the entire multisample study, although it may not be
equal to the sample size computed by the "correct"
method (i.e., the method that takes into account the
multisample nature of the problem).

   Comparing Survival Distributions. Several publications have dealt with sample size and power calculations pertaining to the comparison of exponential survival distributions (9,13,15). Each reference contains extensive tables and examples of computations.
   Tables 5A and 5B and 6A and 6B (13) can be used to
compute the power of the F-test for comparing two exponential survival distributions in the presence of
right censoring, where the null hypothesis is $H_0:\mu_1=\mu_2$
and μ_1 and μ_2 are the respective median survival
times. Exponential survival is frequently encountered
in practice and can sometimes be justified on theoretical grounds. In all circumstances the use of a
statistical method which is based on a parametric
model should be justified. The use of the tables requires knowledge (or estimation) of the ratio of the
larger to the smaller median survival time (ρ) under
the desired alternative hypothesis and the number of
uncensored observations in each treatment group
(n_1, n_2) at the time of statistical analysis. Tables
5A and 5B correspond to $\rho=1.5$ (a 50% increase in median survival) and Tables 6A and 6B correspond to
$\rho=2.0$ (a doubling of median survival). Tables labeled
"A" are for one-sided tests; tables labeled "B" are
for two-sided tests (P=.05).

Example 5. A randomized trial of two treatments, A and
B, is carried out in order to compare median survival.
One wishes to determine if treatment B can double median survival time. Based on expected patient accrual
and expected median survival in each group (under the
alternative hypothesis of interest) it is estimated
that approximately 50 and 20 patients in each group,

respectively, will be dead (i.e., uncensored) at the time of analysis.

Table 6B (ρ=2.0, two-sided test) shows that with n_1=20 and n_2=50 the power of the F-test, given exponential survival distributions, is 0.76.

For a detailed discussion and more extensive tables, as well as a computational method for estimating the number of uncensored observations, see Lesser and Cento (13).

Note that these power calculations can also be used for comparing time-to-relapse distributions or any distributions where the variable studied is an exponentially distributed waiting time.

General Comments

Questions pertaining to sample size and power are, perhaps, those most frequently asked of the statistician in the designing stages of a clinical trial. Although sample size is an obviously important factor in Phase II and III trials, it is only one factor in determining whether or not a trial should be run. Thus, for example, if a trial of a new and never-before-tested therapy is proposed for a rare type of cancer and few patients are available for such a trial and pooling of patients from other institutions is not feasible, then such a trial should not necessarily be abandoned due to small expected sample size. In such a case, "adequate" sample size may not be attainable but a sample size/power calculation would, at least, provide the clinician and statistician with an idea as to the statistical limitations of such a trial.

TABLES 5A–5B, 6A–6B. Power of F-Test as a Function of Number of Uncensored Observations (n_1, n_2) and Ratio of Medians (ρ)[a]

TABLE 5A.

| | $\rho = 1.5$ | | | | | | | $(P = 0.05$, one-sided test$)$ | | | | | | |

n_1 \ n_2	10	20	30	40	50	60	70	80	90	100	110	120	130	140
10	0.22	0.28	0.31	0.33	0.34	0.35	0.36	0.36	0.37	0.37	0.37	0.38	0.38	0.38
20		0.35	0.41	0.45	0.47	0.49	0.50	0.51	0.52	0.53	0.53	0.54	0.54	0.55
30			0.47	0.52	0.55	0.58	0.60	0.61	0.62	0.63	0.64	0.65	0.66	0.66
40				0.56	0.61	0.64	0.66	0.68	0.69	0.71	0.72	0.73	0.73	0.74
50					0.65	0.68	0.71	0.73	0.75	0.76	0.77	0.78	0.79	0.80
60						0.72	0.74	0.77	0.79	0.80	0.81	0.82	0.83	0.84
70							0.77	0.80	0.82	0.83	0.84	0.85	0.86	0.87
80								0.82	0.84	0.85	0.87	0.88	0.89	0.89
90									0.86	0.87	0.89	0.90	0.90	0.91
100										0.89	0.90	0.91	0.92	0.93
110											0.91	0.92	0.93	0.94
120												0.93	0.94	0.95
130													0.95	0.95
140														0.95

TABLE 5B.

| | $\rho = 1.5$ | | | | | | | $(P = 0.05$, two-sided test$)$ | | | | | | |

n_1 \ n_2	10	20	30	40	50	60	70	80	90	100	110	120	130	140
10	0.14	0.19	0.22	0.23	0.24	0.25	0.26	0.26	0.27	0.27	0.27	0.27	0.28	0.28
20		0.24	0.29	0.33	0.35	0.37	0.39	0.40	0.41	0.41	0.42	0.42	0.43	0.43
30			0.34	0.39	0.43	0.45	0.48	0.49	0.51	0.52	0.53	0.54	0.54	0.55
40				0.44	0.48	0.52	0.54	0.56	0.58	0.60	0.61	0.62	0.63	0.64
50					0.52	0.56	0.59	0.62	0.64	0.66	0.67	0.68	0.70	0.70
60						0.60	0.63	0.66	0.69	0.70	0.72	0.73	0.75	0.76
70							0.67	0.70	0.72	0.74	0.76	0.77	0.79	0.80
80								0.72	0.75	0.77	0.79	0.80	0.82	0.83
90									0.77	0.80	0.81	0.83	0.84	0.85
100										0.82	0.83	0.85	0.86	0.87
110											0.85	0.87	0.88	0.89
120												0.88	0.89	0.90
130													0.90	0.91
140														0.92

TABLE 6A.

							n_2								
n_1		10	20	30	40	50	60	70	80	90	100	110	120	130	140
	10	0.45	0.57	0.62	0.65	0.66	0.67	0.68	0.69	0.69	0.70	0.70	0.70	0.71	0.71
	20		0.70	0.78	0.81	0.84	0.85	0.86	0.87	0.88	0.88	0.89	0.89	0.89	0.90
	30			0.85	0.89	0.91	0.93	0.94	0.94	0.95	0.95	0.96	0.96	0.96	0.96
	40				0.92	0.95	0.96	0.97	0.97	0.98	0.98	0.98	0.98	0.98	0.98
	50					0.96	0.97	0.98	0.98	0.99	0.99	0.99	0.99	0.99	0.99
	60						0.98	0.99	0.99	0.99	0.99	1.00	1.00	1.00	1.00
	70							0.99	0.99	1.00	1.00	1.00	1.00	1.00	1.00
	80								1.00	1.00	1.00	1.00	1.00	1.00	1.00
	90									1.00	1.00	1.00	1.00	1.00	1.00
	100										1.00	1.00	1.00	1.00	1.00
	110											1.00	1.00	1.00	1.00
	120												1.00	1.00	1.00
	130													1.00	1.00
	140														1.00

$\rho = 2.0$ ($P = 0.05$, one-sided test)

TABLE 6B.

							n_2								
n_1		10	20	30	40	50	60	70	80	90	100	110	120	130	140
	10	0.32	0.45	0.51	0.54	0.56	0.57	0.58	0.59	0.60	0.60	0.61	0.61	0.61	0.61
	20		0.58	0.67	0.73	0.76	0.78	0.79	0.81	0.82	0.82	0.83	0.83	0.84	0.84
	30			0.76	0.82	0.85	0.88	0.89	0.90	0.91	0.92	0.92	0.93	0.93	0.93
	40				0.87	0.90	0.92	0.94	0.95	0.95	0.96	0.96	0.97	0.97	0.97
	50					0.93	0.95	0.96	0.97	0.97	0.98	0.98	0.98	0.99	0.99
	60						0.97	0.98	0.98	0.99	0.99	0.99	0.99	0.99	0.99
	70							0.98	0.99	0.99	0.99	0.99	1.00	1.00	1.00
	80								0.99	0.99	1.00	1.00	1.00	1.00	1.00
	90									1.00	1.00	1.00	1.00	1.00	1.00
	100										1.00	1.00	1.00	1.00	1.00
	110											1.00	1.00	1.00	1.00
	120												1.00	1.00	1.00
	130													1.00	1.00
	140														1.00

$\rho = 2.0$ ($P = 0.05$, two-sided test)

[a]Reproduced from Lesser and Cento (13).

247

IMPLEMENTATION OF CLINICAL TRIALS

The Protocol

Once a clinical trial has been designed and all interested parties are in agreement with the details of the design, a protocol is drafted. The protocol should be a detailed specification of how the trial is to be conducted. Table 7 (8) lists the main subject headings that should appear in a well-written protocol. Stanley et al. (18) discuss protocol writing and give an example of a complete protocol.

TABLE 7. Subject Headings for a Protocol[a]

---

1. Introduction and scientific background for the study
2. Objectives of the study
3. Selection of patients
4. Design of the study (including schematic diagram)
5. Treatment programs
6. Procedures in event of response, no response, or toxicity
7. Required clinical and laboratory data
8. Criteria for evaluating the effect of treatment
9. Statistical considerations
10. Informed consent
11. Record forms
12. References
13. Study chairman or responsible investigator and telephone number

---

[a]Reproduced from Gehan and Schneiderman (8), in: Cancer Medicine (2nd ed.), James F. Holland and Emil Frei III, eds., Philadelphia, Lea & Febiger, (1982).

The protocol is then submitted to the hospital's institutional review board (IRB) which is generally made up of hospital staff, including physicians, nurses, scientists, lawyers, clergy, laymen, administrators, and statisticians, who review each new protocol and evaluate it for its ethical and scientific merit. At some institutions the latter consideration may be handled by a separate mechanism. The review board will either approve or disapprove the protocol; frequently, approval is granted conditionally upon the inclusion of certain modifications to the protocol.

Once a protocol has been approved, the statistician needs to assist in finalizing data collection procedures, including coding forms, if appropriate. If the trial is randomized, it is the statistician's responsibility to set up the randomization procedure.

Randomization

Generally, only two procedures for randomizing patients are advised: the "envelope method" and the "telephone method". The envelope method refers to the random placement of treatment assignments in individual, sealed envelopes; when a patient is to be randomized the clinician opens the next envelope in sequence to determine the next patient's treatment assignment. The telephone method involves the clinician placing a telephone call to the statistics or central coordinating office and having the treatment assignment given to him over the phone.

Generally, the latter method is preferable since it is virtually impossible for the clinical staff to avoid even an unconscious bias in carrying out the procedure; it also allows for the randomization results of many protocols to be recorded in one central location. One disadvantage is that the telephone method requires that staff (usually, secretarial) be available to randomize patients and to send out written confirmations of the randomizations. This can be time consuming when there are many protocols running concurrently.

The main advantage of the envelope method is that a patient can be randomized at any time of day or night, as long as there is access to the envelopes. This is especially crucial for protocols involving patients who are apt to be admitted to the hospital on an emergency basis, perhaps at night, and need to be randomized at a time when the statistics department is closed.

Randomization, in itself, does not assure that treatment groups will be comparable with respect to important prognostic factors. In trials of small to moderate sample size one may wish to "stratify" patients on given prognostic factors and then randomize patients separately within each stratum. This will assure that each of those prognostic factors will be represented in (approximately) the same proportion in each treatment arm.

In order to realize approximately equal numbers of patients on each treatment arm, a technique known as "blocking" can be used. In a two-arm trial, randomization in blocks of size n (where n is an even number) will assure that after every n patients have been randomized, n/2 will have been assigned to each of the two arms. A discussion of stratification and blocking techniques can be found in (12).

Follow-up on the Progress of the Trial

After a trial has begun, the statistician should play an important role in monitoring its progress. The statistician and his data management staff should monitor the trial in order to insure the timely entry and correctness of data. Monitoring should also focus on patient accrual, to determine whether the number of patients entering the trial is in agreement with the number expected. When patient accrual appears to be substantially below original expectations, the protocol's principal investigator should be notified and action should be taken, when possible, to increase accrual. If accrual is far above projections, then it may be possible to terminate the trial sooner than anticipated and the principal investigator should also be made aware of this situation.

Major and frequent violations of a protocol (by patient or physician) can have a devastating effect on the outcome of the trial and the conclusions drawn from it. For this reason, a trial must be monitored on a frequent basis so that protocol violations can be identified and, when possible, corrected. Two important types of violations are the deviation from proposed treatment plan (e.g., incorrect drug dose, drug administration on the wrong day) and the failure to carry out scheduled diagnostic tests which are specified in the protocol (e.g., patient does not receive chest X-ray 6 weeks after start of treatment). All violations should be reported to the principal investigator on a regular basis.

Interim reports on the therapeutic results of the trial are also important. Since frequent interim statistical analyses of clinical trial data can affect Type I and II error rates, the statistician should participate in any decisions to prematurely terminate the trial based on interim results.

Finally, the statistician and the clinical staff should regularly meet to review the progress of the protocol. Careful monitoring of the trial in this way will increase the likelihood that the study will serve its intended purpose.

REFERENCES

1. Brown, B. W., and Herson, J. (1980), STPLAN: A Computer System for Performing Statistical Calculations Needed to Plan a Study, The University of Texas System Cancer Center, M. D. Anderson Hospital and Tumor Institute, Houston, Texas.

2. Burdette, W. J., and Gehan, E. A. (1970), _Planning and Analysis of Clinical Studies_, Thomas, Springfield, Illinois.

3. Cochran, W. G., and Cox, G. M. (1957), _Experimental Designs_ (2nd ed.), Wiley, New York.

4. Cohen, J. (1969), _Statistical Power Analysis for the Behavioral Sciences_, Academic Press, New York.

5. Davies, O. L., ed. (1967), _The Design and Analysis of Industrial Experiments_ (2nd ed.), Hafner Publishing Company (Longman Group Limited), New York.

6. Fleiss, J. L. (1981), _Statistical Methods for Rates and Proportions_ (2nd ed.), Wiley, New York.

7. Gehan, E. A. (1961), The determination of the number of patients required in a preliminary and a follow-up trial of a new chemotherapeutic agent, _Journal of Chronic Diseases_ 13: 346–353.

8. Gehan, E. A., and Schneiderman, M. A. (1982), Experimental design of clinical trials, in: Holland, J. F., and Frei, E., III, eds., _Cancer Medicine_ (2nd ed.), Lea and Febinger, Philadelphia, pp. 531–553.

9. George, S. L., and Desu, M. M. (1974), Planning the size and duration of a clinical trial studying the time to some critical event, _Journal of Chronic Diseases_ 27: 15–24.

10. Gross, A. J., and Clark, V. A. (1975), _Survival Distributions: Reliability Applications in the Biomedical Sciences_, Wiley, New York.

11. _Guidelines for the Clinical Evaluation of Antineoplastic Drugs_ (1981), U.S. Department of Health

and Human Services, Food and Drug Administration, Washington, D.C.

12. Lee, E. T. (1980), Statistical Methods for Survival Data Analysis, Lifetime Learning Publications Belmont, California.

13. Lesser, M. L., and Cento, S. J. (1981), Tables of power for the F-test for comparing two exponential survival distributions, Journal of Chronic Diseases 34: 533-544.

14. Miller, A. B., Hoogstraten, B., Staquet, M., and Winkler, A. (1981), Reporting results of cancer treatment, Cancer 47: 207-214.

15. Pasternack, B., and Gilbert, J. P. (1971), Planning the duration of long-term survival time studies designed for accrual by cohorts, Journal of Chronic Diseases 24: 681-700.

16. Peto, R., Pike, M. C., Armitage, P., Breslow, N. E., Cox, D. R., Howard, S. V., Mantel, N., McPherson, K., Peto, J., and Smith, P. G. (1976; 1977), Design and analysis of clinical trials requiring prolonged observation of each patient, British Journal of Cancer, Part I, 34: 585-612; Part II, 35: 1-39.

17. Schoenfeld, D. (1980), Statistical considerations for pilot studies, International Journal of Radiation Oncology, Biology, Physics 6: 371-374.

18. Stanley, K., Stjernsward, J., and Isley, M. (1981), The Conduct of a Cooperative Clinical Trial, Springer-Verlag, Berlin. (Recent Results of Cancer Research Series, No. 77).

CHAPTER 8
Data Management and Quality Control
JUDITH R. O'FALLON

INTRODUCTION

For the purposes of this chapter, data management
is defined as systems for generating, collecting, recording, storing, retrieving, and reporting study data.

It is safe to say that data management has not been
one of the more glamorous topics of discussion among
statisticians, although it is more highly regarded
among computer scientists. To statisticians, however,
it is a topic of vital importance, especially in the
conduct of clinical trials, where the data are produced and recorded over relatively long periods of
time. To use a homely example, data management is
rather like brushing one's teeth: something that everyone must do but hardly ever talks about, and that
is capable of resulting in serious physical and financial damage if not performed regularly and properly.

This work was supported by National Cancer Institute
Grants CA-15083 and CA-25224.

Most of the data management papers in the statistical/computer science literature deal primarily with the special difficulties encountered by coordinating centers for multi-institutional cooperative trials, rarely giving detailed consideration to the difficulties encountered by the participating institutions at the local level. Among those that do contain insights that might be helpful at the local level are references 1-3, 6-8, and 11-14. References 4, 5, and 9 contain detailed discussions of various data management problems encountered in clinical trials conducted by single institutions.

Because this book is designed primarily for statisticians and others with a background in statistics who are currently involved in clinical cancer research but are not part of an established biostatistics group, discussion in this chapter will be restricted to considerations of those aspects of data management pertinent to the conduct of single-institution clinical trials. Some of the questions addressed are: Which data items should be included in the research files? How should data collection forms be designed? How should data collection procedures be developed? What staffing is required for adequate quality control? What materials and procedures should be developed for quality control purposes? How should the data be edited? How should reports be developed? What other procedures are needed for the proper functioning of clinical trials?

The following discussion assumes the existence of a well-developed protocol for each clinical trial. Aspects of study design and development which sometimes arise during design of data management systems will not be discussed in this chapter.

DATA ITEM SELECTION

There are certain practical problems that frequently occur when data items for research files are

not selected wisely. For example, items needed for
reports and analyses are never collected, or after
the study is already under way the investigators discover that desired items cannot be collected for a
variety of reasons, or too many unnecessary items are
requested, with the result that the data collectors
get overwhelmed or the computer file becomes unmanage-
able.

Most of these difficulties arise because investigators responsible for the conduct of the clinical trial
fail to distinguish between data required for reports
and analyses and data required for patient-care purposes. The needs of the study must be balanced
against the existing procedures of the institution,
which presumably have limited flexibility. To minimize mistakes in selecting data elements for research
files, it may be helpful to consider carefully the
following questions:

Which items will really appear in the reports and
analyses planned for the study?

For example, will the data analyses use each individual WBC (white blood cell) count and each individual daily dose of medication or only the WBC nadir and total dose?

In what form is the information most easily and accurately obtained?

For example, date of birth is likely to be more accurately obtained than age, and height and weight
are more easily obtained and verified than is body
surface area (a measure of body size), which must
either be computed from a complex formula involving
height and weight or looked up in tables indexed by
height and weight.

Who must record each item?

Some items, such as tumor measurements, can be obtained and recorded only by the physicians. Others, such as toxicities that occur while the patient is being treated, are best observed and recorded by the treatment nurses or technicians. Certain types of preliminary information (e.g., height and weight) may be routinely obtained and recorded by a receptionist. Research personnel such as data managers can collect and record only information that has previously been recorded somewhere in the medical records by clinical personnel.

To identify the items required for an adequate but economical research data file, investigators should first develop a detailed plan for the study analysis. It often proves useful to write a preliminary version of the manuscript expected to be produced at the end of the study. This approach may also be applied usefully to all anticipated reports and should limit item selection to those needed to generate the reports and analyses. It is essential, however, to identify the secondary data items needed to verify the research items. For example, the WBC nadir can be identified only if all the individual WBC counts taken were recorded somewhere in the patient chart; and tumor response can be assessed only if the tumor measurements at each evaluation were recorded. Those responsible for the conduct of the clinical trial must ensure that these items are also obtained and recorded by the appropriate study personnel. Finally, it should be a matter of regular practice to develop a list of standard research data items that can be used in subsequent studies to help reduce the chances of forgetting key data. It should be updated regularly, preferably after each study analysis.

FORMS DESIGN AND TESTING

Many difficulties can arise when the data collection forms and/or the procedures for using them are not well designed. If the data collectors are uncertain about where responsibility for recording some of the items lies, information can be irretrievably lost or, because of duplicate effort, so contradictory as to be useless. If the forms are confusing or difficult to fill out, there may be errors in the recorded data, time wasted in recording data, or even reluctance to enter patients into the study. If the data collection forms are incompatible with available computer-entry methods, new forms must be designed which are computer compatible, and all the collected data must be transcribed from the old forms to the new ones. When key items are inadvertently omitted from the forms, intended reports and/or analyses cannot be produced. If insufficient space is allotted for recording an item, or a decimal point is omitted, that item may be recorded inconsistently or without sufficient precision.

To minimize mistakes in designing forms and the procedures necessary for their use, consideration should be given to the following questions:

How will the data be entered into the computer?

Will they be keypunched or entered through a CRT (cathode ray tube) terminal? Will they be entered into a computer at all? [There are some experienced researchers trained in precomputer days who find certain manual methods of data analysis (e.g., McBee cards, index cards with data items along the edges) more efficient than computerized methods.]

Which items will be collected by whom? When? Where will they be recorded initially?

Some of the items required for the research file

(e.g., site of primary lesion, histology) may be
routinely collected and recorded in the patient
chart during the normal course of patient-care procedures. Other items (e.g., weight, detailed laboratory values) may be observed during the normal
patient-care procedures but not consistently recorded anywhere as part of the permanent records.
Still other items (e.g., summary measures such as
performance score) may be observed or used only in
research settings.

Are certain types of format more familiar or more comfortable for the data recorders?

The medical personnel responsible for filling out
portions of the research forms may well have decided preferences for certain styles of format (e.g.,
fill-in-the-blanks in a sentence layout) and resistance to other styles (e.g., write the answers
in rows of boxes). Also, if these personnel are
already involved in other clinical trials, they may
have an easier time with the forms for the new
study if they resemble forms they are already using
for the older studies.

What technology, if available, should be used to design the forms?

Some computer systems have packages available for
forms design, and word-processing equipment may
ease and simplify forms development and revision.
However, some users of such sophisticated technologies have found that ease of design may be offset
by a tendency to develop inefficient procedures for
using the technology. In particular, the number of
iterations to make minor revisions may increase
sharply, leading to higher development costs.

There are several key steps in the development of
data collection forms and procedures.

First, investigators should select the computer to
be used to store the data and choose the data-entry
method after giving careful consideration to the cost
and convenience of (a) data entry, (b) managing the
files, and (c) retrieving and analyzing the data.

Note. Unfortunately, it sometimes happens that the
most efficient, cost-effective method of entering and
storing the data produces computer files which are
structurally incompatible with the statistical package
available and/or optimal for use in analyzing the data.   Thus, the two "best" systems cannot be used together without acquiring an interface program to
transform the data from the input files into data
properly structured for the analysis files.

Next, accurate information must be obtained regarding existing patient-care procedures for (a) examining
and treating patients, (b) recording observations in
the patient chart, and (c) transferring key documents
such as X-rays and the patient chart itself to those
who need them (e.g., physicians for dictating corre-
spondence, financial personnel for billing purposes,
research personnel for data collection).
    Then decisions must be made as to which items
should be collected by each study participant.

Note. It is vital to assign to medical personnel only
those items that cannot be collected by anyone else.
In general, physicians and nurses properly consider
their patient-care responsibilities to be more important than their data-collection responsibilities and
will act accordingly whenever the two conflict.   Furthermore, the chance for such conflict increases in
direct proportion to the number of data items assigned
to the medical personnel.

At this point the study coordinators should possess sufficient information to develop realistic procedures for collecting and recording all research data and the supporting data needed for verification of the research data.

Note. Logically, the data collection procedures must be developed before the data collection forms can be designed.

The next step is to design the data collection forms themselves with the following considerations in mind:

1. All items which are the responsibility of one collector should be grouped together as much as possible -- in a separate form, if possible; otherwise, in one or two clearly identifiable sections (perhaps shaded in a distinctive color) of a common form.
2. The format with which a given data collector must work should be as "comfortable" as possible.
3. All data items required for the study should be located somewhere on the forms.
4. The keys to all required codes should be located as conveniently as possible on the set of forms.
5. The research data items should be entered into the computer directly from the forms; it should not be necessary to copy them onto a second set of forms for computer entry purposes.

Once designed, the forms should be checked by knowledgeable computer personnel (e.g., programmer, keypuncher) for computer compatibility. Finally, both forms and procedures should be tested on several patients to discover any shortcomings, then revised as appropriate. If both forms and procedures are

subjected to adequate testing and review before mass
production, there will be relatively few problems in
that area of the study.

Note. Some medical researchers have found it useful
to develop dual-purpose forms for both patient-care
and research purposes. In general, such forms feature: structured format to minimize missing data and
to permit computer entry directly from the document;
color coding to highlight items for which physicians
have primary data collection responsibility; and data
items that have proved useful in several types of
studies. Illustrations of the dual-purpose forms used
at one medical center are given in reference 10.

DATA COLLECTION: PERSONNEL, MATERIALS, PROCEDURES

Once the study coordinators have agreed on data
collection forms and procedures, they must deal with
the larger issues of study conduct and data generation, which greatly influence the quality and quantity
of research data collected. If procedures for identifying appropriate study candidates and for managing
study patients, as well as for collecting data, are
not properly designed or monitored, problems can develop which severely damage the integrity of the
study.

For example, failure to identify eligible study
patients can result in reduced accrual and possibly
unrecognized biases. On the other hand, ineligible
patient entries constitute a waste of resources. Appointment scheduling violations often lead to damaged
evaluation information, and violations in the scheduling of laboratory or radiologic examinations can reduce the evaluability of patients. Failure to make a
required observation or failure to record a required
observation may damage patient evaluability. Failure
to administer treatments according to protocol

specifications may result in severe waste of resources. Failure to conduct off-study follow-up properly
can lead to missing or incorrect evaluation information and possibly even to loss of patients to further
follow-up.

Many of these problems can be minimized -- perhaps
even eliminated altogether -- by a careful choice of
quality control personnel, procedures, and materials.

Personnel

In clinical trials, useful quality control personnel are study assistants, appointment secretaries, and
(eventually) senior data managers.

Study assistants are research personnel who assist
the medical personnel in the conduct of clinical trials in much the same way as laboratory technicians
assist laboratory researchers. Some of the functions
they perform effectively are to:

1. Help set up materials for randomization, quality
   control, and the scheduling of appointments and
   laboratory/radiologic tests.
2. Help identify eligible study candidates.
3. Help physicians with the materials and procedures required to enter individual patients into
   suitable studies.
4. Schedule appointments and associated tests according to protocol specifications.
5. Remind medical personnel to make and record certain observations required by protocol.
6. Collect and record study data.
7. Edit the research forms.
8. Enter the data into the computer (especially via
   CRT terminals).
9. Collect follow-up data.
10. Help with the conduct of quality control studies.
11. Help with the generation of reports and analyses.

Appointment secretaries are secretaries trained to schedule patients' appointments with physicians and to order the appropriate laboratory/radiologic tests associated with each appointment according to protocol specifications.

Senior data managers are technical supervisors with responsibility to train and oversee the performance of the study assistants, improve systems and procedures for data collection, and monitor the quality of the research data.

In hiring for quality control positions, it is often a successful strategy to recruit from among current employees of the medical center and to train them for the positions. Familiarity with the institution is often more of an asset than formal qualifications for the job. People who have the innate ability to do a job but lack the formal qualifications are usually more satisfied with the position for a longer period of time than is someone who comes to the position fully qualified.

Essential characteristics to look for in potential candidates for quality control positions are meticulous attention to detail and the abilities to think logically, act independently, and work confidently in a quasi-advisory role with medical personnel. Study assistants should have at least a high school education. Senior data managers should combine these qualities with an aptitude for systems development, proven personnel skills, extensive experience as a study assistant, and a strong desire for continuing education.

For groups that are just beginning to conduct clinical trials, the various phases of quality control staffing can be identified according to 4 levels:

Level 1. Acquire one part-time study assistant with remaining duties as oncology nurse, medical secretary, receptionist, tumor registrar, laboratory technician, or clerk.

Level 2. Expand duties to full-time position or

hire a full-time study assistant.

Level 3. Hire additional study assistants, and ap-
point an experienced one as group leader. Possibly
encourage specialization among the study assistants
(e.g., one having primary responsibility for lung and
brain studies, another for breast and sarcoma studies).

Level 4. Develop a senior data manager from the
group of study assistants.

The amount of work that a single study assistant
can reasonably be expected to handle properly is obviously a function of a number of factors: the number
of different studies assigned, the number of patients
in those studies, the speed with which the data are
accrued, and the amount of time spent assisting medical personnel with aspects of study management. Consequently, it is difficult to give even reasonably
precise estimates of an appropriate study assistant
work load. However, the following rules of thumb are
based on experience with study assistants at one medical center where there are separate secretaries to
handle the appointments:

Study assistants who spend 50% of the time recording and editing data can usually manage the data
for 5-10 studies having a total of 50-125 active
patients. Study assistants who spend full time recording and editing data can usually manage 10-20
studies having a total of 100-200 active patients.

Materials

It has often proved helpful to develop special materials to aid the medical personnel in the conduct
of the study.
Perhaps the single most useful quality control document is the protocol abstract (Figure 1). This

3/6/79
Rev. 1/22/80

ONCOLOGY RECORD – PROTOCOL DATA
MAYO CLINIC, ROCHESTER, MINNESOTA

REG NO _ _ _ _ _

NAME _ _ _ _ _

P.S. _ _ _ _

PROTOCOL NUMBER 7 8 — 7 0 — 0 3

NAME OF PROTOCOL PALA and AMSA in Advanced Malignant Melanoma

DATE OF RANDOMIZATION: ___ MO ___ DAY ___ YR

TREATMENT ASSIGNED

A. PALA
B. AMSA

DRUG ABBREVIATION

PALA = N-(phospho-noacetyl)-L-aspartate

AMSA = 4'-(9-acridinylamino) methanesulfon -m-aniside

STRATIFICATION FACTORS	1	2
Performance Score	0-1	2-3
Dominant Disease	Visceral	Non-Visceral
Metastatic Disease	Meas.	Eval.
Prior Chemo.	Yes	No

DESCRIPTIVE FACTORS

Prior Rx	Prior PALA	Prior AMSA

RANDOMIZATION SCHEMA

Prior AMSA or WBC ≤ 4,100 or PLT ≤ 130,000 ——→ A = PALA

Prior PALA ——————→ B = AMSA

All Other ——→ R ——→ A —⟨ Prog ——→ B
⟨ REGR ——→ Cont. Rx —⟨ Prog ——→ OFF STUDY
B ⟨ Prog ——→ A

ELIGIBILITY CRITERIA

PRO:
Histologic Proof
Meas. or Eval. Mets.
Incurable by Surgery
Informed Consent
P.S. 1-3

CON:
PALA: Creat. >2.0 or Direct Bilirubin↑
AMSA: WBC ≤ 4100 and/or PLT ≤ 130,000
Creat. ≥ 2.0 or Direct Bilirubin↑
P.S. of 4
Prior Rx with PALA or AMSA
Prior Chemo ≤ 3 wks.
6 wks. for Nitrosourea or Mito-c
Major Surgery ≤ 3 wks.
Active Uncont. Infect.
Prior R∅ to 15% of Bone Marrow ≤ 4 wks.

Tests/Procedures	Prior to Initial or Subseq. Rx	Wkly During Interval Between Rx
History, Exam, Tumor Measurements	X	
Hematology WBC	X	X (AMSA)
PLT	X	X (Only)
HGB	X	
Chemistry Group	X	
Chest X-ray	X	
Other tests as Indicated	X	

266

Dosage and Schedule

Regimen	Agent	Days Admin.	Dosage & Route	Approx. Eval. & ReRx Intervals from Day 1 Rx
A	PALA	1	5 gm/m², IV over 90 min.	q. 3 wks.
B	AMSA	1	See 7.2, IV over 60 min. in 500 ml 5% D/W	q. 4 wks.

Initial AMSA Dosage

Condition	Initial AMSA Dose Level
P.S. = 0-1	120 mg/m²/d
P.S. = 2-3	90 mg/m²/d
Prior chemo. & whole abdomen or pelvic R8 regardless of P.S.	90 mg/m²/d
SGOT >60	75 mg/m²/d
Creatinine 1.6-1.9	↓50%

Anticipated Toxicities

Nausea
Vomiting
Diarrhea
Mouth Soreness
Hair Loss
Depression of Blood Counts
Fever
Skin Rashes
Allergic Reactions
Impairment of Liver or Nerve Function

Dosage Adjustments Based on Clinical and Laboratory Observation

Based on Interval Toxicity	Agent	Dosage Change
WBC nadir ≥ 3500 and/or PLT nadir ≥ 100,000	AMSA	↑10%
WBC nadir 1500-2000 and/or PLT nadir 50,000-75,000	AMSA	↓25%
WBC nadir ≤ 1500 and/or PLT nadir ≤ 50,000	AMSA	↓50%
Gastrointestinal - Stomatitis, Diarrhea, Proctitis		
Mild	PALA	Zero
Moderate	PALA	↓33%
Severe	PALA	↓67%
Dermatitis		
Mild	PALA	Zero
Moderate	PALA	↓33%
Severe	PALA	↓67%
At Scheduled Re-Treatment		
WBC ≤ 3500 and/or PLT ≤ 100,000	AMSA	Delay Rx until WBC ≥ 3500 & PLT ≥ 100,000 & ↓Dose 20%
SGOT >60	AMSA	75 mg/m²/d
GI and/or Dermatologic	PALA	Delay Rx until toxicity has abated & ↓20%
Creatinine		
If initial dose was decreased because Creat. > 1.5 and no toxicity observed	PALA	↑50% (once)
Creatinine 1.6-1.9	PALA	↓50%
Creatinine ≥ 2.0	PALA	STOP

Figure 1. The protocol abstract that is inserted into the medical record of each patient in the study.

267

document, designed to be inserted into the patient-
care record of every patient in the study for ready
reference, summarizes virtually all the information
contained in the protocol which is needed for patient
management purposes. Specifically, in a standardized,
structured format are given the eligibility criteria,
study treatments, covariates (including stratification
factors) expected to be involved in the analysis, randomization schema, tests and procedures required by
protocol at each of the patient evaluations, treatment
details, and anticipated toxicities. Before a clinical trial opens, a protocol abstract is prepared for
it, duplicated in quantities appropriate to the expected size of the study, and filed with the consent
forms. Then whenever a patient signs the consent
form, a copy of the protocol abstract is inserted into
the patient-care chart, where it is available for
ready reference to all medical personnel dealing with
the patient during the course of the study.

It has also proved useful to develop a booklet of
protocol abstracts, which can be carried in the physician's jacket pocket for reference in dealing with
potential candidates for studies. In a small ring-
binder are placed abbreviated (containing only information required to answer the patient's questions regarding the study), reduced copies of the protocol
abstracts for those studies which are open for patient
accrual. Whenever a potential study candidate is encountered, the physician uses the protocol abstract
booklet to help identify an appropriate study for the
candidate and to explain the relevant details of the
study to the patient.

Procedures

There are several procedures which have proved useful in improving the conduct of clinical trials.

To improve patient accrual and help identify biases
in sample selection, it may be beneficial to monitor
the surgical listings and/or pathology reports

generated at the medical center each day to identify
possible candidates for clinical trials. If possible,
try to identify the reasons why entry into study
failed to occur (e.g., no study for which patient was
fully eligible, patient refused, patient was never ap-
proached concerning study treatment). Another approach is to keep logbooks of the patients seen by
the medical personnel participating in the studies and
to note the eventual disposition of each.

To reduce the number of ineligible patient entries,
two different procedures have been used successfully.
If randomization is performed by phone at a central
location, the randomization assistant checks the eligibility requirements one-by-one before entering the
patient into the study and performing the randomization. Otherwise, the attending physician or study
assistant is required to fill out an eligibility
checklist to be filed with the on-study data forms.

To help identify potential biases introduced by
data changes, a good procedure is to require that all
corrections to the research forms be made by crossing
out (not erasing) the "wrong" item and inserting the
"right" information nearby. Also, a log of the reasons for all changes should be kept.

Similarly, to help identify potential biases introduced by patient "withdrawal" or "cancellation," require that all changes to the randomization books be
made by crossing out (not erasing) the original randomization information and that a log of the reasons
for each elimination be kept.

DATA EDITING PROCEDURES

It is essential that the information recorded on
the research forms be verified by extensive cross-
checking with the records in the patient chart. Study
assistants usually do such checking conscientiously
and thoroughly, catching inconsistencies that are often missed by medical personnel, who tend to "read

into" the recorded data information they expect to
see. However, it is very helpful to have physicians
review the research forms promptly, too, as they are
frequently able to identify medical inconsistencies,
missing information, and treatment/evaluation violations recorded on the forms. When statisticians also
review the forms, especially those for the first few
patients entered into the study, most misunderstand-
ings about the importance and coding of data items
can be caught early and corrected before substantial
damage to the research file occurs. Thus, it is helpful to have clerical personnel, physicians, and statisticians involved in the manual editing of the data,
especially in the early stages.

While a set of forms is being edited, it is useful
to check off the principal items and to record all major and selected minor violations on a special form
designed for this purpose. At the same time it is
usually convenient to code all items that require coding for computer entry. For quality control purposes,
it is best that such coding be assigned to trained
personnel (e.g., study assistants) rather than to the
medical personnel responsible for collecting the raw
data.

Valuable data editing can be accomplished during
computer entry. If the data are entered into the computer via CRT terminals, it is usually easy to apply
various range and logic checks to the individual items
as they are keyed in. However, such checks will permit many kinds of keying errors (e.g., transposing two
digits, hitting a key once too often) to pass undetected if the resultant error falls within the limits
of the checks. If the data are to be keypunched, keying errors of all types will be virtually eliminated
if the keypunching system incorporates procedures for
data verification (e.g., the data are keypunched independently by two operators and compared for discrepancies). Range and logic checks, however, must be
incorporated into an edit/update program which is run
separately.

For sets of studies or for individual studies of
sufficient size, it is sometimes beneficial to develop
programs for editing the data by computer. Such computerized data-edit programs, if well designed, may
be helpful in managing large or complex data sets because they can automatically check computations
(e.g., body surface area, total dose level), the consistency of interrelated items entered into the file
at different times (e.g., values of the tumor response
variable as a function of time), and the consistency
of items with complex interrelationships (e.g., the
decision to remove a patient from study because of
severe toxicity). Such computerized data-edit programs can reduce the amount of manual editing required
and so can be invaluable when there is a shortage of
clerical personnel. The drawback, unfortunately, is
that they are difficult and expensive to develop.

MONITORING DATA QUALITY

Throughout the conduct of a clinical trial, the
data in the research files should be monitored regularly. One particularly cost-effective method of doing so is to develop computerized listings of key data
items for the study and then to generate them regularly (e.g., monthly, quarterly) depending on the rate
of patient and/or data accrual. Such a list typically
includes patient identification information, treatment
arm, dates of major events (beginning and end of
treatment, progression, death), and patient condition
at each evaluation (tumor response, performance status, hematologic nadirs, and toxicity information).
If there is no computerized data-edit program
available, these listings should be examined regularly
by the study assistant, statistician, and senior data
manager (if there is one) to identify errors, missing
values, and inconsistencies in the data (e.g., highly
unlikely patterns of tumor response in the data for a
single patient collected over time). If there is a

computerized data-edit program available, the listings
can be used as convenient reference materials to identify data problems flagged by the edit program with
error messages (which are, unfortunately, often difficult to interpret). Whether or not there is a computerized data-edit program, these listings serve a major
need for a concise, compact reference that summarizes
all major data items for all study patients. Furthermore, such listings have the potential to alert investigators to developing problems that can be missed
in the periodic processes of data editing, computer
entry, and running of the computerized data-edit program, especially if the latter is done on subsets of
the data.

In addition to regular monitoring of key listings,
it is important to conduct quality assessment studies
occasionally to compare, for random samples of study
patients, the data in the computer files with the data
in the original documents (e.g., the patient chart)
and on the research forms. The study assistant for
the study can usually do the detailed checking under
the direction of the senior data manager or the statistician responsible for the study.

Another convenient method of quality assessment is
to examine the routine reports, which are usually
generated on a regular basis for reporting to coinves-
tigators and funding sources. A careful examination
of the data summaries constituting the report can frequently suggest the existence of subtle data problems
previously undetected. For example, an unexpectedly
high frequency in the use of a legitimate but rarely
used code can lead to the discovery of a misunder-
standing on the part of the coder or the medical personnel responsible for collecting the raw data.

Another equally convenient method of quality monitoring is to use the information acquired during the
data cleanup prior to interim analyses to assess the
quality of the data collection systems, recording procedures, and personnel performance.

It can be a most enlightening experience for a

statistician to visit the areas where patients involved in a clinical trial are treated and evaluated,
where the raw data are recorded, and where the data
are coded and edited. Observing the actual operation
of the systems that produce the research data may lead
to ways to improve them and to assess the dependabili-
ty of certain data items in the research file.

Finally, it can be helpful to invite outside experts to observe and evaluate the data management system. Such experts can often see problems of which the
study participants were completely unaware.

DEVELOPMENT OF REPORTS

Many difficulties can arise during the development
of reports for a single clinical trial, depending on
the personalities of the investigators involved. Such
difficulties can be greatly compounded when reports
must be developed for sets of related clinical trials
conducted by multiple investigators, often representing several disciplines. When several experienced
investigators are involved in multiple trials, two
especially costly problems often arise: Either each
investigator wants a different format for virtually
identical content, or they request minor format changes frequently, usually every time the reports are run.
In both cases, such heavy demands are made on the programming staff that either the programmers are tied
up with reports development, with little time left for
other programming duties, or additional programmers
must be hired and development costs soar.

In developing reports for clinical trials, individually or in sets, investigators should keep the following considerations in mind:

1. What are the reporting requirements of the funding source?
2. What information should be shared with all participants in the study, and what should be given

only to the small group of investigators who are
responsible for the practical and ethical conduct of the study?
3. What is the optimal strategy for data retrieval
in the given system of hardware and software?
In particular, how much programmer time will be
required to write the reports in each of the
available programming languages? What personnel
will be required to run the reports programs in
each of the available systems? What is the expected cost of producing the reports in each of
the systems? How often must the reports be generated? How many revisions can reasonably be
expected?

To minimize the costs and headaches encountered in
developing reports for clinical trials, certain strategies might be helpful:

1. Develop an all-purpose general report containing
all the information to be shared with a general
audience.
2. Develop separate special reports containing all
additional information to be shared with special
audiences (e.g., the funding source or the committee responsible for overseeing the conduct of
the study).
3. Persuade investigators to accept report formats
readily produced with existing software rather
than special formats requiring considerable programmer effort to produce.
4. Write initial drafts and revisions of reports in
the languages of existing software packages
(e.g., SAS, SPSS) rather than in a more efficient but complex programming language (e.g.,
PL/1).
5. Try to develop standardized report formats for
sets of similar studies which can be applied to
new studies more easily and can eventually be

programmed in a more complex language for increased running efficiency.

OTHER PROCEDURES ASSOCIATED WITH DATA MANAGEMENT

There are several additional procedures that must be developed for most clinical trials. Among the most important are, of course, the randomization procedures, but since these procedures are discussed in detail in the chapter on design and implementation of clinical trials (Chapter 7) they will be omitted here.

Procedures for Safety Monitoring

Notification procedures should be devised to guide the actions of medical personnel whenever they encounter a suspected case of lethal or life-threatening toxicity. Furthermore, study assistants should be trained to look for clues to such toxicities, and notification procedures should be developed for them. All participants in the study should be reminded periodically of the details of the notification procedures, as they tend to forget them because they are used so rarely.

Procedures for Breaking Codes in Blinded Studies

Before the study opens, basic guidelines regarding what constitutes "sufficient" reason for revealing a treatment assignment to blinded study participants should be formulated and the chain of authority regarding decisions to break codes should be agreed on.

Procedures for Obtaining Off-Study Follow-Up Information

Early in the study, decisions must be made concerning the amount of follow-up information to collect on a regular basis after the patients have gone "off-study" (i.e., are no longer being treated or evaluated according to the protocol for the study). For example, do the investigators wish to collect detailed information regarding the subsequent stages of disease experienced by each patient? Long-term toxicities? Subsequent treatment? Quality of life measures? Or will they be satisfied to know only whether the patient is alive or dead? Obviously, such decisions must take into consideration the budget and the availability of personnel to conduct the necessary follow-up. (Of course, policies regarding off-study follow-up ought to be spelled out in the protocol -- but often they are not.)

Once these policy decisions have been made, procedures must be developed to collect the desired data. In particular, materials for conducting follow-up (e.g., letters, questionnaires, texts of phone communications) should be developed and approved. Furthermore, procedures must be developed to protect off-study patients from being contacted too frequently (it can be annoying to the patient and embarrassing to the investigator if, for example, the patient is sent a follow-up form letter just a few days after having had a long talk with the investigator on the phone). Because such procedures must govern the actions of all study participants, they should be clearly communicated to all involved in the study.

Procedures for Training Study Personnel

Responsibility for training study personnel should be assigned at the beginning of the project. Manuals and other training materials should be developed as rapidly as possible, not only to improve the efficiency of training new personnel, but also to serve as reference materials and documentation of procedures for experienced personnel. It is helpful if training procedures include periodic refresher sessions for experienced personnel, particularly if there are several studies being conducted simultaneously or the conduct of a single study requires several years for completion.

Communication Procedures

Decisions regarding methods of communication to be used among the study participants should be made before the study opens. For example, will there be regularly scheduled meetings to discuss the conduct of the study? Regularly scheduled conference calls? Newsletters? How often should they take place? Once these decisions have been made and commitments to honor these communication responsibilities have been obtained from all major study participants, responsibility for organizing and publicizing the communication sessions should be clearly allocated.

DISCUSSION

Designing an adequate data management and quality control system for clinical trials is a complex and time-consuming task that involves making decisions about data elements to be included in the research file, hardware and software to be used to manage the data, procedures to be used for collecting data and monitoring data quality, design of data collection forms and reports, and personnel to be assigned responsibility for data collection and quality control. As such, it must be regarded as a major project in its own right.

To design a good data management system requires considerable knowledge about (a) existing systems and procedures for treating patients, recording medical observations, and transferring key medical documents, (b) reporting requirements, (c) appropriate analyses, (d) available computer resources, (e) available personnel, and (f) human relations. Consequently, it is probably optimal to assign the responsibility to a multidisciplinary team consisting of a statistician,

a programmer, a systems analyst, and, if possible, a
computer-oriented physician -- at least one of whom is
wise in the ways of human nature.

A well-designed, smoothly functioning data management and quality control system pays dividends in max-
imizing the amount of usable data available for analysis, reducing stress on data collection and analysis
personnel, and increasing the speed and efficiency of
generating reports and analyses. Such a system is
well worth the professional effort required initially
to develop it.

REFERENCES

1. Bonadonna, G., and Valagussa, P. (1978), The lo-
   gistics of clinical trials, Biomedicine 28: 43-48.

2. Breslow, N. E. (1978), Perspectives on the statistician's role in cooperative clinical research,
   Cancer 41: 326-332.

3. Evans, J. T. (1979), Internal monitoring: Patient
   study management at the clinic, Clinical Pharmacology and Therapeutics 25: 712-716.

4. Hopwood, M. D., Mabry, J. C., and Sibley, W. L.
   (1980), A First-Order Characterization of Clinical
   Trials, Rand, Santa Monica, California.

5. Hopwood, M. D., Mabry, J. C., and Sibley, W. L.
   (1980), The Role of General Clinical Research Centers in Clinical Trials: A Characterization with
   Recommendations, Rand, Santa Monica, California.

6. Karrison, T. (1981), Data editing in a clinical
   trial, Controlled Clinical Trials 2: 15-29.

7. Knatterud, G. L. (1981), Methods of quality
   control and of continuous audit procedures for

controlled clnical trials, Controlled Clinical
Trials 1: 327-332.

8. Kronmal, R. A., David, K., Fisher, L. D.,
   Jones, R. A., and Gillespie, M. (1978), Data management for a large collaborative clinical trial
   (CASS: Coronary artery surgery study), Computers
   and Biomedical Research 11: 553-566.

9. MacLachlan, M. (1979), Never Say Lost! National
   Surgical Adjuvant Project for Breast and Bowel
   Cancer, Pittsburgh.

10. O'Fallon, J. R., Golenzer, H. J., Taylor, W. F.,
    Hu, T., Offord, J. R., Bill, J., and Moertel, C. G.
    (1980), Data quality control for a data management
    system for multiple clinical trials, ASA 1980 Pro-
    ceedings of Statistical Computing Section, 66-75.

11. Peto, R. (1978), Clinical trial methodology, Bio-
    medicine 28: 24-36.

12. Stanley, K., Stjernsward, J., Isley, M. (1981),
    The Conduct of a Cooperative Clinical Trial,
    Springer-Verlag, Berlin. (Recent Results of Can-
    cer Research Series, No. 77).

13. Staquet, M., Sylvester, R., Machin, D.,
    van Glabbeke, M., de Grauwe, G., Wennerholm, A.,
    Tyrrell, J., Renard, J., de Pauw, M.,
    Eeckhoudt, D., Tyrrell, J., and Tagnon, H. J.
    (1977), The E.O.R.T.C. data center, European Jour-
    nal of Cancer 13: 1455-1459.

14. Williams, O. D. (1979), A framework for the quali-
    ty assurance of clinical data, Clinical Pharmacol-
    ogy and Therapeutics 25: 700-702.

CHAPTER 9

Statistical Software: Data Base Management, Statistical Packages, and Graphics

DAVID W. BRAUN, Jr.

INTRODUCTION

Modern statistical analysis would be most difficult without the use of computers. Advances in computing have made it possible to implement statistical procedures that were formerly not practical on computational grounds. But every advance in computing has also made it possible to collect and process ever more complex data sets. These large and complex data sets require powerful statistical procedures for appropriate analysis.

This chapter presents a discussion of the computer software available for managing data, for statistical analysis, and for graphical analysis and presentation. The intent is to provide the information necessary for a statistician to gain access to the computational tools he needs to analyze the complex data sets with which he is faced. With a small budget, a statistician can do quite a bit of data management, statisti-

This work was supported by National Cancer Institute Grant CA-08748.

cal analysis, and graphical presentation by himself.
This chapter is not a comparison of software, but
rather a presentation of a range of software and how
it may be used.

USING A COMPUTER SYSTEM

For a statistician who is involved in biomedical
research, but is not part of an established biostatistics group, there are 3 main areas that must be budg-
eted for. The first is for computer access (computer
time). It is strongly recommended that one begin with
a time-sharing account at a local university. At an
academic computing facility, computer time is relatively cheap compared with commercial time-sharing
rates, there is a wide range of software available,
and perhaps most importantly, there is help available
from graduate students, faculty members, and other
users. Computer time is typically sold by the hour;
the cost can range anywhere from $250 to $1000 per
hour. An hour of computer time yields a lot of computation. It would be unusual if a statistician involved in clinical trials, for example, used more than
10 hours of computer time in a year.
Many organizations such as hospitals have a computer that is used mainly for financial problems, such as
payroll and patient accounts. A statistician at such
an organization would be well advised to still consider time-sharing at an academic computing facility. A
business systems computer facility seldom has much in
the way of statistical or mathematical software, and
help is often not available to the extent common at
a university.

Equipment

To connect to an outside computer, a terminal and
an acoustic coupler are needed. This is the second
budget item. The first terminal obtained by a

statistics group should probably be a printing terminal; this type of terminal provides a paper record of
all time-sharing transactions. Subsequent terminals
can be of the screen type; they are smaller, quieter,
and less expensive. An acoustic coupler provides a
means of connecting a terminal to a standard telephone, and thus to the computer. Usually, acoustic
couplers transfer data at a rate of 300 baud (approximately 30 characters per second). More expensive
acoustic couplers can transfer data at 1200 baud. The
only special supplies needed are paper and ribbons
for the printing terminals.

It would seem at first that outright purchase of
terminals is the least expensive approach, but a maintenance contract must be purchased at the same time,
and owning the terminals is very inflexible. Leasing
terminals is more expensive, but maintenance is included in the cost of the lease. At the end of a
lease period, one can change terminals and/or leasors,
and one can usually upgrade a terminal midlease with
no penalty.

As a guide to costs, a DEC LA120 printing terminal
can be purchased for $2500, or leased for $100 per
month. A Lear Siegler ADM screen terminal can be
purchased for $600 or leased for $50 per month.
Acoustic couplers rarely break down and so should be
purchased; they cost between $300 (300 baud) and $700
(1200 baud). One should also inquire about installa-
tion charges when buying or leasing a terminal.

Data Entry

The cost of data entry into the chosen computer
system is the final major item of cost for the statistician. The simplest approach is direct entry through
the keyboard of the terminal, but for large data sets
this approach is not practical. A common solution is
to copy the data onto forms that are suitable for keypunching. Commercial keypunching services will transfer the data from forms to cards or magnetic tape for

between 15 and 40 cents per card (80 characters of data). Less common approaches are direct key-to-disk and mark-sensitive forms. Data entry can be a major expense, but it is a cost that can often be billed separately to the clinical investigator for whom the statistical analysis is being performed.

Time-Sharing Activities

In practice, performing any sort of procedure using a statistical software package through a time-sharing account involves bringing together many parts. Having arranged for a time-sharing account and installed a terminal and an acoustic coupler, one must become familiar with the procedures of the computing facility. This involves learning the job control language (JCL) needed to run a procedure, arranging to have data on cards or tape entered into the computer, obtaining the telephone numbers for computer access, recorded messages, and telephone consultants, and finding out how to retrieve output and plots. It is necessary to become an expert in the use of a text editor, which is needed to create, save, and modify a user job. Finally, one needs to become even more of an expert in the chosen statistical package: How does one perform a logistic regression, for example; what options are there to control the analysis and control the output, and how are missing values to be handled? This last point is crucial. It is axiomatic that medical data sets always have missing data, so the chosen statistical package/procedure must be able to handle missing values.

The steps in a computer-based analysis are as follows: The data should be collected in a rectangular form, so that for each patient there is a fixed set of values such as survival time, hematology and biochemistry values, and treatment. The data are entered into a computer, either directly from the keyboard if the data set is small, or from punched cards or magnetic tape if the data set is large. The text editor

is used to build the job, including job control language and the command language of the statistical
package. The job is then submitted to run against
the data. The output of the job is retrieved at the
terminal if it is short, or from the output room of
the academic computing center if it is long. Finally,
the results should be carefully examined to ensure
that the analysis that was anticipated is in fact the
analysis that was performed, in other words, that
there are no gross or subtle bugs (errors) in the
program. Although it may seem like a lot of steps,
it all becomes quite routine after a few weeks.

STATISTICAL PACKAGES

Statistical software packages have many advantages
over other approaches to statistical analysis. There
are many data management and statistical features included in these packages, and they are very widely
used, which tends to eliminate bugs. They are well
supported by the organizations that developed them,
with ample documentation in user's manuals. In addition, many of the package implementors will provide
onsite training sessions, and it is very easy to find
experienced users.

It is much less costly to use the statistical packages than to embark on a large-scale programming effort. There is a good analogy: When an investigator
presents a problem and it is not immediately obvious
that the statistical procedures right at hand apply,
there is a temptation for the statistician to start
developing new methodology at his desk. The efficient
statistician does a literature search first; if nothing appropriate is found, the literature search is expanded to encompass related fields such as psychiatry
and reliability. It is the same for statistical software. If a needed procedure does not seem to be
available, the efficient computer user will search for
software, or will try to "fool" an existing package

into performing the required calculations. It is very
wasteful to reprogram what already exists.

One of the overhead costs that one must pay when
using a statistical package is the need to define
variables, name the variables, label the variables,
label the values of those variables, set valid ranges,
and define missing values. However, this file setup
is only done once, since one can form what is typically called a "save file" or a "working file." One
of the nice features of some of these packages is that
once a save file has been created by one package,
another package can work directly on that save file.
It should be noted that when using a time-sharing system, the cost of these packages is already figured into the time charge; there is never a separate charge
for using specific software.

For anyone who has been using one of these packages, for anyone who is an expert, it is well worthwhile
to periodically reread the user's manual. There are
often features and options that do not seem useful at
first, and so one forgets about them, but as one gains
experience with collaborative research it is possible
to really put these powerful statistical packages to
work.

What follows are some general remarks about a number of software packages. Further details can be
found at the end of the chapter (Appendices 1-10),
including the address and telephone number of each
vendor.

SAS (see Appendix 1)

SAS (Statistical Analysis System) is easily the
favorite of statisticians, with more than 2500 instal-
lations. One disadvantage of SAS is that it is only
available on IBM 360/370 equipment or other manufac-
turer's compatible equipment. One of the best features of SAS is that intermediate results are available for further analysis. For example, having performed a regression one can save the residuals, and

treat the residuals as data in a subsequent analysis. This is difficult or impossible to do using some of the other packages.

It should be noted that recently SAS has been discovered by the business community, or perhaps SAS has discovered that there is a very large market in the business community. It is being advertised less as a statistical package and more as a data management and report writing tool. In time, SAS will be proportionally less of a statistical package and more of a general purpose package.

SPSS (see Appendix 2)

SPSS (Statistical Package for the Social Sciences) is a well-liked software system; it is not only the most widely used statistical package, but is probably the most widely used applications package in the world. It can be found everywhere; one advantage that it has over SAS is that it is available for most mainframes and large minicomputers. The statistical capabilities are very wide; it is in no way restricted to the statistical procedures found in a social sciences environment.

BMDP (see Appendix 3)

The mathematics underlying the procedures in BMDP (Biomedical Computer Programs: P-Series) is excellent, and so is the documentation. One disadvantage to BMDP is that each procedure is accessed separately; this is a problem in an environment in which many kinds of analyses are to be performed repeatedly. An example might be where an interim analysis must be run every 3 months and the form of that analysis is well known. Using packages like SPSS and SAS one can put together a procedure file that does it all, save it, and rerun it every time the data is revised. With BMDP this requires more work, because the procedures are accessed separately.

The statistical capabilities are very wide. An interesting feature is a procedure for analyzing the patterns of missing values and also looking for outliers. These are the sorts of things that ought to be done when taking a first look at a set of data.

Minitab (see Appendix 4)

Minitab, a popular package, is ideally suited for students. It is quite easy for nonstatisticians and for people without much background in computer science to use it. Although Minitab is continually being expanded, the range of statistical procedures is not as broad as with the other packages presented so far, and the options and control features are not as rich.

P-STAT (see Appendix 5)

P-STAT (Princeton Statistical Package) is available for most mainframe computers. It can be accessed both in batch mode and interactively, and it can read and write BMDP and SPSS save files. This feature is especially useful if SPSS or BMDP is being used as the primary package, but there is a procedure in P-STAT that is desirable and it is worthwhile to learn enough of P-STAT command language to use it occasionally. One very nice aspect of P-STAT is that it has probably the best cross-tabulation procedure of all the packages. It allows great control of the format of the output; it is possible to slice data according to many variables and still have it appear on a single page.

OSIRIS IV (see Appendix 6)

OSIRIS IV is best known to statisticians working in survey research, since the statistical procedures emphasize the analysis of survey data. It is designed to handle large data sets; a thousand questionnaires pose no problem when processed using OSIRIS IV, and it can handle hierarchical data structure, which is a

feature many of the other packages do not have. Its
error checking and correcting features are excellent.

Going beyond Statistical Packages

Going beyond the facilities provided by the statistical packages involves a substantial cost, far more
than has been required so far. In particular, specialized staff is required to do more than is reasonable for the statistician to do by himself.

There are two routes that can be taken. The first
involves the use of data base management systems, developed for situations when the data set is not rectangular (i.e., rows of patients by columns of variables). The other route is to program in a higher
level computer language, almost certainly FORTRAN.
The advantage to selecting FORTRAN is the vast number
of computer programs that have already been written in
it. The procedures provided in a statistical package
may be limiting, whereas in programming there are almost no limits; whatever is desired can be programmed
exactly. The next two sections detail what is involved in following each of these routes.

DATA BASE MANAGEMENT SYSTEMS

Data can often not be easily collected in a rectangular form suitable for statistical analysis. The
power of the computer can be used to process the data
after they have been collected to satisfy the requirements of the specific question at hand. What follows
is an extended example of the kind of situation where
a data base management system makes it possible to
analyze nonrectangular data. In this case patients
are treated with a drug; a dose is given, say, 3 times
per week, and the dosage is increased over time, perhaps to a maximum tolerated dose. This might be a
Phase I study of a drug. In addition, the extent of
disease is evaluated biweekly in order to monitor the

effect of the drug, that is, to determine if there has
been an objective response. Finally, in managing the
patient, signs and symptoms are recorded routinely
(temperature and blood pressure); not surprisingly
because of the nature of an escalating drug dose
study, the signs and symptoms are recorded more frequently following each drug dose, because the drug may
very well have an effect on temperature and blood
pressure.

The important point concerning a study like this is
that not only are there different kinds of data collected according to different schedules, but in practice the schedules as presented cannot be followed
rigidly. To say that a dose is going to be given 3
times a week is a guide; certainly for medical reasons
it may be necessary not to escalate the dose, or to
delay treatment for a time because of the condition of
the patient. And patients may have personal reasons
for missing a dose. Although the schedule is 3 times
per week, the data cannot be forced into that format.

Biweekly evaluation of extent of disease is another
schedule that may not be realized in practice. Because of competing demands on the hospital house
staff, quite often the extent of disease will not be
evaluated as often as planned. If, on the other hand,
a patient's disease is progressing rapidly, the extent
of disease may be evaluated more often.

The fact that signs and symptoms are recorded in
relation to the schedule of drug dose will also make
for very uneven data.

There are some easy questions that can be answered
with the data set described, if the computer processing can be restricted to only one of the 3 data
types. It is not difficult to analyze average dose;
it is not difficult to do a tabulation of extent of
disease; it is not difficult to extract typical blood
pressure readings. There are hard questions that can
be asked of a data set like this. A question such as
how the dosage of the drug affects blood pressure requires linking together, by date, the dose records and

the many signs and symptoms records that were collected on that date.

A more difficult question is whether disease response is related to the drug, or to the escalation of the drug dosage, or to cumulative drug dose. Not only is it difficult to link these records, but in some sense the answer to the question requires an algorithm, one that may have been previously provided by a physician. A rectangular data set is often the summarization of a nonrectangular data set, where the summarization was done by a highly trained, thinking human being. When nonrectangular data is collected for computer processing, implicitly the computer must now do the summarization. As a simple example, suppose temperature is to be analyzed in relation to the dosage of the drug. Does a patient's temperature go up with a dose of the drug? A clinician knows that a patient who has recently received a blood transfusion will experience a high body temperature, independent of any drug. A computer program linking drug records and temperature records may not have transfusion data available to it, and may not have been instructed to exclude these "spurious" temperature spikes in any case.

Taking on the job of data aggregation is an enormous responsibility because data aggregation is so complex. Data base management systems do provide the ability to store, process, and retrieve complex data. The data can be looked at on many levels and across levels. The algorithms for data aggregation can be very involved, but they are only sensitive to anticipated exceptions. They cannot be expected to replace judgment.

The programming language associated with these data base management systems is complex and difficult to master. Data base management systems make it possible to analyze complex data; they do not make it easy. And since they do not make it easy, specialized staff is required: computer programmers or data base administrators. This is a large expense. So far in this

chapter, a few thousand dollars is all that was required to get a terminal and access to an academic
computing facility that supported statistical packages. A programmer or data base administrator can command the salary of a professional statistician. Furthermore, some data base management systems are so expensive that academic computing facilities cannot
afford them.

Some Data Base Management Packages

Some of the best known data base management systems
are System 2000, TOTAL, ADABAS, and RAMIS II; these
systems are very powerful indeed. A system like
ADABAS provides a query language for asking questions
of the data base; there are facilities for report
writing; the system can be interfaced with modules
written in other computer languages; variables can be
stored in inverted lists for easy processing. But
ADABAS costs $100,000. RAMIS II is $12,000 to
$24,000.

These packages are advertised as being nonprocedural; often the command language is very much like English. But the nonprocedural language only applies to
relatively straightforward queries. With medical data, queries are often complicated because therapy is
an art as well as a science. These data base management systems also have a procedural language that must
be accessed for the more complicated types of retrieval. Use of this language is just like programming in
any other high level language like FORTRAN, and that
is why specialized staff is so necessary.

A Useful General Package: SIR (see Appendix 7)

A somewhat specialized data base management system
is SIR (Scientific Information Retrieval). This system is nowhere nearly as powerful as the other commercial packages, but, on the other hand, it does not
cost anywhere nearly as much. A commercial installa-

tion of SIR is less than $6000; a degree granting in-
stitution can obtain SIR for $2000. Because of the
low cost, academic computing facilities are making SIR
available to time-sharing users.

SIR is designed to handle hierarchical data struc-
tures. The example of dose records, extent of disease
records, and signs and symptoms records is one where
SIR excels. Other examples are cooperative trials
among institutions or program projects where data from
participating laboratories are brought together in a
central repository for analysis.

Data are stored as variables within records. This
is a less powerful approach than treating each variable separately, but there are savings in the ease and
reduced cost of processing data. One disadvantage to
SIR is that only one job can access the data base at
one time. This is not a constraint if the data base
is primarily a tool of the statistician; it is a serious constraint if many people need to access information at the same time. SIR supports a procedural retrieval language, has a report writing feature, and
provides many levels of access security. The most
useful feature of SIR from the point of view of the
statistician is that after collapsing data into a rectangular form, SIR can directly create an SPSS or BMDP
save file.

In an environment where one of the major statistical packages is used heavily, SIR is a natural choice
as a data base management system for data that will
eventually be subject to statistical analysis.

FORTRAN PROGRAM LIBRARIES

There is another area that is of great interest to
workers in biostatistics. To get involved in the community that is trading software on methods that have
not yet found their way into the major packages, a
statistician must utilize FORTRAN. FORTRAN programming provides access to libraries of mathematical,

statistical, and graphical subroutines, and to software associated with the latest statistical literature. If it is clear from a scientific publication
that the statistical results were obtained on a computer, it is almost certain that the program was written in FORTRAN. Contacting the author will often produce a copy of the program. A statistician can derive
full benefit from new developments by acquiring the
available relevant software. In a sense, FORTRAN programming allows one to keep up with the current literature.

Example of a FORTRAN Library: IMSL (See Appendix 8)

     The first package of FORTRAN routines to consider
is IMSL (International Mathematical and Statistical
Libraries). This organization has a blue ribbon advisory board to make sure that the mathematical and
statistical routines are correct and that they reflect
the current literature. If a better way to decompose
a matrix is developed, very often it will be found in
IMSL quite soon. There are a great many procedures in
the library ranging from analysis of variance to finding zeros of functions. This library is available for
almost all machines that support FORTRAN. It costs
less than $1200 and can be found at most academic com-
puting facilities.

Graphics Packages

     Another aspect of getting into FORTRAN programming
is that graphics is now more accessible. There are 3
kinds of graphics. Analysis graphics are used by the
person who generated the graph to gain an insight into
the data. A printer plot is often adequate, and the
major statistical packages do printer plots very well.
Presentation graphics are used to present results to
others when there is someone there to explain the
graph; a pen plotter is a good choice for this kind of
graph. Publication graphics go into statistical or

medical papers. Many journals now accept computer
graphics, saving the high cost of manual art work.

Self-contained commercial graphics packages are not
cheap. For example, DISPLAA and TEL-A-GRAF of ISSCO
cost $25,000 each. A recent development is that the
latest versions of SAS and SPSS include access to
parts of DISPLAA and TEL-A-GRAF. High quality bar
graphs and pie charts will soon be available to the
time-sharing community.

NCAR (see Appendix 9)

Another approach to graphics is to employ a programmer to use packages of FORTRAN subroutines to develop the necessary graphs. An example package is
NCAR, a library that draws maps, contour plots of
functions, and perspective views. This package is not
as well supported as some of the other packages discussed. In practice, discrepancies between the user's
manual and the program will be found, and there are
still some bugs in the programs. This is typical of
software obtained for free or for little cost; getting
it to work in a different hardware environment may
take a lot of work by a programmer.

GR-Z (see Appendix 10)

Another graphics package is GR-Z from Bell Laboratories, which is a source of some very high quality
software. A good feature of GR-Z is that there are
high-level routines that use a lot of default values,
so that a user can get a basic chart with a small number of subroutine calls. There are intermediate routines that provide more control of scaling, location
of labels, and plot size. Finally, there are low-
level routines that provide almost total control of
the chart, at the expense of a great number of subroutine calls. Extensive documentation is available.

SUMMARY

Wherever one is located, a real possibility to be considered is access to an academic computing facility through a computer terminal. Without a great cost, the statistician can make use of powerful software to solve his data management and statistical analysis problems. The most direct approach is to select one of the major statistical packages, become expert in that package, and use it as much as possible.

The next step of moving to a data base management system or to doing FORTRAN programming is very expensive because of the specialized staff required. It is not a move that should be undertaken lightly.

A quite common fixture in the hospital environment is the minicomputer. With an in-house minicomputer one can install statistical or mathematical packages, but it is unlikely that all of the software found at an academic computing facility can be installed. It may be a mistake to compromise the statistical analysis for the sake of using a nearby minicomputer.

As a group grows in staff and budget, it may be possible to justify bringing outside computing activities in-house, on a "super" minicomputer, such as the DEC VAX 11/780 or on a small mainframe computer like the DEC 20. These are very powerful machines that can support many of the software packages described above. The critical issue is the total software cost, which now must be born by a single department or institution, not spread among a large user community.

BIBLIOGRAPHY

Much of the literature on statistical software can be found in the first 3 references.

Computer Science and Statistics: Annual Symposium on the Interface.

American Statistical Association, Proceedings of the Statistical Computing Section.

SAS Users Group, Proceedings of the Annual SUGI Conference.

Ivor, Francis, ed. (1979), A Comparative Review of Statistical Software: Exhibition of Statistical Program Packages, The International Association for Statistical Computing, Netherlands.

Schmid, C. F., and Schmid, S. E. (1979), Handbook of Graphical Presentation (2nd ed.), Wiley, New York.

APPENDIX 1. SAS

ADDRESS   SAS Institute Inc.
                                 P.O. Box 8000
                                 Cary, NC   27511

TELEPHONE   (919) 467-8000

GENERAL REMARKS   Can read SPSS, BMDP and OSIRIS
                                    save files
                                 Available for IBM 360/370 only
                                 Written in PL/1

OVERALL CAPABILITIES   Some error checking features
                                 Good file handling
                                 Report writer
                                 Intermediate results available
                                    for analysis

TABLE OF CONTENTS   Analysis of variance for bal-
                                    anced data
                                 Autoregression
                                 BMDP interface
                                 Canonical correlation
                                 Bar charts (histograms), pie
                                    charts, star charts
                                 Cluster analysis
                                 Contents and history of SAS da-
                                    ta set
                                 BMDP, Data-Text, OSIRIS, SAS72,
                                    SPSS file conversion
                                 Copying SAS data sets
                                 Correlation analysis
                                 Listing, deleting, and renaming
                                    SAS data sets
                                 Deleting SAS data sets
                                 Discriminant analysis
                                 Duncan's multiple range test
                                    (two versions)
                                 Interactive and batch editing

of SAS data sets
Factor analysis
Defining formats to print value
   labels
Frequency and cross-tabulation
   tables
Categorical analysis
Introduction to the general
   linear models procedure:
   simple regression, multiple
   regression, analysis of co-
   variance, response surface
   models, weighted regression,
   polynomial regression, par-
   tial correlations, multivari-
   ate analysis of variance
Guttman scaling
Matrix language
Means and other descriptive
   statistics
Nearest neighbor discriminant
   analysis
Nested analysis of variance
Nonlinear regression
One-way analysis of variance on
   ranks
Listing, deleting, and renaming
   PDS members
Copying load modules and li-
   braries
Randomized plans for experi-
   ments
Printer plotting
Printing SAS data sets
Routing procedure output to
   disk or tape
Probit analysis
Ranking
Releasing unused space at the
   end of a data set

All possible regressions
Linear combinations of coeffi-
cients and data values
Sorting SAS data sets
Printing source library con-
tents
Spectral analysis
Standardization
Stepwise regression
Summary statistics
Ordinary least squares, two-
stage least squares, limited
information maximum likeli-
hood, 3-stage least squares,
seemingly-unrelated regres-
sions
Copying tape volumes
Printing contents of tape vol-
umes
t-tests
Univariate descriptive statis-
tics, including percentiles
Variance component analysis
Multidimensional scaling
D. R. Cox's life-table regres-
sion model (two versions)
Quick check of input data
Print oversized text
Display contents of FORMAT li-
braries
Print mailing labels and other
line-printer forms
Least squares and maximum likelihood analysis for geneti-
cists
Cluster analysis on the units
of a transaction flow table
Subset an indexed sequential
data set
Normality tests

Linear model using least abso-
lute values criterion
Logistic multiple regression
(two versions)
One-way ANOVA on ranks
Analyze OPSCAN/100 output
Compute percentiles
Contour plots
Nonparametric regression for
censored data
Schematic plots
Test differences between sur-
vival curves
Convert TPL tables to SAS data
sets
Time-series cross-section re-
gression

EXTENSIBILITY   Yes: FORTRAN or PL/1

GRAPHICS   Yes: ISSCO

APPENDIX 2. SPSS

ADDRESS	SPSS Inc. Suite 3000 444 North Michigan Avenue Chicago, IL 60611
TELEPHONE	(312) 329-2400

GENERAL REMARKS	Most widely used statistical
	    package
	Available for most mainframes
	    and large minicomputers
	Written in FORTRAN

OVERALL CAPABILITIES	Some error checking features Basic file handling Report writer

TABLE OF CONTENTS	Descriptive statistics and one-
	    way frequency distributions
	Producing descriptive statis-
	    tics for aggregated data sets
	Contingency tables and related
	    measures of association
	Description of subpopulations
	    and mean difference testing
	Bivariate correlation analysis:
	    Pearson correlation, rank-
	    order correlation, and scat-
	    tergrams
	Partial correlation
	Multiple regression analysis
	Special topics in general line-
	    ar models
	Analysis of variance and co-
	    variance
	Discriminant analysis
	Factor analysis
	Canonical correlation analysis

Guttman scale
Reliability
Report generator
Spectral analysis of time se-
ries
Smallest space analysis
Summary tables
Survival analysis
Tetrachoric correlation coeffi-
cients
Generalized 3-stage least
squares
Jöreskog factor analysis
Cross-tabulation tables for
multiple response variables
Nonlinear regression
Nonparametric statistical tests
Digital (CalComp) plotting
Multivariate analysis of vari-
ance and covariance

EXTENSIBILITY   Yes, although very difficult

GRAPHICS   Yes: ISSCO

APPENDIX 3. BMDP

ADDRESS	BMDP Statistical Software, Inc. P.O. Box 24A26 Los Angeles, CA 90024
TELEPHONE	(213) 825-5940

GENERAL REMARKS	The "original" statistical
	  package (1961)
	Excellent underlying mathemat-
	  ics
	Excellent documentation
	Available for most mainframes
	Written in FORTRAN

OVERALL CAPABILITIES	Each procedure accessed sepa- rately Error detection features

TABLE OF CONTENTS	Multipass transformation
	Simple data description
	Detailed data description, in-
	  cluding frequencies
	Single column frequencies, nu-
	  meric and nonnumeric
	Comparison of two groups with
	  t-tests
	Description of groups (strata)
	  with histograms and analysis
	  of variance
	Multiway description of groups
	Histograms and univariate plots
	Bivariate (scatter) plots
	Two-way frequency tables; meas-
	  ures of association
	Two-way frequency tables; empty
	  cells and departures from in-
	  dependence
	Multiway frequency tables; the

log-linear model
Missing value correlation
Description and estimation of
missing data
Multiple linear regression
Stepwise regression
All possible subsets regression
Regression on principal compo-
nents
Polynomial regression
Nonlinear regression
Derivative-free nonlinear re-
gression
Maximum likelihood estimation
Stepwise logistic regression
One-way analysis of variance
and covariance
Analysis of variance and co-
variance, including repeated
measures
General mixed model analysis of
variance
General mixed model analysis of
variance; equal cell sizes
Nonparametric statistics
Cluster analysis of variables
Cluster analysis of cases
Block clustering
k-means clustering of cases
Factor analysis
Canonical correlation analysis
Partial correlation and multi-
variate regression
Stepwise discriminant analysis
Life tables and survival func-
tions

EXTENSIBILITY   No

GRAPHICS   No

APPENDIX 4. Minitab

ADDRESS   Minitab Project
                            215 Pond Laboratory
                            University Park, PA   16802

TELEPHONE   (814) 865-1595

GENERAL REMARKS   Very easy to use; ideal for
                               students
                            Interactive
                            Available for most mainframes
                               and minicomputers
                            Written in FORTRAN

OVERALL CAPABILITIES   Range of statistical procedures
                               is not as broad as with SPSS/
                               SAS/BMDP
                            Options and control are more
                               limited

TABLE OF CONTENTS   Plots and histograms
                            Random number generation
                            Sorting
                            Descriptive statistics
                            Regression
                            Probability functions
                            Mann-Whitney test
                            Analysis of variance
                            Correlation
                            Walsh averages
                            Chi-square test
                            Contingency tables
                            Time series
                            Exploratory data analysis

EXTENSIBILITY   Yes

GRAPHICS   No

APPENDIX 5. P-STAT

ADDRESS	P-STAT, Inc.
	P.O. Box 285
	Princeton, NJ 08540
TELEPHONE	(609) 924-9100
GENERAL REMARKS	Interactive and batch
	Available for most mainframes
	Written in FORTRAN
OVERALL CAPABILITIES	Easy to learn and use
	Good file manipulation abilities
	Error detection and correction
	Can read and write BMDP/SPSS save files
TABLE OF CONTENTS	Frequency distributions, plots, and histograms
	Cross-tabulation
	Chi-square
	F-tests
	t-tests
	Pearson product moment correlations
	Regression
	Principal components
	Iterative factor analysis
	Backwards-stepping multiple discriminant analysis
	Multivariate analysis of variance
EXTENSIBILITY	No
GRAPHICS	No

APPENDIX 6. OSIRIS IV

ADDRESS	Institute for Social Research Box 1248 Ann Arbor, MI 48106
TELEPHONE	(313) 764-4417
GENERAL REMARKS	Developed for survey data
OVERALL CAPABILITIES	Rectangular and hierarchical files Excellent error checking features Available for IBM 360/370 only Written in FORTRAN
TABLE OF CONTENTS	Checking and correcting datasets Displaying datasets Building and modifying structural datasets Transforming datasets Frequency distributions and associated statistical measures Correlation and regression analysis Analysis of variance Multivariate analysis using ordinal and nominal predictors Factor analysis and multidimensional scaling Cluster analysis Sampling error analysis
EXTENSIBILITY	No
GRAPHICS	No

APPENDIX 7. SIR

ADDRESS   Scientific Information
                                    Retrieval, Inc.
                                 P.O. Box 1404
                                 Evanston, IL   60201

TELEPHONE   (312) 475-2314

GENERAL REMARKS   Hierarchical data base manage-
                                    ment system
                                 Available for most mainframes
                                 Written in FORTRAN

OVERALL CAPABILITIES   Ready interface with SPSS and
                                    BMDP
                                 Data stored as variables within
                                    records
                                 Only one job at a time can ac-
                                    cess the data base

TABLE OF CONTENTS   File security
                                 Schema definition
                                 Batch data input and management
                                 Data retrieval by case or rec-
                                    ord
                                 Report generator
                                 Utilities
                                 Interactive mode

EXTENSIBILITY   No

GRAPHICS   No

APPENDIX 8. IMSL

ADDRESS   IMSL, Inc.
                         Sixth Floor, NBC Building
                         7500 Bellaire Boulevard
                         Houston, TX   77036

TELEPHONE   (713) 772-1927

GENERAL REMARKS   FORTRAN subroutine library
                         Blue ribbon advisory board
                         Subroutines reflect the current
                           literature
                         Available for most mainframes
                           and minicomputers

OVERALL CAPABILITIES   Covers the most common mathe-
                           matical and statistical top-
                           ics
                         Consistent style of calling
                           arguments

TABLE OF CONTENTS   Analysis of variance
                         Basic statistics
                         Categorized data analysis
                         Differential equations; quad-
                           rature; differentiation
                         Eigensystem analysis
                         Forecasting; time series;
                           transforms
                         Generation and testing of ran-
                           dom numbers
                         Interpolation; approximation;
                           smoothing
                         Linear algebraic equations
                         Mathematical and statistical
                           special functions
                         Nonparametric statistics
                         Observation structure; multi-
                           variate statistics

Regression analysis
Sampling
Utility functions
Vector, matrix arithmetic
Zeros and extrema; linear pro-
    gramming

GRAPHICS   No

APPENDIX 9. NCAR

ADDRESS   Software Distribution
                            National Center for Atmospheric
                              Research
                            P.O. Box 3000
                            Boulder, CO   80307

TELEPHONE   (303) 494-5151

GENERAL REMARKS   FORTRAN subroutine library

OVERALL CAPABILITIES   General package for plotting
                              graphs and maps
                            Will drive a variety of plot-
                              ting devices

TABLE OF CONTENTS   Draws and annotates curves or
                              families of curves
                            Software dashed line package
                              with labeling capability
                            Halftone (gray scale) pictures
                              from a two-dimensional array
                            Iso-valued surfaces (with hid-
                              den lines removed) from a 3-
                              dimensional array
                            High quality software charac-
                              ters
                            Simplest software characters
                            Movie titling package
                            Three-dimensional display of a
                              surface (with hidden lines
                              removed) from a two-
                              dimensional array
                            Plots a representation of a
                              vector field flow of any
                              field for which planar vector
                              components are given on a
                              regular rectangular lattice,
                              displaying both field

direction (via lines of flow
containing arrowheads and
feathers) and field magnitude
(based on distance between
those flow lines)

Continental outlines and political boundaries in various
projections

Provides 3-space line drawing
capabilities, with entry
points equivalent to the line
drawing entry points of the
system plot package

Two-dimensional velocity field
displayed by drawing arrows
from the data locations

Provides a clipping capability
for lines extending outside a
user-defined window, thus allowing part of a picture to
be plotted without distortion
or overwriting near the edge
of the picture

APPENDIX 10. GR-Z

ADDRESS   Bell Laboratories
                           600 Mountain Avenue
                           Murray Hill, NJ   07974

TELEPHONE   (201) 582-7330

GENERAL REMARKS   FORTRAN subroutine library

OVERALL CAPABILITIES   High-, intermediate- and low-
                              level routines
                           Sensible default values
                           Extensive documentation

PLOTTING CAPABILITIES   Scatterplots
                           Box plots
                           Contour plots
                           Bar charts
                           Spiral seasonality plots

Part V

Statistical Methodology

CHAPTER 10

Estimation in Survival Analysis: Parametric Models, Product-Limit and Life-Table Methods

BYRON W. BROWN, Jr.

In many clinical studies of cancer, the basic observation on each patient is the time elapsed from
one well-defined event, for example, diagnosis, to
another well-defined event, for example, death. This
would be called a waiting time. Other examples of
waiting time variables that are encountered in clinical cancer studies are the following:

Time elapsed from
{
diagnosis
start of treatment
remission of symp-
toms
    or
progression of dis-
ease
}
to
{
death
recurrence of symp-
toms
visceral occurrence
of disease
    or
progression/recur-
rence
}

At first glance, statistical analysis of waiting
times may seem to present no unusual problems. In
fact, however, two difficulties arise. First, waiting
time distributions are positively valued and most are
very highly skewed in the positive direction. This
positive skewness suggests the use of transformations
or nonparametric procedures to reduce the influence
of the infrequent extraordinarily long waiting time,

317

and to provide better approximations by asymptotic
theory.

The second statistical difficulty is the presence
of censoring. In many clinical studies it is necessary or, at least, desirable to analyze the data for a
group of patients before all the patients have experienced their terminating event. For example, suppose
the waiting time is to be defined as time from diagnosis to death. A patient diagnosed two years prior to
the time of analysis and still surviving would present
a censored value of two years. We know the waiting
time for the patient will be two years plus an unde-
termined further amount. The observation is said to
be right censored. Right censoring is typical of
clinical cancer studies and presents problems in statistical analysis not discussed in many standard
courses in statistical application and theory.

Before discussing some estimation procedures for
censored waiting time data, some concepts and notation
commonly used in this area should be introduced.
Again, we think of the waiting time as the time from
diagnosis to death, and we denote this time by t.
Thus, t is the time of death as measured from diagnosis, or, equivalently, the length of survival. Then
the following functions can be defined:

Distribution function = $F(t)$ (1)
    = P(death by time t)

Survival function = $S(t) = 1-F(t)$ (2)
    = P(surviving past time t)

Density function = $f(t) = F'(t) = -S'(t)$ (3)

Conditional density = $f(t)/S(t_0)$
    = probability density, given survival to $t = t_0$ (4)

$$\left.\begin{array}{c}\underline{\text{Rate function}}\\\underline{\text{Hazard function}}\\\underline{\text{Force of mortality}}\end{array}\right\} = h(t) = f(t)/S(t) \qquad (5)$$

Note that the hazard function can be interpreted as
the conditional density, at t, conditional on surviving to t. In other words, $h(t) \cdot \Delta t$ is approximately
the probability of dying between t and $t+\Delta t$, given
survival to t.

If the preceding differential equation defining the
hazard function is solved, by integrating both sides
of the equation with respect to t, the following basic
relationship is obtained:

$$S(t) = \exp[-\int_0^t h(u)du] \ . \tag{6}$$

The actuaries and demographers have estimated survival functions (birth to death) from population data.
Their methods date from the 17th century. They base
their estimates on the number of people at risk at
age t, and the number of those people at risk who die
at that age. These figures are readily available for
most developed countries, where census figures show
the numbers of people at risk of death at each age,
and death certificate figures show the numbers of people dying at each age. The ratio of deaths per year
to persons at risk, at age t, provides an estimate of
h(t) and from h(t), the estimate of S(t) is readily
calculated, using equation 6.

Waiting time data from a clinical study present
estimation problems that are quite different from
those of the actuary. Figure 1 depicts a small set
of fictitious data, illustrating the nature of waiting
times in a typical randomized clinical study. Patients are admitted to the study sequentially through
calendar time. They are randomly assigned to one of
the two treatment arms, called A and B, and then followed to death. The vertical line at the fortieth
month might be the time set for analysis of the study.
In that case, the second, seventh, and tenth patients
would still be alive and would contribute censored
data points, since the investigator would not know
how much longer those patients would survive.

Figure 2 shows the same data, regrouped by treat-

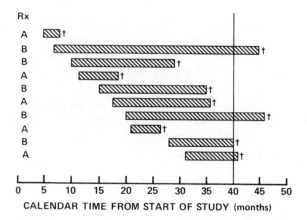

Figure 1. Survival times for 10 cancer patients randomly assigned to treatments A and B (hypothetical data).

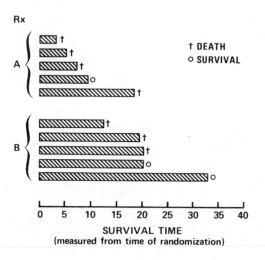

Figure 2. Survival times from time of randomization for 10 cancer patients, assuming termination of study at t = 40.

320

ment assignment, and plotted against time of survival, from study entry. The censored data points are distinguished from the deaths, assuming the time of analysis to be the fortieth month of the study.

The data for a series of patients, for which some observations are censored, are often listed with plus signs attached to the censored values. For example, the data in Figure 2 would be listed as follows:

Treatment A: 3,   7, 18,   5,   9+
Treatment B: 12, 19, 20, 20+, 33+

Note that there are 4 deaths and one survival among the 5 patients randomly assigned to treatment A, and 3 deaths and 2 survivals among the patients assigned to treatment B. Note also that there is a marked tendency for longer survival in the B group.

The survival function for each treatment group can be estimated by a nonparametric method called the Kaplan-Meier (4) or product-limit method. Like the sample cumulative distribution estimate, the Kaplan-Meier method assigns a probability mass to each observed value or time of death. However, the masses are not all equal. They are calculated as conditional probabilities of death, given survival to each observed time of death, d_i/n_i, where n_i is the number surviving and thus at risk of death at the ith observed death time, and d_i is the number of deaths occurring at this time. Then the unconditional probability of surviving past the ith death time is the product of the conditional probabilities of surviving the times up to and including the ith death time. The arithmetic is simple and is illustrated in Table 1 for the data of treatment A. The general formula is as follows:

$$\hat{S}(t) = \prod_{t_j \le t} \frac{n_j - d_j}{n_j} ,$$

TABLE 1. Illustration of the Calculation of the Kaplan-Meier or Product-Limit Estimate of the Survival Function for the Data for Treatment A in Figure 2

t	No. at risk (n)	No. died (d)	Probability at t of dying (p)	not dying (q)	Probability of surviving past time t ($\hat{S}$)
3	5	1	$\frac{1}{5}$	$\frac{4}{5}$	$\frac{4}{5} = .8$
5	4	1	$\frac{1}{4}$	$\frac{3}{4}$	$\frac{4}{5} \cdot \frac{3}{4} = .6$
7	3	1	$\frac{1}{3}$	$\frac{2}{3}$	$\frac{4}{5} \cdot \frac{3}{4} \cdot \frac{2}{3} = .4$
18	1	1	$\frac{1}{1}$	$\frac{0}{1}$	$\frac{4}{5} \cdot \frac{3}{4} \cdot \frac{2}{3} \cdot \frac{0}{1} = 0$

where the product is over all observed death times, t_j, such that $t_j \leq t$. Note that this method yields a step function, with steps down proportional to the proportion of deaths at t_j among those surviving and thus at risk at t_j. In tracing the calculations in Table 1 it is easy to see that if the set of data were uncensored the product-limit method would produce the complement of the familiar sample cumulative distribution function, with n steps of $1/n$ for a sample of n distinct uncensored death times.

Figure 3 shows the Kaplan-Meier survival curves for the two treatment groups. It is customary to denote the censored observations on the curve by some sort of tick mark or other symbol such as the small circles used in the figure. Note that if the largest observation in a sample is censored, as in the treatment B group, the survival curve will not come down to zero, thus leaving the remaining portion of the curve undefined. The smooth curve will be discussed later.

When the data set is quite large, little will be

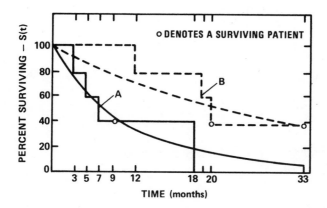

Figure 3. Kaplan-Meier and exponential estimates of survival curves for treatments A and B.

lost by grouping the observations by time interval and using one or another method patterned more closely after the methods used by the actuaries in computing survival curves for insurance computations. The method used most frequently is called the Berkson-Gage (2) procedure. It is illustrated in Table 2 for a set of data on 374 cancer patients which appears in Armitage's text (1). The waiting time is from operation to death or point of analysis if the patient has not died. The times are grouped into intervals of one year. The number of deaths in each interval is shown in column 2 and the number of censored observations in the interval is shown in column 3. Column 4 shows the number of persons alive and under observation at the start of each interval, and column 5 shows the same number reduced by half of the censored observations. The conditional probability of death in the interval is then estimated as the number of deaths divided by this estimated number at risk. The complement is then the estimated probability of survival, and the product of these for all intervals preceding and including the interval yields an estimate of the survival function at the end of the specified inter-

TABLE 2. Life Table Calculations for Patients with a Particular Form of Malignant Disease[a]

Interval since operation, years j-1 to j	Last reported during this interval		Living at start of interval ℓ_j	Adjusted number at risk $n_j = \ell_j - w_j/2$	Estimated probability of death $p_j = d_j/n_j$	Estimated probability of survival $q_j = 1 - p_j$	Percentage of survivors after j-1 years[b]
	Died d_j	Alive w_j					
0-1	90	0	374	374.0	0.2406	0.7594	100
1-2	76	0	284	284.0	0.2676	0.7324	75.9
2-3	51	0	208	208.0	0.2452	0.7548	55.6
3-4	25	12	157	151.0	0.1656	0.8344	42.0
4-5	20	5	120	117.5	0.1702	0.8298	35.0
5-6	7	9	95	90.5	0.0773	0.9227	29.1
6-7	4	9	79	74.5	0.0537	0.9463	26.8
7-8	1	3	66	64.5	0.0155	0.9845	25.4
8-9	3	5	62	59.5	0.0504	0.9496	25.0
9-10	2	5	54	51.5	0.0388	0.9612	23.7
10-	21	26	47	-	-	-	22.8

[a] Adapted from Berkson and Gage (2) and Armitage (1).

[b] $100 S_{j-1} = 100 \prod_{i \leq j-1} q_i$.

val. By convention, we let q_0 and S_0 both equal one.

It is easy to see that the Berkson-Gage method will be identical to the Kaplan-Meier method if the intervals are allowed to become infinitesimally small so that the necessity for grouping is obviated.

For either method of estimation, Greenwood's formula for the standard error of $S(t)$ is as follows:

$$S.E.[\hat{S}(t)] = \hat{S}(t) \left(\sum_{t_j \le t} \frac{p_j}{n_j \cdot q_j} \right)^{\frac{1}{2}} , \qquad (7)$$

where the p_j, q_j, and n_j are as given in Table 1 or Table 2. Note that for the Kaplan-Meier method $p_j/n_j q_j$ is simply $d_j/n_j(n_j-d_j)$. If there are no ties in times of death, then all d_j equal one so that $p_j/n_j q_j$ is simply $1/n_j(n_j-1)$.

Sometimes the shape of the survival function can be described in parametric form, that is, in explicit mathematical form with one or several unspecified parameters or constants. If so, there may be an important advantage in making use of this information, for simplicity and also because a reduction in the standard errors for the survival curve and its characteristics will usually be achieved.

The simplest, yet widely used, parametric model for waiting time data is the exponential curve. It flows from an assumption of constant hazard or force of mortality. Focusing on waiting time to death, we assume that the conditional probability of death in the interval $(t, t+\Delta t)$, given survival to time t, does not depend on how long the survival, t. We denote this constant hazard by θ; using the notation of equation 5,

$$h(t) = \theta .$$

From equations 1 through 6, it then follows that

$$S(t) = \exp(-\theta t)$$

and

$$f(t) = \theta\exp(-\theta t) \ .$$

It is easily verified that the mean (μ) and median (t_{50}) for the distribution are:

$$\mu = 1/\theta \ ,$$

and

$$t_{50} = \ln 2/\theta \ .$$

Table 3 lists 6 parametric models commonly used in the analysis of waiting time data. The first is

TABLE 3. Commonly Used Parametric Models

---

1. Exponential $h(t) = \theta$ (constant)
   $S(t) = \exp(-\theta t)$

2. Weibull $h(t) = \theta t^{\beta}$ (monotonic or constant)
   $S(t) = \exp[-(\theta/\beta)t^{\beta+1}]$

3. Gompertz $h(t) = \theta\exp(\beta t)$ (monotonic or constant)
   $S(t) = \exp\{(\theta/\beta)[\exp(\beta t)-1]\}$

4. Gamma $h(t)$ (monotonic or constant)

5. Log normal $h(t)$ increases to max, then decreases

6. Cure model $S(t) = \pi S_1(t)+(1-\pi)S_2(t)$
   π = the probability of cure;
   S_1 is the survival function for cures and S_2 for noncures; they might be of any specified parametric form.

---

the exponential, having one parameter and a constant
hazard function. The second, third, and fourth have
two parameters each, with hazard functions that can
be constant (yielding the exponential as a special
case) or can either increase or decrease monotonically
through time. The log normal has a hazard function
that increases to a maximum and then decreases. For
large coefficients of variation the log normal distribution approximates the exponential distribution.

The cure model, the sixth in Table 3, was proposed
by Berkson and Gage (3). They took $S_1(t)$ to be known
from vital statistics data for the general population,
and took $S_2(t)$ to be an exponential imposed on the
same background hazard, thus leaving two parameters
to be estimated from the sample data, the cure rate
(π) and an exponential hazard (θ) due to the uncured
disease they were studying.

Estimation for any parametric model usually employs
likelihood methods. The likelihood function for a set
of data with some right censored values has two components, one for the uncensored values and the other for
the censored values. Denoting the uncensored values
by t_i, i = 1, 2, ..., d, and the censored values by
t_i, i = d+1, d+2, ..., n, the likelihood function can
be written:

$$L = \prod_{i=1}^{d} f(t_i) \prod_{i=d+1}^{n} S(t_i) \ .$$

The likelihood is maximized with respect to the parameters in the expression, usually by differentiating
the log likelihood and solving the equations resulting
from setting the derivatives equal to zero. The
standard errors for the resulting maximum likelihood
estimates are obtained from the estimated Fisher information.

We will illustrate the method for the simplest
case, the one parameter exponential model. The likelihood is:

$$L = \prod_{i=1}^{d} \theta\exp(-\theta t_i) \prod_{i=d+1}^{n} \exp(-\theta t_i) \ .$$

The log likelihood, LL, is:

$$LL = d\cdot\ln\theta - \theta\sum_{i=1}^{n} t_i \ .$$

Differentiating LL with respect to θ yields the estimator for θ:

$$\hat{\theta} = d/ \sum_{i=1}^{n} t_i \ .$$

The Fisher information, I, is the negative of the expected value of the second derivative of LL with respect to θ:

$$I = -E\left(\frac{\partial^2 LL}{\partial\theta^2}\right) = E(d)/\theta^2 \ .$$

The standard error of $\hat{\theta}$ will be approximately $I^{-\frac{1}{2}}$, and we estimate I by substituting d for E(d) and $\hat{\theta}$ for θ, obtaining:

$$S.E.(\hat{\theta}) = \hat{\theta}/\sqrt{d} = \sqrt{d}/\Sigma t \ .$$

Note that there is some reason for basing inference on $\ln \theta$ rather than on θ. First $\ln \hat{\theta}$ will be more nearly normal in distribution than $\hat{\theta}$, and the asymptotic variance does not depend on θ. The standard error for $\ln \hat{\theta}$ is:

$$S.E.(\ln \hat{\theta}) = 1/\sqrt{d} \ .$$

To illustrate the calculations we compute the estimate of the survival curve for treatment A in Figure 2. The 5 observations are 3, 7, 18, 5, and 9+. We have:

$$\hat{\theta} = 4/[3+7+18+5+9] = 0.0952 ,$$

$$\text{S.E.}(\hat{\theta}) = 0.0952/\sqrt{4} = 0.0476 .$$

On the log scale the results are:

$$\ln \hat{\theta} = -2.3514 ,$$

$$\text{S.E.}(\ln \hat{\theta}) = 1/\sqrt{4} = 0.50 .$$

The maximum likelihood estimates of S(t) for treatments A and B are shown by the two smooth curves in Figure 3.

If we were interested in estimating the value of S(t) for treatment A at t = 12, with confidence limits, we would use:

$$\hat{S}(12) = \exp(-12\hat{\theta}) = 0.3191 .$$

For computing the confidence limits, we use $\ln \hat{\theta}$ and then transform back to the $\hat{S}$ scale. The transformation required is a double log transformation and the results are as follows:

$$\ln[-\ln \hat{S}(12)] = \ln 12 + \ln \hat{\theta} = 0.1335$$

$$\text{S.E.}\{\ln[-\ln \hat{S}(12)]\} = 0.50$$

$$95\% \text{ confidence limits} = 0.1335 \pm 1.96(0.50)$$

$$= -0.8465 \text{ to } 1.1135 .$$

Transforming back by exponentiating, changing the sign, and then exponentiating again, we have the following limits for S(12):

$$0.0476 < S(12) < 0.6512 \ .$$

For comparison we compute the limits for the Kaplan-Meier estimate, using Greenwood's formula, equation 7. From Table 1 we see that $\hat{S}(12) = 0.40$. The standard error using equation 7 is:

$$\text{S.E.}[\hat{S}(12)] = 0.40(1/5\cdot4 + 1/4\cdot3 + 1/3\cdot2)^{\frac{1}{2}} \ ,$$

$$= 0.2191 \ .$$

The limits could be computed as $\hat{S} \pm 1.96 \text{S.E.}$ or $0.40 \pm 1.96(0.2191)$, yielding lower and upper values of $0 < S(12) < 0.8294$. Thus, the limits for the nonparametric procedure are markedly, and typically, wider than those obtained by the parametric procedure.

Estimation for the more complex models in Table 3 is more difficult than for the simple exponential. Each of the others has two or more parameters, thus involving a system of likelihood equations. None of the models leads to a system that can be solved explicitly in closed form. Therefore, iterative methods are needed and a computer is highly desirable, to solve the equations, to compute the elements of the Fisher information matrix, and to invert the matrix (the last especially when the number of parameters exceeds two).

One of the most difficult problems facing the applied statistician is the choice of an inference procedure from the many that might be applicable for the problem at hand. Even in the example we have studied, namely, estimating the survival curves for treatments A and B, we could choose the nonparametric Kaplan-Meier procedure or we could choose to use one of a number of parametric models. A little simulation study will be presented here to illustrate some of the procedures that might be employed in settling on an approach, and to exemplify a common phenomenon, namely, that the choice of model is not so critical as one might fear.

Consider the cure model, the sixth in Table 3. Let the cure rate be $\pi = 0.40$; let the cures have a hazard rate of zero [i.e., $S_1(t) = 1$] and let the noncures have an exponential survival function with a median survival time of 12 months [and, thus, a hazard rate of $(\ln 2)/12 = 0.0578$]. Thus, the model is:

$$S(t) = 0.40 + 0.60 \exp(-.0578t) . \qquad (8)$$

The survival function is shown as the smooth curve in Figure 4. Note that the curve decreases exponentially, at the rate of $\theta = 0.0578$, to a cure rate asymptote of 0.40.

Using this cure rate model a set of sample data can be generated. We assume that 20 patients are admitted

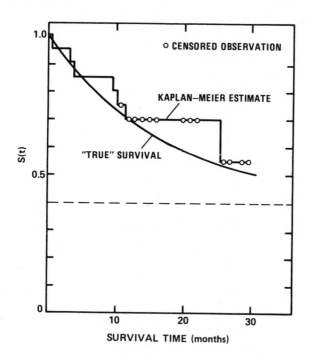

Figure 4. Cure rate model and Kaplan-Meier estimate based on the set of simulated data in Table 4.

to the study, one each successive month, and that the
study lasts for 30 months, so that the potential
follow-up periods for the successive patients are 30,
29, 28, ..., 11, respectively. The potential follow-
up times are listed in Table 4. A single uniform random number is chosen for each patient, and the corresponding survival time is obtained by inverting the
formula for the survival curve, equation 8, or, equivalently, reading from the smooth curve of Figure 4 the
abscissa values corresponding to the random values on
the ordinate scale. Of course, any patient with a

TABLE 4. Simulated Data for the Cure Rate Model
in Equation 8 of the Text

Potential follow-up	Random no.	Survival time	Observed
11	.356	Cure	11+
12	.026	Cure	12+
13	.327	Cure	13+
14	.230	Cure	14+
15	.069	Cure	15+
16	.130	Cure	16+
17	.729	10.4	10.4
18	.710	11.4	11.4
19	.900	3.2	3.2
20	.016	Cure	20+
21	.555	23.4	21+
22	.361	Cure	22+
23	.745	9.6	9.6
24	.986	0.4	0.4
25	.881	3.8	3.8
26	.056	Cure	26+
27	.360	Cure	27+
28	.535	25.8	25.8
29	.214	Cure	29+
30	.024	Cure	30+

random number value less than or equal to 0.40 is a
cure and automatically a survival. The random numbers
and the survival times are listed in the second and
third columns of Table 4. Since certain of the patients had survival times beyond their potential
follow-up times, for example, the patient with potential follow-up time of 21 months, the observations for
such patients would be censored at the time of study
end, that is, at the end of their follow-up periods,
as would the patients who were cured. Of course, the
investigator would not be able to distinguish between
cured patients and those uncured but still surviving
(at least not without further follow-up). The actual
data available to the investigator are listed in column 4 of Table 4.

The data in Table 4 will be analyzed in several
ways, with the view that the investigator does not
know the form of the survival curve and simply wants
to estimate the survival curve, with due caution for
his ignorance of the real underlying distribution.
One alternative is to use the nonparametric Kaplan-
Meier procedure. The calculations are exhibited in
Table 5 and the estimate of the survival curve is
shown in Figure 4.

An alternative procedure would be to use the simple
exponential model. However, the investigator might
hesitate to use this model without some reassurance
that the model is an adequate description of the form
of the underlying survival curve for this situation.
To obtain such assurance the investigator could use a
richer model that has the exponential model as a
special case, and then determine whether the richer
model yields important further information not comprehended by the simple exponential model.

One such richer model that has been used by a few
workers is the linear hazard model,

$$h(t) = \alpha + \beta t \; .$$

The model is appealing for our purposes because a test

TABLE 5. Calculation of Kaplan-Meier Curve

Times of death	No. at risk	No. dying	$\hat{q}$	$\hat{S}$	$\dfrac{1}{n(n-1)}$	S.E.
0.4	20	1	.949	.949	.0026	.048
3.2	19	1	.947	.899	.0029	.067
3.8	18	1	.944	.848	.0033	.080
9.6	17	1	.941	.798	.0037	.089
10.4	16	1	.938	.749	.0042	.097
11.4	15	1	.933	.699	.0048	.102
25.8	5	1	.800	.559	.0500	.149

for $\beta = 0$, say by likelihood methods, would be a reasonable test of whether the hazard is constant (i.e., the survival function is exponential) or is changing through time.

Another model might be the two parameter cure model, the model actually used to generate the data (though this would be unknown to the investigator). Again, $\pi = 0$, that is, no cures, would correspond to the exponential model.

Results obtained in estimating the survival function under the 3 models are shown in Table 6. The survival curves estimated by the 3 parametric methods are shown in Figure 5, along with the Kaplan-Meier estimate, and the actual model used to generate the data. Note in Table 6 that for the linear hazard approach $\hat{\beta}$ is negative, suggesting that the hazard does decrease with time (as indeed it does for the cure model), but $\hat{\beta}$ is only a quarter of a S.E. from zero, not close to significant. The cure model itself does fairly well, the estimate of π being very close to the "true" value of 40%, with a S.E. that strongly suggests that the cure rate is not zero. However, when one looks at the graphical representations in

TABLE 6. Results for Three Models, Using
the Data of Table 4

---

1. Exponential:

$$\hat{\theta} = 7/320.6 = .0218$$
$$\text{S.E.}(\hat{\theta}) = .0083$$

2. Linear hazard: $h(t) = \alpha + \beta t$

$$\hat{\alpha} = .0253 \qquad \hat{\beta} = -.000168$$
$$\text{S.E.}(\hat{\alpha}) = .0134 \quad \text{S.E.}(\hat{\beta}) = .000463$$

3. Cure model: $S(t) = \pi + (1-\pi)\exp(-\theta t)$

$$\hat{\pi} = .377 \qquad \hat{\theta} = .0420$$
$$\text{S.E.}(\hat{\pi}) = .193 \quad \text{S.E.}(\hat{\theta}) = .0202$$

Figure 5, the agreement among the 3 parametric
estimates, along with the Kaplan-Meier estimate, is
striking. In fact, the log likelihood values for the
3 parametric approaches were computed and are almost
identical, namely, -33.77, -33.71, and -33.71, respectively, suggesting most clearly that there is nothing
to be gained by use of the two richer models. The exponential model is quite adequate as a description of
the data at hand.

This little simulation study cannot furnish a basis
for generalization, but broader experience does repeatedly suggest that the exponential distribution can
be quite adequate for a wide range of applications in
cancer survival analysis. Experience suggests that
the choice of model may not be as critical as the com-
pulsive statistician might fear. The use of parametric models with few parameters, usually no more
than two (often the simple one parameter exponential
will do), may well be safe. The gain in power over

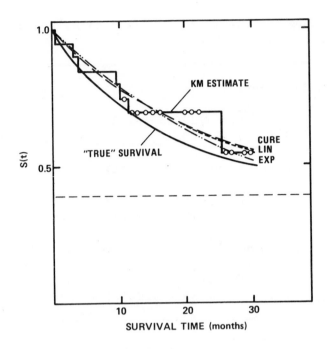

Figure 5. The Kaplan-Meier estimate and 3 parametric estimates of the survival curve, based on the data of Table 4.

the more conservative nonparametric approach can be substantial, and the risk of serious misspecification of the model will be minimal. [Some recent analytical work of Miller (5) in a technical report graphically demonstrates the gain to be had.]

In conclusion, it should be noted that much has been written in recent years on the analysis of censored data as encountered in clinical trials, especially in investigations of cancer therapy. Over the past decade this has been an area of wide and intense statistical research. We are fortunate that much of this work has recently been gathered together in several important books devoted to the subject. Although the references to such work have not been made specifically in the present exposition, except in a few instances, the selected bibliography will furnish the interested statistician with key books, and with references to certain of the more innovative papers and papers that opened up new areas or furnish reviews of certain general areas of interest and research in survival analysis with censored data.

REFERENCES

1. Armitage, P. (1971), Statistical Methods in Medical Research, Wiley, New York.

2. Berkson, J., and Gage, R. P. (1950), Calculation of survival rates for cancer, Proceedings of Staff Meetings, Mayo Clinic 25: 250.

3. Berkson, J., and Gage, R. P. (1952), Survival curve for cancer patients following treatment, Journal of the American Statistical Association 47: 501-515.

4. Kaplan, E. L., and Meier, P. (1958), Nonparametric estimation from incomplete observations, Journal of the American Statistical Association 53: 457-481.

5. Miller, R. G., Jr. (1981), What Price Kaplan-Meier? Technical Report No. 71 (R01 GM21215), Division of Biostatistics, Stanford University, Stanford, California.

BIBLIOGRAPHY

Books

Elandt-Johnson, R. C., and Johnson, N. L. (1980), Survival Models and Data Analysis, Wiley, New York.

Gross, A. J., and Clark, V. A. (1975), Survival Distributions: Reliability Applications in the Biomedical Sciences, Wiley, New York.

Jordan, C. W., Jr. (1952), Life Contingencies, The Society of Actuaries, Chicago.

Kalbfleisch, J., and Prentice, R. L. (1980), The Statistical Analysis of Failure Time Data, Wiley, New York.

Lee, E. T. (1980), Statistical Methods for Survival Analysis, Lifetime Learning Publications, Belmont, California.

Mann, N., Schafer, R., and Singpurwalla, N. D. (1974), Methods for Statistical Analysis for Reliability and Life Data, Wiley, New York.

Miller, R. (1981), Survival Analysis, Wiley, New York.

Spiegelman, M. (1968), Introduction to Demography, Harvard University Press, Cambridge, Massachusetts.

Papers

Aitken, M., and Clayton, D. (1980), The fitting of exponential, Weibull and extreme value distributions to complex censored survival data using GLIM, Applied Statistics 29: 156–163.

Cox, D. R. (1972), Regression models and life tables, Journal of the Royal Statistical Society, Series B 34: 187–220.

Crowley, J., and Hu, M. (1977), Covariance analysis of heart transplant survival data, Journal of the American Statistical Association 72: 27–36.

Johansen, S. (1978), The product limit estimator as maximum likelihood estimator, Scandinavian Journal of Statistics 5: 195-199.

Link, C. L. (1979), Confidence intervals for the survival function using Cox's proportional hazard model with covariates, Technical Report No. 45 (R01 GM21215), Division of Biostatistics, Stanford University, Stanford, California.

Littel, A. S. (1952), Estimation of the T-year survival rate from follow-up studies over a limited period of time, Human Biology 24: 87-116.

Nelson, W. (1972), Theory and applications of hazard plotting for censored failure data, Technometrics 14: 945-966.

Schoenfeld, D. (1980), Chi-squared goodness-of-fit tests for the proportional hazards regression model, Biometrika 67: 145-153.

Zippin, C., and Armitage, P. (1966), Use of concomitant variables and incomplete survival information in the estimation of an exponential survival parameter, Biometrics 22: 665-672.

CHAPTER 11

Inference in Survival Analysis: Nonparametric Tests to Compare Survival Distributions

STEPHEN W. LAGAKOS

INTRODUCTION

This chapter describes nonparametric statistical
tests for the comparison of two or more groups on the
basis of time until some critical event referred to
as survival time. Common examples of "survival times"
in clinical trials are time to remission, relapse, or
death from disease.

From a technical point of view, the testing problem
is different from ones encountered in more standard
situations. For one thing, survival data are right
skewed, often extremely so. More importantly, some
observations are right censored, and represent only a
lower bound for the survival time of interest. As a
result of these complications, classical statistical
methods do not directly apply to survival data.

The goal of this chapter is to discuss some of the
commonly used nonparametric tests for comparing two or
more groups, as well as their properties and

This work was supported by National Cancer Institute
Grants CA-00505 and CA-23415.

limitations. The first section reviews notation, censoring, and parametric approaches. The next section introduces a family of nonparametric tests in terms of 2x2 contingency tables. This way of presenting the tests facilitates their construction and elucidates their properties. The section thereafter shows how the same family of tests also arises from a likelihood score function, from which large-sample behavior can be examined. In the final two sections the properties of the tests are considered and several extensions are mentioned. It should be emphasized that the methods considered here by no means represent all nonparametric tests, but only the subset that has found the greatest use in clinical trials and other biomedical situations.

PRELIMINARIES

Suppose T is a nonnegative continuous random variable representing survival time. The cumulative distribution function of T is denoted $F(t)$. The complement of F is called the survivor function, and is denoted $S(t)$. The distribution of T can also be characterized by the hazard function, $h(t)$, defined by

$$h(t) = \lim_{\Delta t \to 0+} (\Delta t)^{-1} P(t \leq T < t + \Delta t \mid T \geq t) .$$

It is easily demonstrated that F, S, and h are related by

$$h(t) = \frac{F'(t)}{1 - F(t)} = -\frac{S'(t)}{S(t)} ,$$

$$S(t) = \exp[-\int_0^t h(u)du] ,$$

and

$$-\ln\ S(t)\ =\ \int_0^t h(u)du\ .$$

In many situations, it is easiest to study survival distributions using hazard functions. For example, health statistics are often recorded in terms of numbers of individuals at risk and failing during regular time intervals. This leads naturally to consideration of h(t). Also, for many types of survival data h(t) [or ln h(t)] varies relatively slowly with t, making it suitable as a starting point for models.

As indicated above, the analysis of survival data is complicated by the presence of censored observations. A common situation arising in clinical trials that leads to censoring is illustrated in Figure 1.

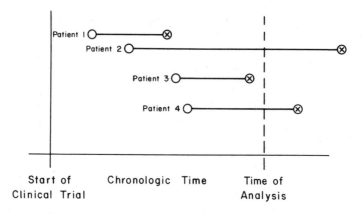

Figure 1. Schema indicating how censored observations can arise in a clinical trial (O = time of entry; ⊗ = time of failure; survival time = elapsed time between entry and failure).

Patients accrue into the trial at various points in chronologic time, and the data are analyzed at some later point. Survival time is measured from entry into the trial until failure. Complete (i.e.,

uncensored) observations arise when failure occurs before the time of analysis. If patients have not
failed by that time, their survival time is censored.
In the figure, patients 1 and 3 have uncensored survival times, while patients 2 and 4 have censored
times. Formally, the observed time for a subject is

$$U = \min(T,Y) , \tag{1}$$

where T is the actual (sometimes unobserved) survival
time, and Y is the "potential" censoring time, that
is, the time between entry to the trial and the time
of analysis. U is uncensored if and only if $T \leq Y$.
    Censoring can occur in other ways. For example,
survival times are sometimes censored due to patients
lost to follow-up, toxic side effects, and refusal of
therapy. Virtually all statistical methods that accommodate censoring assume (either implicitly or explicitly) that it is noninformative, that is, an observation that is censored at t provides only the information that survival time exceeds t, no more or no
less. If censoring is informative, ordinary methods
are inappropriate and can give misleading results
(see, e.g., 9).
    Although censored observations prevent the direct
application of inference methods such as least
squares, they pose no particular difficulty for like-
lihood-based inferences. The likelihood function for
F based on a set of independent realizations for equation 1 is proportional to

$$L(F) = [\Pi F'(t_i)]\{\Pi [1-F(s_j)]\} , \tag{2}$$
$$\quad i \qquad j$$

where the t_i and s_j represent the uncensored and censored times, respectively. Thus, if a parametric approach is adopted, equation 2 simplifies to a function
of one or more parameters which can be analyzed using
standard likelihood techniques.

To illustrate, consider the exponential distribution with parameter $\lambda > 0$. We have

$$S(t) = 1-F(t) = \exp(-\lambda t)$$

and

$$h(t) = \lambda \ .$$

The exponential distribution plays a central role among survival distributions, analogous to the role of the Gaussian distribution in classical statistics. The constant hazard function reflects the memoryless property of the exponential distribution. For example, the expected additional lifetime for a subject surviving until time t is λ^{-1}, independently of t. The mean, median, and variance of the exponential distribution are λ^{-1}, $(\ln 2)\lambda^{-1}$, and λ^{-2}. As an indication of the large dispersion of the exponential distribution, note that for T_1, T_2 exponential with $E(T_2)$ = $1.5E(T_1)$, we have $P(T_2>T_1)$ = 0.6. That is, in comparing two treatment groups in which median (or average) survival in one is 50% greater than the other, the chances that a patient with the better treatment will outlive one with the poorer treatment are only 0.6.

The likelihood function for the exponential distribution is, from equation 2,

$$L(\lambda) = \lambda^r \exp(-\lambda W) \ ,$$

where r is the number of uncensored times and $W = \Sigma t_i + \Sigma s_j$, the total observed time. The resulting MLE is $\hat{\lambda} = r/W$, and the negative inverse of the second derivative of $\ln L$ is λ^2/r. Because $\ln \lambda$ tends to be more normally distributed than λ in small samples, it is customary to base inferences about $\hat{\lambda}$ on the approximate pivotal (19)

$$\frac{\ln \hat{\lambda} - \ln \lambda}{\sqrt{1/r}} .$$

An approximate test of the equality of two exponential samples can thus be obtained by regarding

$$\frac{\ln \hat{\lambda}_1 - \ln \hat{\lambda}_0}{\sqrt{\dfrac{1}{r_0} + \dfrac{1}{r_1}}} .$$

as a standard normal deviate.

Our objective in this chapter is to review non-parametric tests, so we will not dwell on the exponential or other parametric models. For a more thorough discussion of these see Zelen (19) or Kalbfleisch and Prentice (7), and the following chapter.

A FAMILY OF NONPARAMETRIC TESTS

Suppose we wish to compare two treatment groups denoted by 0 and 1. For group 0 there are M independent realizations of equation 1, with T and Y having cumulative distribution functions $F_0(t)$ and $G_0(t)$, respectively. For group 1 there are N observations, with distribution functions $F_1(t)$ and $G_1(t)$. The hypothesis of treatment equality is H: $F_0(t)=F_1(t)$ for all t. Equivalently, we can express H by $S_0 = S_1$ or $h_0 = h_1$. The censoring functions G_0 and G_1 are equal in many randomized clinical trials, but can be unequal in some situations. None of the tests we describe requires for its validity that $G_0 = G_1$.

Suppose $t_1 < t_2 < \ldots < t_J$ are the distinct times of failure from among the M + N patients. We can summarize the data by considering the information relevant to each t_j in a 2x2 contingency table:

Treatment group	Failures at t_j		At risk at t_j-0
0	m_j	M_j-m_j	M_j
1	n_j	N_j-n_j	N_j

The quantities m_j and n_j are the number of patients that fail at t_j, and M_j and N_j are the number that are alive and on-study just before t_j (termed "at risk" at t_j).

Suppose now that H holds and that we consider the distribution of n_j conditional on the 4 marginal counts. The conditional null distribution of n_j, given the marginals, is the hypergeometric distribution, that is, from a finite population of M_j+N_j items of which m_j+n_j have a particular characteristic (in this case failures at t_j), we select a sample of size N_j and observe the number n_j that have the characteristic. Accordingly, the null conditional expectation and variance of n_j are

$$E_j = \frac{N_j(m_j+n_j)}{M_j+N_j} \qquad (3)$$

and

$$V_j = \frac{M_j N_j (m_j+n_j)(M_j+N_j-m_j-n_j)}{(M_j+N_j-1)(M_j+N_j)^2} . \qquad (4)$$

Suppose $w_1, w_2, \ldots, w_J$ are some known constants. If we regard $n_1, n_2, \ldots, n_J$ as independently normal with moments given by equations 3 and 4, it follows that $\Sigma w_j(n_j-E_j)$ is also normal. Hence

$$Q(w) = \frac{[\Sigma_j w_j(n_j-E_j)]^2}{\Sigma_j w_j^2 V_j} \qquad (5)$$

has the χ_1^2 distribution under H. Alternatively,

$$\sum_j w_j(n_j-E_j)/ (\sum_j w_j^2 V_j)^{\frac{1}{2}}$$

is $N(0,1)$ under H. In truth, the n_j are neither normal nor independent, but they can be regarded as such as a convenience in thinking about $Q(w)$, which asymptotically is χ_1^2 under H.

Two specific members of this family of tests play a prominent role in survival analyses. The first is when $w_j = 1$ for each j, resulting in the proportional hazards (PH) test:

$$Q_{PH} = \frac{(O-E)^2}{V} ,$$

where $O = \sum n_j$ is the observed number of failures on treatment 1, $E = \sum E_j$ is an expected number, and $V = \sum V_j$. The PH test, or variations of it, is also referred to as the log-rank, Mantel-Haenszel, generalized Savage, and exponential order scores test. (See, for example, reference 11.) The second important special case is when $w_j = M_j+N_j$, whereupon equation 5 reduces to Q_{GW}, the so-called generalized Wilcoxon (GW) test. Variations of this test have also been referred to as Gehan's test, Gilbert's test, and Breslow's test. A more detailed discussion of these may be found in Kalbfleisch and Prentice (7). The PH and GW tests are used so routinely in the analysis of survival data that a recent article determines critical values for the more significant of Q_{PH} and Q_{GW} (17).

To illustrate the tests, we consider the leukemia data analyzed by Gehan (4). Table 1 lists 42 times to remission of disease, half from patients receiving the drug 6-MP and half from patients receiving no treatment (controls). The remission times are in weeks, and those censored are indicated with a +. Figure 2 gives the Kaplan-Meier (8) nonparametric estimates of S_0 and S_1, and clearly suggests a treat-

TABLE 1. Results of a Leukemia Study: Times of Remission (Weeks) of Leukemia Patients[a]

Sample 1 (drug 6-MP)[b]	6+, 6, 6, 6, 7, 9+, 10+, 10, 11+, 13, 16, 17+, 19+, 20+, 22, 23, 25+, 32+, 32+, 34+, 35+
Sample 0 (control)	1, 1, 2, 2, 3, 4, 4, 5, 5, 8, 8, 8, 8, 11, 11, 12, 12, 15, 17, 22, 23

[a]Adapted from Gehan (4) and Freireich et al. (3).
[b]A + sign indicates censored observation.

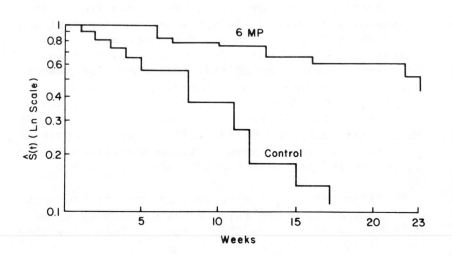

Figure 2. Survival plots of data in Table 1.

ment difference. Table 2 carries out the calculation of E_j and V_j for $j = 1$ ($t=1$) and $j = 16$ ($t=22$). The values of E_j and V_j for all distinct failure times are given in Table 3.

To compute the proportional hazards test we simply sum the E_j, n_j, and V_j from each table. This gives $E = 19.25$, $O = 9$, and $V = 6.28$. The two-sided chi-square statistic therefore equals

$$Q_{PH} = \frac{(9-19.25)^2}{6.28} = 16.7 \ ,$$

giving an approximate significance level of $P = P(\chi_1^2 \geq 16.7) < .001$. (A one-sided test is probably more appropriate in this situation, but for simplicity we hereafter discuss only the two-sided versions of the tests.) The generalized Wilcoxon test is obtained by weighting $n_j - E_j$ by $w_j = N_j + M_j$. This gives

$$\sum_j w_j (n_j - E_j) = -269.22 \ ,$$

$$\sum_j w_j^2 V_j = 5481.68$$

so that

$$Q_{GW} = \frac{(-269.22)^2}{5481.68} = 13.2 \ ,$$

with a corresponding significance level of $P(\chi_1^2 \geq 13.2) < .001$.

DERIVATIONS OF TESTS FROM COX'S REGRESSION MODEL

In the previous section we constructed a family of tests from the perspective of 2x2 tables. In this section the tests are derived from a regression model for the hazard function (1).

TABLE 2. Calculation of E_j and V_j for j=1 and j=16

At $t_1 = 1$			
Treatment	Failures		At risk
0	2	19	21
1	0	21	21
Total	2		42

$n_1 = 0; \ E_1 = \dfrac{21}{42}\cdot 2 = 1; \ V_1 = \dfrac{(21)(21)(2)(40)}{(41)(42)^2} = 0.49$

At $t_{16} = 22$			
Treatment	Failures		At risk
0	1	1	2
1	1	6	7
Total	2		9

$n_{16} = 1; \ E_{16} = \dfrac{7}{9}\cdot 2 = 1.56; \ V_{16} = .30$

Suppose z is a binary indicator of whether a patient is in group 0 or 1. Cox's model postulates that the hazard function for a subject with covariate z is

$$h(t|z) = h_0(t)\exp(\beta z) , \qquad (6)$$

where β is an unknown parameter. That is, the hazard functions for the two groups are $h_0(t)$ and $\exp(\beta)h_0(t)$, and hence are proportional. The hypothesis of treatment equality is given by $\beta = 0$, while $h_0(t)$ plays a role of a "nuisance" function.

TABLE 3. Calculations of E_j and V_j for Data in Table 1

t_j	N_j+M_j	n_j+m_j	N_j	n_j	E_j	V_j
1	42	2	21	0	1.00	0.49
2	40	2	21	0	1.05	0.49
3	38	1	21	0	0.55	0.25
4	37	2	21	0	1.14	0.48
5	35	2	21	0	1.20	0.47
6	33	3	21	3	1.91	0.65
7	29	1	17	1	0.59	0.24
8	28	4	16	0	2.29	0.87
10	23	1	15	1	0.65	0.23
11	21	2	13	0	1.24	0.45
12	18	2	12	0	1.33	0.42
13	16	1	12	1	0.75	0.19
15	15	1	11	0	0.73	0.20
16	14	1	11	1	0.79	0.17
17	13	1	10	0	0.77	0.18
22	9	2	7	1	1.56	0.30
23	7	2	6	1	1.71	0.20
				9	19.25	6.28

The analysis of equation 6 is based on a partial likelihood function (2). The overall likelihood can be written as a product of two terms,

$$L(\beta,h_0) = L_1(\beta)L_2(\beta,h_0) \ ,$$

where L_1 depends only on β. Since β seems to be inextricably tied up with h_0 in L_2, Cox proposes ignoring it. He shows that for purposes of inference about β, it is valid to act as if $L_1(\beta)$ is the actual likelihood. Others (e.g., 6) have further justified the use of L_1. The functional form of $L_1(\beta)$ is

$$L_1(\beta) = \prod_j \left[\frac{\exp(\beta z_j)}{\sum_{\ell \in R_j} \exp(\beta z_\ell)} \right] \qquad (7)$$

where R_j indexes the patients at risk at t_j and z_j is the value of z for the subject that fails at t_j. When there are tied failure times, the jth term in equation 7 is modified to be the product of such terms for each failure at t_j. This corresponds to Peto's (12) "rough probability" convention for handling ties. Other methods for ties have also been proposed (7). Censored observations can be incorporated into equation 7 also, and do not change the explicit form of the partial likelihood function.

Suppose we wish to assess the hypothesis H: $\beta = 0$ of treatment equality. One approach is to use the likelihood score function,

$$S(0) = \frac{\partial \ln L_1(\beta)}{\partial \beta}$$

evaluated at $\beta = 0$. Taking logarithms and differentiating $L_1(\beta)$ we get

$$S(0) = \sum_{j=1}^n (n_j - E_j) \ ,$$

which is the square root of the numerator of Q_{PH}. An estimated variance for $S(0)$ is obtained from the sample information

$$\frac{-\partial^2 \ln L_1(\beta)}{\partial \beta^2}$$

evaluated at $\beta = 0$. This turns out to be very similar, though not exactly equal, to the denominator of Q_{PH}. Thus, we see that for all practical purposes, Q_{PH} also arises as the score test from Cox's model. Because of this, it can be shown to be near optimal when the treatments being compared have proportional hazard functions.

Now suppose we modify equation 6 to be

$$h(t|z) = h_0(t)\exp[\beta z w(t)] \; . \qquad (8)$$

This corresponds to a hazard ratio

$$h(t|z=1)/h(t|z=0) = \exp[\beta w(t)] \; ,$$

which is not independent of time. When $\beta = 0$ the treatments are equivalent, but when it is not their hazards need not be proportional. If we again use a partial likelihood, the resulting score statistic for $\beta = 0$ is (10)

$$S(w) = \sum_j w_j (n_j - E_j) \; ,$$

where $w_j = w(t_j)$. This corresponds to the numerator of $Q(w)$. Thus, we see that $Q(w)$ defines a test which is particularly suited to alternatives of the form of equation 8.

In theory, we now have the machinery to design a test that is particularly suited to any specific alternative. In practice, however, one seldom has any feel for the shape of $w(t)$. As a result, it has been customary to use the PH test or, if early differences are particularly important, the GW test.

PROPERTIES OF TESTS

In this section we consider how the family of tests behaves for specific alternatives to H: $h_0(t) = h_1(t)$. The aim is to provide intuition for the properties of the tests, and the presentation is rather heuristic. For simplicity we assume there are no ties.

Let us reconsider the 2x2 tables discussed previously, but now without assuming that h_0 and h_1 are equal. Conditional on N_j, M_j, and $n_j + m_j (=1)$, the expectation of $n_j - E_j$ is

$$\frac{N_j h_1(t_j)}{M_j h_0(t_j) + N_j h_1(t_j)} - \frac{N_j}{M_j + N_j} = k_j \left[\frac{h_1(t_j)}{h_0(t_j)} - 1 \right] , \quad (9)$$

where $k_j = M_j N_j / \{ (M_j + N_j) [N_j h_1(t_j)/h_0(t_j) + M_j] \}$. The sum of these expectations over j is

$$\sum_j k_j \left[\frac{h_1(t_j)}{h_0(t_j)} - 1 \right] . \quad (10)$$

Although this is not the true expectation of O-E, it can be regarded as such to see the behavior of Q_{PH} when h_0 and h_1 are not proportional. It can be shown that equation 9 is asymptotically the noncentrality parameter of the limiting normal distribution of O-E (15). Furthermore, when $G_0 = G_1$ and treatment differences are small, the k_j are approximately equal.

To evaluate Q_{PH}, suppose first that $h_0 = h_1$. Then equation 10 becomes zero, indicating that under H we would expect small values of Q. Next suppose $h_1(t)/h_0(t) = \exp(\beta) > 1$. Then each bracketed term in equation 9 approximates $\exp(\beta) - 1 > 0$ and so the sum is positive. Thus, large values of Q_{PH} would be expected when h_0 and h_1 are unequal and proportional. When h_0 and h_1 are not proportional, but $h_1(t)/h_0(t) > 1$ for every t, each sum in the brackets is still positive. In this case Q_{PH} is not the optimal test, since the optimal test would give greater weight to those t where $h_1(t)/h_0(t)$ is larger. Nevertheless, it is clear that Q_{PH} will have reasonably good power over the broad class of alternatives for which $h_1(t) > h_0(t)$ for all t.

Now suppose not only that h_0 and h_1 are nonproportional but that they cross. Then the terms in equation 9 for which $h_1(t)/h_0(t) > 1$ will tend to cancel out those for which $h_1(t)/h_0(t) < 1$. Hence, Q_{PH} can take a value close to zero, signaling no treatment difference, even though h_0 and h_1 are quite different. Note that h_0 and h_1 can cross while the corresponding

F_0 and F_1 do not. Gill (5) has shown that Q_{PH} is consistent as long as F_1 and F_0 do not cross.

It is helpful to examine a few hypothetical situations in terms of both the hazard and survivor functions. In Figure 3a, the survivor functions, plotted on a log scale, move apart and then together. This corresponds to crossing hazards and hence Q_{PH} can have poor power. In Figure 3b the survival functions are initially equal and then diverge. This corresponds to hazards that are at first equal and later unequal. It is clear that the PH test will "waste power" in this situation because it utilizes positive weight in a region (small t) where h_0 and h_1 are very nearly equal. A better test would have been one with small (or zero) weights for early t, and large weights for larger t. In Figure 3c the survivor curves at first move apart and then become parallel. This corresponds to converging hazard functions. In this situation a test such as Q_{GW} would have been better than Q_{PH} in that it would place greater weight on earlier differences.

From the preceding discussion, it is clear that a statistical test for proportionality of hazards can be very useful. We will briefly describe one graphical and one formal method of checking for proportional hazards.

Suppose that $h_0(t)$ and $h_1(t)$ are proportional, that is, $h_1(t) = \exp(\beta)h_0(t)$. Then we have

$$\int_0^t h_1(u)du = \exp(\beta)\int_0^t h_0(u)du$$

which is equivalent to

$$-\ln S_1(t) = \exp(\beta)[-\ln S_0(t)]$$

which is equivalent to

$$\ln[-\ln S_1(t)] = \beta + \ln[-\ln S_0(t)] \ .$$

Hence, if $\hat{S}_0$ and $\hat{S}_1$ are estimates of S_0 and S_1 which

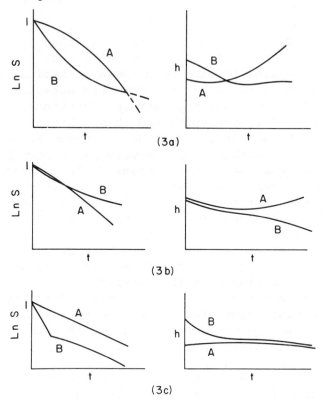

Figure 3. Various nonproportional hazard situations.

are not based on proportional hazards, a log(-log) plot of $\hat{S}_0$ will tend to be parallel to a log(-log) plot of $\hat{S}_1$ when $h_0(t)$ and $h_1(t)$ are proportional. Figure 4 displays such a plot based on Kaplan-Meier estimates for the data in Table 1. The approximately parallel appearance of the curves suggests that $h_1(t)$ and $h_0(t)$ are approximately proportional. Hence, we can be confident that Q_{PH} is an appropriate, and perhaps nearly efficient, test for this situation.

Next consider a formal test for proportional hazards. Any two hazard functions can be expressed

$$h_1(t) = h_0(t)\exp[\beta zw(t)] \ .$$

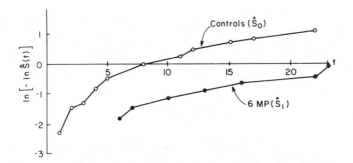

Figure 4. Graphical check of proportional hazards for data in Table 1.

The hazard ratio is thus

$$\frac{h_1(t)}{h_0(t)} = \exp[\beta w(t)] \ .$$

Since the form of $w(t)$ is not usually known, it is reasonable to approximate it by the first two terms of the Taylor series expansion of w about 0, that is, $w(t) \cong c_1 + c_2 t$. This gives

$$h(t|z) \cong h_0(t)\exp(\beta_1 z + \beta_2 zt) \ .$$

An approximate hypothesis of proportional hazards is then H_2: $\beta_2 = 0$ and one of treatment equality is H: $\beta_1 = \beta_2 = 0$. We can assess H_2 using the partial likelihood score statistic

$$\frac{\partial \ln L_1(\beta_1,\beta_2)}{\partial \beta_2} \ .$$

evaluated at $\beta_2 = 0$ and $\beta_1 = \hat{\beta}_1$. If this test supports hypothesis H_2, then Q_{PH} can be used to test H_1: $\beta_1 = 0$ (given $\beta_2 = 0$). If not, we need not even test H_1 since H_2 is a necessary condition for H. Alternatively, H can be tested in a single step by using $(\hat{\beta}_1, \hat{\beta}_2)$ and its estimated covariance matrix. If h_0 and h_1 are proportional (i.e., $\beta_2 = 0$) this test will, of course, be less powerful than Q_{PH}. This score test for $\beta_2 = 0$ was applied to the data in Table 1 and yielded a significance level of 0.78, which supports the hypothesis of proportional hazards.

EXTENSIONS

The results of the previous sections easily generalize in several respects, some of which will now be briefly described.

Comparing Three or More Groups

Suppose there are k+1 "treatment" groups to be compared (k≥1). These groups might represent actual treatments, or the k+1 levels of some categorical variable. The data at t_j can be represented in a (k+1)x2 contingency table with entries:

Treatment group	Failures at t_j		At risk at t_j-0
0	n_{0j}	$N_{0j}-n_{0j}$	N_{0j}
1	n_{1j}	$N_{1j}-n_{1j}$	N_{1j}
2	n_{2j}	$N_{2j}-n_{2j}$	N_{2j}
.	.	.	.
.	.	.	.
.	.	.	.
k	n_{kj}	$N_{kj}-n_{kj}$	N_{kj}
Total	$n_{\cdot j}$	$N_{\cdot j}-n_{\cdot j}$	$N_{\cdot j}$

The analogs of n_j, $\underline{E}_j$, and V_j are

$$\underline{n}_j = (n_{1j}, n_{2j}, \ldots, n_{kj})', \quad \underline{E}_j = (E_{1j}, E_{2j}, \ldots, E_{kj})',$$

where

$$E_{ij} = N_{ij} n_{\cdot j} / N_{\cdot j} \; ,$$

and

$$V^{(j)} = [v_{i\ell}^{(j)}] \; ,$$

where

$$v_{i\ell}^{(j)} = \frac{n_{\cdot j} N_{ij} (N_{\cdot j} - n_{\cdot j})(N_{\cdot j}\delta_{i\ell} - N_{\ell j})}{(N_{\cdot j}-1)N_{\cdot j}^2}$$

and δ is the Kronecker delta. If $\underline{O}$, $\underline{E}$, and V denote
the sums, over j, of $\underline{O}j$, $\underline{E}j$, and $V^{(j)}$, it follows that
the generalized proportional hazards statistic

$$Q_{PH}^{(k)} = (\underline{O}-\underline{E})\,'V^{-1}(\underline{O}-\underline{E})$$

is approximately χ_k^2 under the hypothesis H: $h_0(t)=$
$h_1(t)=\ldots=h_k(t)$. This result generalizes to allow
weights w_j in the obvious way (18).

In some situations the k+1 treatment groups have
a natural ordering so that it would be appropriate to
have a test for H that is particularly oriented toward
alternatives of the form

$$K: \; h_0(t) \leq h_1(t) \leq \; \ldots \; \leq h_k(t) \; .$$

For example, the k+1 categories might correspond to
patient performance status which, if associated with
survival time, would be expected to correspond to a
trend effect. Suppose $\underline{c} = (c_0, c_1, \ldots, c_k)\,'$ are weights
satisfying $c_0 < c_1 < \ldots < c_k$. Then we would expect $\underline{c}\,'(\underline{O}-\underline{E})$
to be close to zero under H and large and positive un-
der K. An appropriate χ_1^2 test statistic is thus

$$Q_{Tr}^{(k)} = \frac{[\underline{c}\,'(\underline{O}-\underline{E})]^2}{\underline{c}\,'V\underline{c}} \; .$$

Furthermore, the difference, $Q_{PH}^{(k)} - Q_{Tr}^{(k)}$, is approximately χ_{k-1}^2 under H and appropriate for testing for departure from trend (16).

Strata

The PH test can also be used to compare treatments over a heterogeneous population determined by S strata (see, e.g., reference 13). For example, we may wish to compare two treatment groups among patients having various disease stages. One approach is to first consider the S data sets determined by the individual strata and compute an O, E, and V for each (denoted O_S, E_S, V_S). These can then be combined to form the statistic $(O.-E.)^2/V.$, where $O. = \Sigma O_S$, $E. = \Sigma E_S$, and $V. = \Sigma V_S$. This statistic also arises as the score test based on Cox's partial likelihood when the hazard function for a subject receiving treatment z in stratum s is generalized to be $h_s(t)\exp(\beta z)$. That is, the underlying hazard is allowed to vary across strata, but in a way that the treatment hazard ratio over any stratum is $\exp(\beta)$.

Incorporating Mode of Failure

In some clinical trials, failure is classified into one of several categories. For example, clinical trials involving radiation therapy often distinguish disease progression due to a local recurrence from progression due to metastatic spread. This information can be incorporated into the analysis by introducing an indicator variable, say $b \in \{1,2,\ldots,m\}$ that specifies the m types of failure. The outcome for a subject is thus extended from T to the pair (T,b). This situation is commonly referred to as competing risks, even though the categories of b need not compete in any real sense.

The statistical problem now consists of comparing the two treatments with respect to the joint distribu-

tion, say $\Lambda(T,b)$, of T and b. One way of character-
izing $\Lambda(T,b)$ is by the cause specific hazard functions

$$h_j(t) = \lim_{\Delta t \to 0} (\Delta t)^{-1} P(t \leq T < t + \Delta t, b=j \mid T \geq t)$$

for $j=1,2,\ldots,m$. To see that $(h_1,\ldots,h_m)$ characteriz-
es Λ, note that

$$P(t \leq T, b=j) = \int_t^\infty h_j(x) \exp[-H.(x)] dx \ ,$$

where

$$H.(x) = \int_0^x [h_1(u)+\ldots+h_m(u)] du \ .$$

The hypothesis of equality of treatments 0 and 1 can
thus be expressed

$$H = H_1 \cap H_2 \cap \ldots \cap H_m \ ,$$

where

$$H_j : \quad h_j^{(0)}(t) = h_j^{(1)}(t) \ .$$

An important feature of this characterization of Λ is
that standard survival software applies directly. In
particular, H_j can be assessed by any of the two sample tests we have considered by regarding observations
for which $b = j$ as uncensored, and those for which
$b \neq j$ as censored.

Though these computations are simple, the interpretation of competing risk data is more complicated than
that of ordinary survival data. For one, though the
h_j have all the properties of hazard functions, the
corresponding survivor functions

$$S_j(t) = \exp[-\int_0^t h_j(u) du]$$

do not, in general, correspond to any observable random variables (see, e.g., reference 14). Thus, plots of the S_j should not be presented in an analysis unless it is made clear that they cannot be interpreted in the same way as Figure 2. A second important consideration is that analyses should not, in general, consist only of examining a particular risk h_j. It is possible, for example, that $h_1^{(0)}(t) > h_1^{(1)}(t)$ while $h_2^{(0)}(t) < h_2^{(1)}(t)$, and, hence, a comparison based only on h_1 can be misleading. This would occur, for example, if two treatments were in reality equal, but there were classification errors with respect to b that differed for the two treatment groups.

SUMMARY

In this paper we have attempted to provide an overview of a family of nonparametric tests having broad application in problems concerning survival data. The tests evolved from work in the analysis of contingency tables also arise as partial likelihood score tests. Their popularity among statisticians involved in clinical trials and other biomedical problem areas stems from their simplicity, interpretability, efficiency, and robustness.

Most of the discussion in this chapter has focused on the comparison of two treatment groups with respect to time to failure. However, the preceding section indicates that the family of tests generalizes readily to accommodate 3 or more treatment groups, strata, and competing risks.

REFERENCES

1. Cox, D. R. (1972), Regression models and life tables, Journal of the Royal Statistical Society, B34: 187-220.

2. Cox, D. R. (1975), Partial likelihood, Biometrika 62: 269-276.

3. Freireich, E. J, Gehan, E., Frei, E., III, et al. (1963), The effect of 6-mercaptopurine on the duration of steroid-induced remissions in acute leukemia: A model for evaluation of other potentially useful therapy, Blood 21: 699-716.

4. Gehan, E. A. (1965), A generalized Wilcoxon test for comparing arbitrarily singly-censored samples, Biometrika 52: 203-223.

5. Gill, R. D. (1979), Censoring and Stochastic Integrals, Doctoral Thesis, Free University of Amsterdam.

6. Kalbfleisch, J. D., and Prentice, R. L. (1973), Marginal likelihoods based on Cox's regression and life model, Biometrika 60: 267-278.

7. Kalbfleisch, J. D., and Prentice, R. L. (1980), The Statistical Analysis of Failure Time Data, Wiley, New York.

8. Kaplan, E. L., and Meier, P. (1958), Nonparametric estimation from incomplete observations, Journal of the American Statistical Association 53: 457-581.

9. Lagakos, S. W. (1979), General right censoring and its impact on the analysis of survival data, Biometrics 35: 139-156.

10. Lustbader, E. D. (1981), Time-dependent covariates in survival analysis, Biometrika 67: 697-698.

11. Mantel, N. (1966), Evaluation of survival data and two new rank order statistics arising in its con-

sideration, Cancer Chemotherapy Reports 50: 163-170.

12. Peto, R. (1972), Contribution to discussion of paper by D. R. Cox, Journal of the Royal Statistical Society B34: 200-202.

13. Peto, R., Pike, M. C., Armitage, P., Breslow, N. E., Cox, D. R., Howard, S. V., Mantel, N., McPherson, K., Peto, J., and Smith, P. G. (1977), Design and analysis of randomized clinical trials requiring prolonged observation of each patient, British Journal of Cancer 35: 1-39.

14. Prentice, R. L., Kalbfleisch, J. D., Peterson, A. V., Flournoy, N., Farewell, V. T., and Breslow, N. E. (1978), The analysis of failure times in the presence of competing risks, Biometrics 34: 541-554.

15. Schoenfeld, D. (1981), The asymptotic properties of nonparametric tests for comparing survival distributions, Biometrika 68: 316-319.

16. Tarone, R. E. (1975), Tests for trend in life table analysis, Biometrika 62: 679-682.

17. Tarone, R. E. (1981), On the distribution of the maximum of the logrank statistic and modified Wilcoxon statistic, Biometrics 37: 79-96.

18. Tarone, R. E., and Ware, J. H. (1977), On distribution-free tests for equality of survival distributions, Biometrika 64: 156-160.

19. Zelen, M. (1969), Lecture notes on the theory of biometry, State University of New York at Buffalo.

CHAPTER 12
Analysis of Survival Data: Cox and Weibull Models with Covariates

DAVID P. BYAR

INTRODUCTION

In studies of patients with cancer and other diseases, it has long been recognized that certain characteristics of the patient and of his disease may markedly influence survival, but only in the past decade have powerful and flexible statistical methods been available for incorporating these covariates, often referred to as <u>prognostic factors</u>, into the analysis of survival data. Most earlier work evaluated prognostic factors by constructing separate survival curves for different categories of patients. Methods were not available for dealing with more than one variable at a time except by further subcategorization and construction of separate survival curves. Although some work appeared earlier describing the use of parametric survival models based on the exponential survival distribution (e.g., references 2,10,11,18), the most important new development was the publication of the seminal paper of D. R. Cox in 1972 (8). By specifying a proportional hazards model, Cox was able to write a partial likelihood equation that did not depend on the form of the underlying hazard, and thus this approach has been referred to as a semiparametric model. Within the class of proportional hazard models

365

one may also fit fully parametric models such as the
Weibull model. In this chapter, I shall not attempt
a general review of the literature on survival models
incorporating covariate information, which by now has
become rather extensive, but will instead concentrate
on use of the Cox and Weibull models in actual analyses of cancer data. Useful references for further
study are the recent books by Kalbfleisch and Prentice
(12) and Lee (13).

Before discussing these models, it is appropriate
to review our reasons for studying prognostic factors.
One important reason is to understand how a disease
behaves. Is the prognosis similar in men and in wom-
en, is age an important prognostic factor, does the
extent of a tumor or its histologic grade materially
influence the outcome, and are the values of certain
laboratory tests and the results of physical examination significantly correlated with length of survival?
If several of these variables are important, how do
they act together? When these questions have been
answered, we can use the results of our statistical
analysis to predict survival for groups of patients,
a second important goal. A third goal is to enable
us to perform adjusted survival analyses when comparing groups of patients for which imbalances exist in
the distribution of important prognostic factors.
This need arises especially in the analysis of retrospectively collected data, but such analysis can also
be important in interpreting data from randomized
clinical trials when imbalances have occurred by
chance, or if they arise in studying subsets of patients. A fourth goal of analyzing prognostic factors
is to aid us in the design of new studies. Our analyses may tell us how long to expect the patients to
live and how to stratify the randomization in such a
way as to assure balance on the most important prognostic factors.

SCREENING FOR PROGNOSTIC SIGNIFICANCE

Death Rates

In medical studies, it is common for information to
be collected on a large number of variables of possible prognostic importance. Although each variable
could be examined individually by constructing separate survival curves for each category of the variable
(e.g., male vs. female, or age divided into convenient
categories such as 5-year age groups) and/or computing
appropriate test statistics based on death ranks (14),
we have found it convenient to screen variables by
simply computing death rates and testing these rates
for heterogeneity across categories or, if appropriate, for linear trend. In this context, screening
means choosing for further study those variables for
which differences or trends in death rates across
categories are too great to be attributed to chance
effects. This approach requires that all continuous
variables first be categorized. At the first stage
of analysis, the choice of category boundaries is not
too important and should be dictated by convenience
and the amount of data available. A reasonable first
approach is simply to divide the data into 4 or 5
quantiles, although if the data are very abundant,
more categories might be used. After examining the
death rates in each of these categories, we may decide
to lump adjacent categories if their death rates appear to be similar.

The death rate is defined as the number of deaths
(or other events) divided by the total follow-up time
for all the patients in a group, whether or not they
had an event. This simple old-fashioned idea actually
corresponds to the maximum likelihood estimate of the
scale parameter (hazard) for a simple exponential
model. The data are arranged as in Table 1.

The symbols d_i refer to the number of deaths in the
ith category, but they can also be used to represent
other end points. For example, they could refer to

TABLE 1. Screening Death Rates

Category	Number of patients	Number of deaths	Total months follow-up	Death rate
1	n_1	d_1	t_1	d_1/t_1
2	n_2	d_2	t_2	d_2/t_2
.	.	.	.	.
.	.	.	.	.
.	.	.	.	.
k	n_k	d_k	t_k	d_k/t_k
All categories	N	D	T	D/T

deaths from some specific cause (with deaths from other causes being treated as censored observations), or they could represent some other event entirely, such as development of metastasis. For convenience I shall subsequently refer to all events as deaths. The t_i refer to the total follow-up time for all patients in the ith category, $i=1,2,\ldots,k$. Time can be measured in any units, but it is often convenient to use months of follow-up, perhaps multiplied by some appropriate factor (such as 1000) so that the death rates will have conveniently placed decimal points.

Heterogeneity and Trend Tests for Death Rates

If we assume that survival is exponential in each of the categories, we can use score tests based on the derivatives of the log likelihood evaluated under the null hypothesis to test for heterogeneity and trend. These tests are algebraically simple and may be expressed as functions of the observed numbers of deaths, d_i, and the expected number of deaths, e_i, under the null hypothesis that the k death rates are all equal. The e_i are simply obtained by multiplying the total follow-up time in the ith category by the overall death rate estimated by D/T, where D is the sum of the d_i and T is the sum of t_i. Formally,

$$E(d_i) = e_i = t_i(D/T) . \qquad (1)$$

The test for heterogeneity is given by

$$\chi^2_{k-1} = \sum_{i=1}^{k} (d_i - e_i)^2 / e_i \qquad (2)$$

which is distributed approximately as a chi-square with k-1 degrees of freedom.

When the categories are naturally ordered and we have a set of scores S_i, a test for trend in death rates is appropriate and is given by

$$\chi^2_1 = [\sum_{i=1}^{k} S_i(d_i - e_i)]^2 / \{ \sum_{i=1}^{k} S_i^2 e_i - [(\sum_{i=1}^{k} S_i e_i)^2 / \sum_{i=1}^{k} e_i] \} \qquad (3)$$

which is distributed approximately as a chi-square with one degree of freedom. If we do not have reason to use a particular set of S_i, we may test for a simple linear trend by replacing the S_i's in equation 3 by the consecutive integers i=1,2,...,k.

Since the one degree of freedom chi-square for trend is a formal partition of the k-1 degree of freedom chi-square for heterogeneity, the chi-square for trend will always be less than or equal to that for heterogeneity, and it is easy to show that formulas 2 and 3 give the same result when there are only two categories.

The two tests just described are easy to compute and are useful for screening large numbers of vari-

ables as well as for deciding how to combine categories. As a general principle, we include in multivariate survival models only those variables known be-
forehand to be of particular interest, together with
those variables which have small P-values (say less
than 0.05) when screened in this manner. We do not
take these P-values too seriously, both because of the
multiple comparisons problem and because the tests are
based on the assumption of exponentiality. Even if
the data are not exponentially distributed within categories, these tests are still useful as a general
guide in screening large numbers of variables.

SURVIVAL MODELS INCORPORATING COVARIATES

Although it is possible to miss important variables
by studying them one at a time (because their effects
may be confounded by other variables), it is usually
impractical to try to fit a multivariate model using
all candidate variables without some preliminary
screening unless the number of variables under study
is small, say 15 or fewer. We therefore identify a
group of potentially prognostic variables by using
prior information, constructing survival curves for
various categories of patients, or employing the methods described in the previous section. The next step
is to choose a multivariate survival model in order
to evaluate the effects of these variables when they
are studied simultaneously.

In this section we will review the Cox and Weibull
models, discuss the formation of risk groups, and consider some examples based on real data for cancer patients.

The Cox Model

As mentioned in the "Introduction," the Cox model
(8) may be considered a semiparametric proportional
hazards model. The reasons for these qualifying

adjectives will be clear after examining its mathematical form.

Assume that we have n patients assigned to one of two treatments for whom initial covariate vectors, follow-up time, and survival status are known. Although the Cox model may be used for other purposes as well, we will assume for concreteness in presenting the model that our goal is to compare the two treatments while adjusting for possible imbalances in the initial covariate vectors. Let

t_i = the time of death or censoring for patient i, i=1,2,...,n,

y_i = an indicator variable for treatment for patient i (e.g., y_i=0 for treatment A and y_i=1 for treatment B),

$\underline{X}_i$ = a vector of covariates (adjustment variables) for patient i,

α = a parameter representing treatment effect

$\underline{\beta}$ = a vector of regression coefficients for $\underline{X}$.

The hazard at time t is defined as the conditional probability of death in time period $(t+\Delta t)$ given survival until t and is given, for the ith patient, by

$$h_i(t) = \lambda(t)\exp(\alpha y_i+\underline{\beta}'\underline{X}_i) \ . \tag{4}$$

The factor $\lambda(t)$ represents an arbitrary base-line hazard and is sometimes referred to as the "nuisance hazard" because it need not be specified in order to draw inferences about α and $\underline{\beta}$. Since $\lambda(t)$ is an arbitrary function, we say that the Cox model is only semiparametric. Replacing $\lambda(t)$ by a specified function of time results in a fully parametric model as we shall see later with the Weibull distribution. The parametric aspect of the Cox model is the proportional hazards assumption implied by the fact that in equation 4 the full hazard is the product of the nuisance hazard and a function of the covariates (including treatment). Although the function $\exp(\alpha y+\underline{\beta}'\underline{X})$ is

almost always used in practice because it guarantees
that $h(t) \geq 0$ for all values of α and $\underline{\beta}$, other functions
of the covariates could be used and we would still
have a proportional hazards model. The fundamental
assumption is that the covariates taken together have
the same multiplicative effect on the hazard at all
points in time. (This assumption can be relaxed by
making some or all of the covariates functions of
time, so-called "time-dependent covariates," but that
possibility will not be explored further here.)

Having specified the form of the hazard, we may now
turn to the problem of estimating α and $\underline{\beta}$. A partial
likelihood (9) may be written by considering the ob-
served death times as fixed and arguing along the following lines. If all patients were alike and there
were R_i still at risk (not previously dead or censored) at observed death time t_i, then the probability
of death for the particular patient who died would
simply be $1/R_i$. However, the patients are not all
alike, so we must weight the probability for each patient according to his hazard as given by equation 4.
The probability that the particular patient died is
thus his hazard (obtained by substituting his values
for y_i and $\underline{X}_i$ in equation 4 divided by the sum of the
hazards for himself and the other patients at risk at
t_i. Because the nuisance hazard, $\lambda(t)$, is shared by
all patients, it cancels out of this probability and
the contribution to the partial likelihood at each
distinct death time (when there are no tied death
times) is given by

$$\ell_i = \exp(\alpha y_i + \underline{\beta}'\underline{X}_i) / \sum_{j \epsilon R_i} \exp(\alpha y_j + \underline{\beta}'\underline{X}_j) . \tag{5}$$

The notation $j \epsilon R_i$ means that the summation is taken
over all patients at risk at t_i. No contributions to
the partial likelihood are required at the times of
censored observations, but data for patients with censored observation times enter the denominator of the

contributions at death times for as long as the patients with censored times are still at risk. If
there are d distinct death times and no tied death
times, the partial likelihood is given by the product
of the ℓ_i over those i corresponding to the d distinct
death times. By convention, tied death and censoring
times are resolved by assuming that the deaths occur
first so that the patients with censored times are
still considered to be at risk when the deaths occur.

In the case of tied death times, several approaches
have been suggested, but for practical reasons we prefer the simple approach described in Breslow (1) which
has been shown to be approximately correct if there
are not too many ties and if the multiplicity of
deaths at any one time point is not too great. This
approach amounts to making a contribution to the partial likelihood at each death time, whether they are
distinct or not, and assuming that the risk set is the
same for all tied death times. For example, if 3
deaths occur at some time point, the risk set for each
of the 3 contributions to the partial likelihood consists of those 3 patients plus all others at risk at
that time point.

Having now specified the partial likelihood, we may
estimate the parameters α and $\underline{\beta}$ by the maximum likelihood principle using the Newton-Raphson method. The
covariances of the parameter estimates may be estimated by the inverse of the observed information matrix evaluated at the maximum likelihood estimates of
the parameters.

Generally, it will not be necessary or desirable
to retain all the covariates in the vector $\underline{X}$ in the
final analysis. If the number of covariates is modest, say 15 or fewer, one may begin by fitting with
all of them included, then systematically eliminate
variables that do not contribute substantially to our
ability to predict survival. Such a procedure is referred to as a step-down procedure. Alternatively,
we could begin with the variable we thought was most
significant and progressively add variables in order

of their predictive strength until further additions did not result in substantially improved ability to predict survival. This approach is called a step-up procedure. Mantel (15) has argued that when practicable, step-down procedures may generally be preferred over step-up procedures, especially when some variables may act together. Whatever method is used for adding or deleting variables, a useful way to decide if a variable substantially improves our ability to predict survival in the presence of the other variables in the model is to examine the standardized regression coefficient, defined as $\hat{\theta}/S.E.(\hat{\theta})$ for some general parameter θ. These standardized regression coefficients are asymptotically distributed as normal variates with mean 0 and variance 1. In practice we seldom retain variables whose standardized regression coefficients are less in absolute value than 2.0, corresponding roughly to the 5% critical values for a standard normal deviate.

After we have determined the set of important covariates needed for adjustment, we may draw inferences about the treatment parameter   in several ways, all of which are asymptotically equivalent. We may refer $\hat{\alpha}/S.E.(\hat{\alpha})$ to standard normal tables as described above, we may construct a score test, or we may use likelihood ratio tests. A score test is defined as follows. Let:

D = the vector of first partial derivatives of
    the log likelihood with respect to α and $\underline{\beta}$.
-S = matrix of second partial derivatives of the
    log likelihood with respect to α and $\underline{\beta}$.

Then the score test is given by

$$T = D'(\underline{\hat{\beta}}, \alpha=0)S^{-1}(\underline{\hat{\beta}}, \alpha=0)D(\underline{\hat{\beta}}, \alpha=0) \ , \tag{6}$$

where the notation for T is taken to indicate that D and S are evaluated at their null hypothesis values, $\alpha = 0$ (indicating no treatment effect) and $\underline{\beta} = \underline{\hat{\beta}}$, the maximum likelihood values obtained by fitting the model without the term for treatment. The quadratic form T is distributed asymptotically as a chi-square with one degree of freedom because all the elements of D but one are constrained to be zero due to maximum likelihood estimation of $\underline{\beta}$.

The third method, a likelihood ratio test, is performed by using the asymptotic result that minus twice the difference in the log likelihoods for two nested models is distributed as a chi-squared variate with degrees of freedom equal to the difference in the numbers of parameters fitted in the two models. If we let LL represent a log likelihood, then for comparing our two treatments,

$$\chi_1^2 = -2[LL(0,\underline{\hat{\beta}}) - LL(\hat{\alpha},\underline{\hat{\beta}}*)] \ . \tag{7}$$

In this equation the notation $LL(0,\underline{\hat{\beta}})$ represents the log of the maximized likelihood when the treatment term is omitted, while $LL(\hat{\alpha},\underline{\hat{\beta}}*)$ corresponds to the fit including the term for treatment. Note that in general $\underline{\hat{\beta}} \neq \underline{\hat{\beta}}*$.

Of course, these 3 approaches to inference may also be used to assess the importance of the regression coefficients for the covariates. In the case of more than two treatments, say p, we simply introduce p-1 indicator variables to represent the treatment contrasts and the same methods may be employed with only minor modifications.

Finally, we note that $\exp(\hat{\alpha})$ provides a convenient estimate of the summary relative risk of death over time associated with treatment after adjusting for the covariates in $\underline{X}$. Suppose in our previous notation that treatment A represents placebo ($y_i=0$) and treatment B is some new treatment ($y_i=1$). If $R = \exp(\hat{\alpha})$ is less than 1.0, then the data suggest that B is an effective treatment, especially if $\hat{\alpha}$ is judged significant.

This estimate of relative risk will often be very close numerically to the estimate of the summary relative odds proposed by Mantel and Haenszel (16) and discussed elsewhere in this book.

The Weibull Model

The Weibull survival model to be presented here may be viewed as a fully parametric proportional hazards model. The only change from the Cox model just presented is that we assign a functional form to $\lambda(t)$ in equation 4, namely, $\lambda(t) = \exp(\beta_0)kt^{k-1}$. The factor $\exp(\beta_0)$ represents an intercept parameter needed for the Weibull model, but unnecessary for the Cox model. In practice this parameter is introduced into the model by adding a column of ones to the design matrix formed by the $\underline{X}$ vectors. Since the intercept parameter β_0 is shared by all patients, it may be factored out and viewed as part of the nuisance hazard.

The new parameter k is called the shape parameter of the Weibull distribution because it determines the shape of the survival curve by specifying the change in the base-line hazard as a function of time. Specifically, if k = 1.0 the hazard is constant and the Weibull distribution reduces to the exponential distribution; if k>1.0 the hazard increases in time (positive aging); and if k<1.0 the hazard decreases in time (negative aging). Although the Weibull model provides considerable flexibility in fitting data for groups of cancer patients, this flexibility is limited by the fact that for a given value of k the hazard is a monotone function. This means, for example, that if the data suggest that the hazard first increases and then decreases, or the reverse, the Weibull model will not provide an adequate description of the data and either another parametric form should be sought (e.g., the log-normal or the gamma distributions), or the semiparametric Cox model should be used. Some further advice on selecting parametric survival models is given by Byar (2).

The main advantage of the Weibull model is its simplicity, particularly if we wish to estimate survival curves for specified values of y and $\underline{X}$. Although methods are available for the Cox model, they are somewhat more difficult to understand and to implement.

Using the notation of the previous section (except that $\underline{\beta}$ now includes the intercept β_0 and a 1 has been added as the first element of $\underline{X}$ for each patient as discussed above), we may readily write down explicit expressions for the hazard, the survival curve, and the probability density

$$h(t) = kt^{k-1}\exp(\alpha y + \underline{\beta}'\underline{X}) , \qquad (8)$$

$$S(t) = \exp[-\exp(\alpha y + \underline{\beta}'\underline{X})t^k] , \qquad (9)$$

$$f(t) = h(t)S(t) . \qquad (10)$$

The factor $\exp(\alpha y + \underline{\beta}'\underline{X})$ represents the scale parameter of the Weibull distribution and in our applications has been modeled as a function of the covariates (including treatment). In applications explored thus far we have required that the shape parameter be fitted in common for all patients in a given analysis.

Using the definitions just displayed we can write a full likelihood for right censored data providing that the censoring mechanism is independent of the death process (noninformative censoring). Letting $z_i = 0$ if t_i is a censored time, and $z_i = 1$ if t_i is a death time, the likelihood is given by

$$L = \prod_{i=1}^{n} h_i(t_i)^{z_i} S_i(t_i) . \qquad (11)$$

Subscripts have been added to $h(t)$ and $S(t)$ to indicate that they are obtained by substituting the treatment indicator y_i and the covariate vector $\underline{X}_i$ for the ith patient.

As with the Cox model, the parameters α and $\underline{\beta}$ are estimated by maximum likelihood, and one may make

inferences about the parameters using exactly the same
approaches as those discussed above, that is, standardized regression coefficients, score tests, or likelihood ratio tests. Again, the relative risk for
treatment may be estimated by $\exp(\hat{\alpha})$.

Formation of Risk Groups

After fitting any survival model incorporating covariates it is of interest to use the results of the
analysis to divide patients into groups with varying
degrees of risk of death. First, such an exercise
permits us to examine graphically the fit of the model
by comparing the actuarial or Kaplan-Meier survival
curves for each risk group with the curves predicted
by the model based on the patients' covariates. Second, a plot of survival by risk group is an easily
understood method of describing the extent of variation in survival present in a group of patients under
study. Third, forming risk groups permits examination
of treatment differences separately in groups of patients with varying probabilities of death (which may
often be interpreted as representing different degrees
or types of the same disease). The advantage of having fit a multivariate model is that it helps us combine information for possibly many important prognostic variables in assessing summary risk. The risk
groups we form may also be used as stratifying factors
in the design of new studies or to predict survival
for similar groups of patients.

Although the approach we use in forming risk groups
will work for any survival model incorporating covariates, we will illustrate this simple technique with
the Weibull model. After we have estimated α and β,
we may calculate a "personalized hazard" for each patient by substituting his values of y_i and X_i into
equation 8. Forming risk groups of patients with similar death rates is then just a matter of dividing the
patients into groups on the basis of their fitted hazard values. Although these hazard values change in

time (except for the exponential model), if we have
required that all patients have the same shape parameter k, then the rank ordering of the fitted hazards
for any group of patients is invariant over time (excluding the possibility of time-dependent covariates).

Perhaps the simplest way to form risk groups would
be to sort the individual hazards by their magnitudes
and then arbitrarily define risk groups by the quantiles of this ordered list. There are, however, some
disadvantages with this approach. First, two or more
risk groups may have very similar values of risk so
that the groups are not nicely separated. In addition, some risk groups may contain patients with markedly differing hazards. A more satisfactory method
is to classify the patients according to their predicted survival at some specified point in time based on
the fit of the model. For the Weibull model this may
be readily accomplished by choosing a value of t, letting k = $\hat{k}$, and setting S(t) in equation 9 to a desired survival probability, p_ℓ. Letting c_ℓ represent
$(\alpha y + \underline{\beta}'\underline{X})$ in equation 9, we solve for c_ℓ obtaining

$$c_\ell = \ln(-\ln p_\ell / t^k) \ . \qquad (12)$$

We refer to the values c_ℓ obtained for different survival probabilities as cut-points. In this manner we
define g risk groups by determining g-1 cut-points,
and the values of $\hat{\alpha} y_i + \underline{\hat{\beta}}'\underline{X}_i$ for each patient are compared with each c_ℓ to determine risk group membership.
Generally, it is sufficient to form 3 to 5 risk
groups, depending on the amount of data available, the
number of important prognostic variables, and the extent of variation in observed survival times.

The approach just described could be carried out
for the Cox model, but this would require estimation
of the nuisance survival curve up to time t.

Some Examples Using Cancer Data

To illustrate some of the methods just presented we

TABLE 2. Screening Variables for Thyroid Cancer

Variable	Categories	Number of patients	Number of deaths	Total months follow-up	Death rate (x100)	χ² Heterogeneity (P-value)	χ² Trend (P-value)
Age at diagnosis	<30	91	4	5077.5	0.788		
	31-40	79	9	4176.5	2.155		
	41-50	84	25	3746.0	6.674	244.34 (<.00001)	172.99 (<.00001)
	51-60	87	30	3666.5	8.182		
	61-70	119	69	3637.5	18.969		
	>70	47	38	933.5	40.707		
Sex	Female	342	103	15428.0	6.676	16.74 (.0005)	
	Male	165	72	5809.5	12.393		
Cell type[a]	Anaplastic	77	68	760.5	89.415	644.10 (<.00001)	340.38 (<.00001)
	MED or FLD	121	45	4769.5	9.435		
	All other	309	62	15707.5	3.947		
Tumor	Not extended	401	106	18242.5	5.811	92.66 (<.00001)	
	Extended	106	69	2995.0	23.038		
Metastatic sites	None	421	122	19041.5	6.407	149.87 (<.00001)	98.41 (<.00001)
	Single	78	46	2142.0	21.475		
	Multiple	8	7	54.0	129.630		
All patients	--	507	175	--	8.240	--	--

[a]MED, principal cell type is medullary; FLD, principal cell type is follicular less-differentiated. Mixed tumors having any anaplastic component are classified as such.

will consider a set of data for 507 patients with his-
tologically diagnosed carcinoma of the thyroid gland
(5). Since the data were collected for a registry
rather than in a randomized clinical trial, treatment
comparisons were not attempted. Of many variables
studied, those which showed prognostic importance when
screened using death rates are shown in Table 2, arranged in a format like that in Table 1. These variables were then entered into both Weibull and Cox regression models. Age at diagnosis was treated as a
continuous covariate, 0-1 indicator variables were
used to represent sex and tumor extension, a 3-level
variable was used for metastatic sites (0=none, 1=sin-
gle site, and 2=multiple sites), and cell type was
coded as two separate 0-1 variables. The results of
fitting the two models are given in Table 3. The sim-
ilarity of the two fits is remarkable, and it is clear
that the same conclusions would have been reached from

TABLE 3. Comparison of Weibull and Cox Models

Variable	Weibull model		Cox model	
	$\hat{\beta}$	$\hat{\beta}$/S.E.	$\hat{\beta}$	$\hat{\beta}$/S.E.
Sex	0.55865	3.5573	0.52295	3.3266
Age	0.04585	7.5013	0.04439	7.2826
Anaplasia	2.04890	10.3700	1.92250	9.4446
FLD–MED	0.47858	2.4055	0.47010	2.3583
Tumor	0.47704	2.8470	0.45506	2.6840
Met sites	0.67901	4.9541	0.60420	4.4063
Intercept	-7.40150	-17.0430	--	--
Shape[a]	0.80593	4.0505	--	--
LL	-812.1431		-877.7599	

[a]For this parameter we test $(\hat{k}-1.0)$/S.E. rather than
$\hat{k}$/S.E.

either analysis. On the basis of the Weibull fit a
prognostic index for thyroid cancer was proposed
(Table 4). Here for simplicity the Weibull regression

TABLE 4. Proposed Prognostic Index for Thyroid
Carcinoma

Age at diagnosis (in years)
+12 if male
+10 if cell type is medullary or follicular
    less-differentiated
+45 if cell type is anaplastic
+10 if tumor is extended
+15 if there is at least one distant metastatic
    site
+15 in addition to above if there are multiple
    distant metastatic sites

Total score

---

coefficients were divided by the smallest (that for
age) and rounded to the nearest integer. Cut-points
were calculated corresponding to predicted survival
at 3 years of 90, 80, 60, and 20%, allowing the 507
patients in the study to be divided into 5 risk
groups. The survival curves predicted by the model
and actuarial survival curves for the same groups of
patients (Figure 1) demonstrated that the model provides a reasonable fit to the observed data. The sep-
aration of the risk groups is very striking; in the
best risk group there is almost negligible mortality,
while in the worst (where 94% of the patients had anaplastic tumors), mortality was extremely high. Additional insight into the behavior of a disease is often
provided by tabulating the average characteristics of
patients in the various risk groups (for examples of

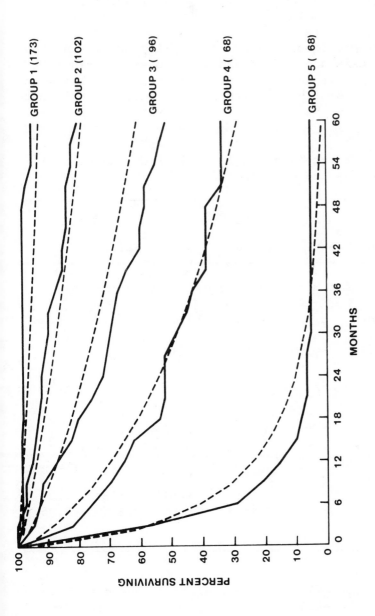

Figure 1. Survival curves predicted by the Weibull model (---) and actuarial survival curves (——) for 5 risk groups of patients with thyroid carcinoma. Numbers of patients shown in parentheses.

383

such tabulations, see references 5, 7, and 17).

Although here the Weibull and Cox analyses were quite similar, this need not always be the case. The Cox model provides greater flexibility in fitting the nuisance hazard and, because it is based on ranks of death times, it is robust with respect to outliers in survival time. The disastrous effect of a single outlier in the Weibull model is illustrated in Table 5.

TABLE 5. Effect of a Single Outlier on the Weibull Model versus the Cox Model

Variable	Coefficient	Weibull Value	Weibull Z	Cox Value	Cox Z
Original fit with one t_i coded as 9999 (N=239)					
Intercept	β_0	-1.5815	-10.05		
Age (0,1,2,3)	β_1	0.1027	1.38	0.2913	4.14
Cell type (0,1)	β_2	-0.1054	-0.66	-0.4495	-2.88
Shape parameter	k	0.5325	-21.07		
Refitted with the outlier removed (N=238)					
Intercept	β_0	-2.7713	-13.04		
Age	β_1	0.3436	4.90	0.3064	4.37
Cell type	β_2	-0.4963	-3.16	-0.4450	-2.85
Shape	k	1.0306	0.52		

(The outlying value was in reality an unknown value code that had escaped notice.) Neither of the two variables studied, age and cell type, was significant in the presence of the outlier, and the shape parameter appeared to be wildly significant compared to the value k = 1.0 for an exponential distribution. The results for the Weibull model after removing the single outlier were markedly different. On the other hand, the two fits for the Cox model were quite similar and were little affected by the outlying survival time. This example is not meant to indicate that the Cox model is better than the Weibull model, but only that care is required in fitting and interpreting parametric models.

We close this section by displaying log survival plots (Figure 2) for risk groups based on fitting the Weibull model for 3 other sets of data [prostate (4), lung (7), and brain (17) cancer] along with a similar plot for the thyroid cancer (Table 2) data. These log survival plots are useful for model selection because, if the survival curves generally plot as straight lines or monotonically increasing or decreasing lines, then the Weibull model may provide an adequate description of the data. We would regard all 4 fits as quite reasonable because we see no systematic deviations between the actuarial and predicted curves. The estimated values for the shape parameters in these 4 examples were 0.806 for the thyroid cancer data, 1.0 for the prostatic cancer data, 1.34 for the lung cancer data, and 1.45 for the brain cancer (malignant glioma) data.

These 4 data sets were not chosen because the Weibull model happened to provide an adequate description of the data; they were simply 4 recent analyses we have performed on reasonably large sets of data with important prognostic factors. The data for prostate, lung, and brain cancer were obtained in randomized clinical trials. For all of these data sets parallel analyses using the Cox model produced very similar results. The observations in this paragraph are meant to suggest that the Weibull model is sufficiently flexible to provide a generally useful tool for analyzing sets of cancer data and that it should not be

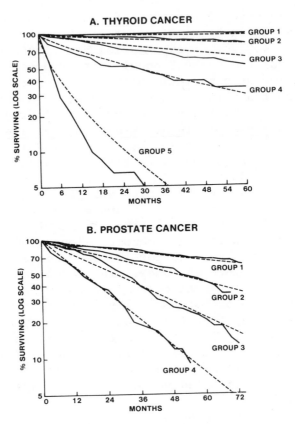

Figure 2 (A-D). Log survival curves predicted by the Weibull model (---) and log actuarial survival curves (——) for risk groups of patients with cancer at 4 different sites: (A) thyroid cancer, (B) prostate cancer, (C) lung cancer, and (D) brain cancer (malignant glioma). Reprinted, in part, by permission of The New England Journal of Medicine, 303: 1328, (1980) (17) .

viewed as a specialized parametric model of limited usefulness.

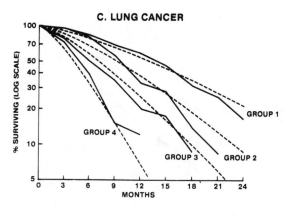

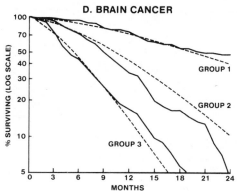

Figure 2 (A-D). (continued)

FITTING INTERACTION TERMS

Interaction terms are needed in regression models whenever the effect of one or more variables on the response depends on the value of one or more other variables. Such interactions may be of two general types: _quantitative_ or _qualitative_. A quantitative interaction is one where the effect on response of a given variable depends on the value of another variable, but only the magnitude of the effect, not its

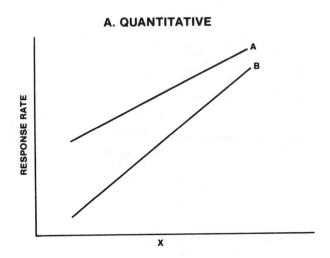

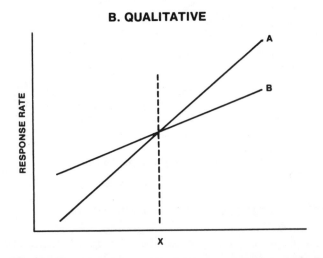

Figure 3. Diagrammatic representation of two types of interactions: (A) quantitative, and (B) qualitative.

sign, is affected. A qualitative interaction, on the other hand, is one in which the sign of the effect of a variable depends on the level of another variable.

These concepts are illustrated in Figure 3 where the
two variables having an interaction are treatment
(represented by two lines labeled A and B) and a single covariate X. In Figure 3A we notice that the difference in response rate for the two treatments depends on the value of X, but the sign is always the
same since treatment A always has the higher response
rate. We therefore call this a quantitative interaction. In Figure 3B, however, the sign of the difference between treatments in response rate depends on
X, so this is a qualitative interaction.

Quantitative interactions are quite commonly encountered in data for treatment of cancer patients.
For example, a treatment for breast cancer may be more
effective in premenopausal than in postmenopausal
women, or a treatment for lung cancer may be more effective for some histologic types than others. Qualitative interactions appear to be less common, but
when present they are important to detect, especially
if they are treatment-covariate interactions, because
they may imply that some patients may benefit by a
treatment that might be harmful for other patients.
We will return to this point after presenting a convenient method for routinely examining sets of data
for significant interactions. When I have asked experienced data analysts if they often encounter important interactions in their analyses, the usual answer
is no. When I ask further if they routinely look for
them, the answer is again usually no. It is no surprise that one seldom finds interactions if one does
not look for them!

The reason that interactions are seldom examined
routinely is that there are potentially too many of
them. Suppose that we have p variables in a regression model. If we model the interactions as products
of all pairs of variates, then there are $p(p-1)/2$ new
terms to be fitted in addition to the main effects,
and even for modest p this can be an unwieldy number
of terms. For example, with $p = 6$, we would need 22
terms in our model if we include all interactions and

main effects plus an intercept. In addition, we would
for most existing computer programs have to augment
the design matrix to fit these extra terms, a lot of
work for so little expected gain. A reasonable way of
avoiding all this extra work and still looking for
important interactions is provided by computing score
tests based on the fit of a model containing only the
main effects. This approach will involve very little
extra calculation and will not require augmentation
of the design matrix.

Suppose we have just fit a model on $\underline{X} = (1, X_1, X_2,$
$\ldots, X_p)$ and we wish to see if another variable $f(\underline{X})$
might be needed in addition to those already in the
model. The new variable $f(\underline{X})$ is a function of one or
more of the elements of $\underline{X}$, such as $X_1 X_2$ or X_3^2. Let

> $\hat{\underline{\beta}}$ = the maximum likelihood regression
> coefficients for $\underline{X}$,
> γ = the regression coefficient for the
> new variable $f(\underline{X})$.

Define

> D = vector of first partial derivatives of the log
> likelihood (LL) with respect to $\underline{\beta}$ and γ,
> $-S$ = matrix of second partial derivatives of the log
> likelihood (LL) with respect to $\underline{\beta}$ and γ.

The score test for the hypothesis that $\gamma = 0$ is given
by the quadratic form

$$Q = D'(\hat{\underline{\beta}}, \gamma=0) S^{-1}(\hat{\underline{\beta}}, \gamma=0) D(\hat{\underline{\beta}}, \gamma=0) \ , \tag{13}$$

where the notation in parentheses indicates that D
and S are evaluated at $\underline{\beta} = \hat{\underline{\beta}}$ and $\gamma = 0$. Q is distributed as a chi-square variate with one degree of free-
dom.

Equation 13 is much easier to compute than it may
appear because if we partition S as shown in Table 6,

TABLE 6. Partitioning of S

	β_0 • • • • • β_p	γ
β_0		
•		
•	R_{11}	R_{12}
•		
β_p		
γ	R_{21}	R_{22}

then

$$Q = (\partial \, LL/\partial\gamma)^2 / (\partial^2 \, LL/\partial\gamma^2 - R_{21}R_{11}^{-1}R_{12}) \, . \quad (14)$$

The great simplification in equation 14 results from the fact that all the elements of D except that for ($\partial \, LL/\partial\gamma$) are equal to zero due to the maximum likelihood estimation of $\underline{\beta}$. In addition, R_{11}^{-1} will already have been obtained in estimating the covariance matrix for $\underline{\hat{\beta}}$, so little extra computation is involved.

Although the approach just presented is valid for any $f(\underline{X})$, we may confine our attention to the single function $f(\underline{X})=X_iX_j$, $i,j=1,...,p$, which allows us to examine (one at a time) the effects of adding all squared terms and two-way product interactions. We may ask our computer program to print only those values of Q exceeding some interesting prespecified value which should depend on the number of main effects in the model and an appreciation of the high probability of obtaining spurious significance at the usual levels for Type I error when making multiple comparisons.

Unfortunately, the test just described cannot distinguish between quantitative and qualitative interactions, and tests capable of this discrimination do not appear to have been developed. The approach is thus first to find convincingly significant interactions and then to examine the data in other ways to find out if they are quantitative or qualitative.

Admittedly, the routine examination of data for interactions belongs more to the area of exploratory data analysis than to formal hypothesis testing because we do not really have prespecified null and alternative hypotheses in mind, we are unsure about the P-values of our results, and we are simply exploring the data for possibly meaningful patterns that might be missed by classical hypothesis testing. For this reason we should regard the results of such analyses as suggestive rather than conclusive. Important results found in this way should be confirmed in other sets of data before they may be believed.

Earlier in this section I pointed out that qualitative treatment-covariate interactions play an especially important role because of their possible implications for the care of patients. When they are present we may speak of an optimal treatment or treatment of choice (2), meaning that our analysis suggests that some patients with a given diagnosis should be treated in one way, but that other patients with the same diagnosis should be treated another way. This means that the choice of treatment depends on the characteristics of the patient. Such a situation is particularly likely to occur if a treatment has a genuine effect on a disease, but has associated toxicity that may outweigh its benefits for some categories of patients.

An example of the treatment of choice concept is provided by a randomized clinical trial of estrogen therapy versus placebo for patients with stage III (local extension) and IV (distant metastases) prostatic cancer (3,4). An earlier study had shown that although an oral dose of 5 mg per day of the synthetic estrogen diethylstilbestrol (DES) had a definite effect on prostatic cancer, its advantages were nulli-

fied by excess cardiovascular mortality in the group
of patients treated with estrogen. In the second
study patients were randomized to placebo or to 0.2,
1.0, or 5.0 mg of DES daily and information relative
to cardiovascular status was collected. Preliminary
analysis showed that the 1.0 and 5.0 mg doses of DES
had similar effects on the cancer and that the 0.2
dose behaved very much like placebo. For this reason
in the analysis I shall present, P refers to the placebo and 0.2 mg DES groups combined (241 patients)
while E refers to the two groups randomized to 1.0 and
5.0 mg of DES daily (242 patients).

An additive exponential survival model (6) was fit
which included a 0-1 indicator for treatment (0=P,
1=E) and 6 pretreatment covariates defined in Table 7.
The response variable was time to death from any
cause. Score tests suggested that stage-grade category and age at diagnosis interacted with treatment,
so these two interactions were added to the design
matrix. The results of the fit for the full model
(Table 8) indicated that the two interaction terms
showed borderline significance in the presence of the
other variables. Note that two of the main effects
involved in the interactions (RX and AG) are not significant. This does not mean that they should be removed from the model because interaction terms cannot
be sensibly interpreted if they are fit in the absence
of their main effects. Fitting interactions without
their main effects is analogous to fitting simple linear regression without an intercept and can lead to
serious misinterpretations.

Dividing the patients into 4 risk groups and plotting the curves predicted by the model versus the actuarial curves for the same groups of patients showed
that the model provided a good description of the data. Loosely speaking, the interpretation of the two
interaction terms is that patients with tumor in the
high stage-grade category should be treated with E
while those of age 75 or more should be treated with
P. A formal decision about the "best" treatment for

TABLE 7. Definitions of Prognostic Variables for Prostatic Cancer

Variable	Symbol	Value	Definitions of the categories
Hemoglobin	HG	0	≥12.0g/100ml
		1	9.0-11.9g/100ml
		2	<9.0g/100ml
Performance status	PF	0	Normal
		1	Limitation of activity
History of cardiovascular disease	HX	0	No
		1	Yes
Gleason stage-grade category	SG	0	≤10
		1	>10
Age at diagnosis	AG	0	≤74 years
		1	75-79 years
		2	≥80 years
Size of primary lesion	SZ	0	$<30 \ cm^2$
		1	$≥30 \ cm^2$

each patient can be made by computing the hazard for each patient both for the treatment he received and for the opposite treatment. His treatment of choice is defined as that associated with the lower hazard. If the treatment of choice for all patients is the same, we conclude that the interactions are only quantitative; if they are not all the same, then we have some evidence for a qualitative interaction, although formally assessing its statistical significance is a

TABLE 8. Final Model with Six Main Effects and Two
Interaction Terms for Prostate Cancer Data

Variable	Regression coefficient[a]	t-value[b]	P-value[c]
Intercept	8.790	4.75	<.0001
HG	8.337	2.71	.0067
PF	11.692	1.98	.0477
HX	9.863	4.48	<.0001
SG	13.433	3.92	<.0001
AG	0.804	0.28	.7794
SZ	17.820	3.19	.0014
RX[d]	-3.105	-1.37	.1707
RX-SG	-8.447	-2.00	.0455
RX-AG	9.975	2.45	.0143

[a]Expressed in deaths per 1000 patient-months.
[b]The t-values are equal to the regression coefficients divided by their estimated standard errors.
[c]All P-values are two-tailed.
[d]RX stands for treatment group. Treatment P was
coded as 0 and treatment E was coded as 1.

currently unresolved problem.
     For this set of data the interactions appeared to
be qualitative, so patients were divided into two
groups according to their optimal treatment and within
each group survival curves were compared according to
the treatments to which the patients had actually been
randomly assigned in order to examine the magnitude
of the interaction. In Figure 4A we see the survival
curves for all patients along with the two-tailed P-
values for the Mantel-Haenszel (MH) and Gehan (G)
tests. Neither test indicates a significant difference in the two curves at P=0.05. In Figure 4B the
comparison of treatments is confined to patients whose

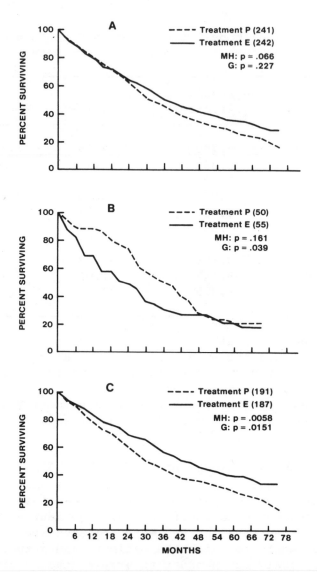

Figure 4. Actuarial survival curves for all causes of death combined with P-values for the Mantel-Haenszel (MH) and Gehan (G) tests. Numbers of patients shown in parentheses. (A) All patients. (B) Patients whose optimal treatment was P. (C) Patients whose optimal treatment was E.

optimal treatment was placebo and of course the placebo group appears to show superior survival. The reverse is true in Figure 4C where treatments are compared for patients whose optimal treatment was E. The P-values quoted in Figures 4B and 4C are of course not valid (they are much too small) because of the biased way in which the groups were formed, but if they were not significant given this bias, we would have to conclude that the qualitative interactions could not be very important. At the risk of overinterpretation we may note that the shapes of the survival curves in Figures 4B and 4C are those we might expect to see if the benefit of estrogen therapy takes a while to appear but continues thereafter, while its undesirable effects appear early. It was in fact known from the previous study that almost all the excess cardiovascular mortality due to estrogen occurred in the first year after treatment was begun.

Although we used only deaths from all causes in our analysis, if our interpretation of the interaction effects is correct, we would expect to see an excess of cardiovascular deaths among patients treated with E whose optimal treatment was P, and an excess of deaths due to prostatic cancer among patients treated with P whose optimal treatment was E. The results in Table 9 provide some confirmation of these expectations, 16 versus 26 cardiovascular deaths in the P and E groups, respectively, for optimal treatment P, and 72 versus 43 cancer deaths for P and E, respectively, among patients whose optimal treatment was E.

CONCLUSIONS

In this chapter I have described simple and practical methods for examining variables for prognostic significance and reviewed why it is important to identify prognostic variables and use them in the design and analysis of cancer studies. We have seen how the Cox and Weibull models may be used to examine the ef-

TABLE 9. Cause of Death by Actual and Optimal Treatment

Optimal treatment:	P		E	
Actual treatment:	P	E	P	E
Alive	11	10	46	72
Dead				
Prostatic cancer	5	5	72	43
Cardiovascular	16	26	45	52
Other causes	18	14	28	20
All patients	50	55	191	187

fects of these variables when they act jointly and I have discussed the detection and interpretation of important interaction terms. The successful implementation of the techniques suggested often depends on many specific decisions about matters such as how reliable the data are, how variables should be coded, and what biases might exist in the data. These matters, while extremely important, have not been dealt with here because they depend heavily on the details of any particular study. The biostatistician can best avoid erroneous analyses and overinterpretation by learning as much as possible about the disease under study through wide reading and talking with substantive experts. With this caveat in mind, the analysis of survival data in heterogeneous populations presents an exciting challenge to the biostatistician, and his methodologic skill may permit him to contribute meaningfully to our growing knowledge about factors that affect the outcome for cancer patients and about the effects of treatment. The rapid and continuing methodologic progress in this field of biostatistics has enabled us to answer a much wider range of questions posed by our physician collaborators than was possible before.

REFERENCES

1. Breslow, N. E. (1975), Analysis of survival data under the proportional hazards model, International Statistical Review 43: 45-57.

2. Byar, D. P. (1977), Analysis of survival data in heterogeneous populations, in: Barra, J. R., et al., eds., Recent Developments in Statistics, North-Holland, Amsterdam.

3. Byar, D. P., and Corle, D. K. (1977), Selecting optimal treatment in clinical trials using covariate information, Journal of Chronic Diseases 30: 445-459.

4. Byar, D. P., and Green, S. B. (1980), The choice of treatment for cancer patients based on covariate information: Application to prostate cancer, Bulletin du Cancer (Paris) 67: 477-490.

5. Byar, D. P., Green, S. B., Dor, P., Williams, E. D., Colon, J., van Gilse, H. A., Mayer, M., Sylvester, R. J., and Van Glabbeke, M. (1979), A prognostic index for thyroid carcinoma. A study of the EORTC Thyroid Cancer Cooperative Group, European Journal of Cancer 15: 1033-1041.

6. Byar, D. P., Huse, R., Bailar, J. C. III, and the Veterans Administration Cooperative Urological Research Group (1974), An exponential model relating censored survival data and concomitant information for prostate cancer patients, Journal of the National Cancer Institute 52: 321-326.

7. Byar, D., Kenis, Y., Van Andel, J. G., de Jong, M., Laval, P., Marion, L., Couette, J. E., and Longueville, J. (1978), Results of an E.O.R.T.C. randomized trial of cyclophosphamide and radiotherapy in inoperable lung cancer: Prognostic factors and treatment results, European Journal of Cancer 14: 919-930.

8. Cox, D. R. (1972), Regression models and life tables, Journal of the Royal Statistical Society, Series B, 34: 187-202.

9. Cox, D. R. (1975), Partial likelihood, Biometrika 62: 269-276.

10. Feigl, P., and Zelen, M. (1965), Estimation of exponential survival probabilities with concomitant information, Biometrics 21: 826-838.

11. Glasser, M. (1967), Exponential survival with covariance, Journal of the American Statistical Association 62: 561-568.

12. Kalbfleisch, J. D., and Prentice, R. L. (1980), The Statistical Analysis of Failure Time Data, Wiley, New York.

13. Lee, E. T. (1980), Statistical Methods for Survival Data Analysis, Lifetime Learning Publications, Belmont, California.

14. Mantel, N. (1966), Evaluation of survival data and two new rank order statistics arising in its consideration, Cancer Chemotherapy Reports 50: 163-170.

15. Mantel, N. (1970), Why stepdown procedures in variable selection? Technometrics 12: 621-625.

16. Mantel, N., and Haenszel, W. (1959), Statistical aspects of the analysis of data from retrospective studies of disease, Journal of the National Cancer Institute 22: 719-748.

17. Walker, M. D., Green, S. B., Byar, D. P., Alexander, E., Jr., Batzdorf, U., Brooks, W. H., Hunt, W. D., MacCarty, C. S., Mahaley, M. S., Mealey, J., Owens, G., Ransohoff, J., II, Robertson, J. T., Shapiro, W. R., Smith, K. R., Wilson,, C. B., and Strike, T. A. (1980), Randomized comparisons of radiotherapy and nitrosourea for the treatment of malignant glioma after surgery, The New England Journal of Medicine 303: 1323-1329.

18. Zippin, C., and Armitage, P. (1971), Use of concomitant variables and incomplete survival information in the estimation of an exponential survival parameter, Biometrics 22: 665-672.

CHAPTER 13
Analysis of Categorical Data: Exact Tests and Log-Linear Models

THOMAS A. LOUIS

INTRODUCTION

Whenever some or all of the components of multi-variate data are categorical, statistical analysis based on discrete data methods is appropriate and powerful. This chapter identifies some of the principal methods, provides examples of their use, and lists additional techniques, with the goals of showing the virtues and drawbacks of log-linear models for discrete data. Important, recent work is in the bibliography. A good background in the subject is provided by Fienberg (6), Gart (7), and Goodman (8), with more advanced topics and detailed examples contained in Bishop, et al. (2), Cox (4), and Haberman (10).

We start by discussing analysis of a 2x2 contingency table, illustrating basic descriptive and inferential concepts, including analysis using exact probability distributions. We then discuss a 3-way table, introducing the Mantel-Haenszel test, and techniques for combining evidence. This discussion leads to an example of the dangers of pooling data.

From this basis we move to a discussion of the characteristics of the log-linear representation, and analysis of residuals from models to assess fit and identify outliers. Two special topics, random effects and Bradley-Terry models, conclude the technical discussion.

THE 2x2 TABLE

Consider some typical data displayed in a 2x2 array, as shown in Table 1. This table displays the

TABLE 1. Smoking for Husbands and Wives for 200 Couples

| | | Wife | | Husband |
		Smoker	Nonsmoker	marginal
Husband	Smoker	54	44	98
	Nonsmoker	36	66	102
	Wife marginal	90	110	200

joint frequency distribution of husband's and wife's smoking status, where, for example, 54 indicates that in 54 of the 200 couples both husband and wife are smokers. By adding across rows we can find the marginal distributions for husbands (98 of 200 smoke) and by adding down columns we find the marginal for wives (90 of 200 smoke).

Our goal is to study the relationship between husband's and wife's smoking status, where the relationship is characterized by the underlying probability distribution: $P_{ij} = P(\text{row } i, \text{ column } j)$. For example, P_{11} is the probability that both husband and wife smoke and we could estimate it by $\hat{P}_{11} = .27$ (54/200).

The two factors are statistically independent if knowledge of one does not change the probability distribution of the other. (That is, the conditional probability distribution of one factor given the other is the same as the marginal distribution of the first factor.) In terms of the underlying probability distribution, if all $P_{ij} > 0$, then the probability that the husband smokes given that the wife smokes is

$$P_{i|j} = P_{ij}/P_{+j} = P_{i+} \quad \text{for all } (i,j) ,$$

$$P_{j|i} = P_{ij}/P_{i+} = P_{+j} \quad \text{for all } (i,j) ,$$

where

$$P_{+j} = \sum_{i=1}^{2} P_{ij} , \text{ etc.}$$

For example, in our table, the observed frequencies indicate that

$$P(\text{husband smokes} | \text{wife smokes}) = \frac{54}{90} = .60$$

which is not equal to the marginal

$$P(\text{husband smokes}) = .49 \ (98/200) .$$

Therefore, husband's and wife's smoking status appear to be associated, with the likelihood of the husband's smoking increasing for wives who smoke. If the observed frequencies accurately reflected the true, underlying probability model, this would say that the variables are statistically dependent. For these data we must assess the strength of evidence.

To avoid the asymmetry in the definition of statistical independence through conditional probabilities and the problem of dividing by zero, independence is defined by

$$P_{ij} = P_{i+} \cdot P_{+j} , \quad \text{all } (i,j) .$$

This definition applies to two-way tables of arbitrary
size (IxJ), and provides the basis for log-linear
analysis. If a cell probability can be computed as
the product of marginals, then its logarithm will be
the sum of the logarithms of the marginal probabilities. Generally, in analogy with the two-way ANOVA,
we can write a saturated model

$$Y_{ij} = \ln P_{ij} = U + U_1(i) + U_2(j) + U_{12}(i,j)$$

$$= Y.. + (Y_i.-Y..) + (Y._j-Y..)$$

$$+ (Y_{ij}-Y_i.-Y._j+Y..) \; , \qquad (1)$$

where, for I rows and J columns,

$$Y_{ij} = \ln P_{ij}, \; i=1,\ldots,I, \; j=1,\ldots,J \; ,$$

$$Y_i. = \frac{1}{J} \sum_{i=1}^{J} Y_{ij} = \frac{1}{J}Y_{i+} \; ,$$

U constrains the sum of the table probabilities,
$U_1(i)$ represents the effect of the ith row,
$U_2(j)$ represents the effect of the jth column, and
$U_{12}(i,j)$ measures dependence: $U_{12}(i,j) \equiv 0$ is equiv-
            alent to independence between rows and col-
            umns.

This model guarantees that all P_{ij} are in the interval [0,1] and add to 1. These goals are accomplished with the same constraints on the subscripted
U-terms as in the usual ANOVA:

$$U_1(+) = U_2(+) = U_{12}(i,+) = U_{21}(+,j) = 0 \; ,$$

where

$$U_1(+) = \sum_{i=1}^{I} U_1(i) \; , \text{ etc.}$$

For the general IxJ table, the degrees of freedom partition:

$$IJ = 1 + (I-1) + (J-1) + (I-1)(J-1) .$$

Note that when the two factors (husband's smoking status, wife's smoking status) are statistically independent,

$$P_{ij} = P_{i+} \cdot P_{+j} .$$

Therefore, in the log scale, the no-interaction model ($U_{12} \equiv 0$), is equivalent to independence. Conceptual justification of log-linear models is based primarily on this equivalence between independence and the standard, no-interaction model.

For Table 1, using equation 1, we can estimate the U's by

$$\hat{U} = -1.4117, \quad \hat{U}_1(1) = 0, \quad \hat{U}_2(1) = -.10035,$$

$$\hat{U}_{12}(1,1) = .2027$$

$$= \frac{1}{4} \ln \left| \frac{54 \cdot 66}{36 \cdot 44} \right| = \frac{1}{4} \ln \hat{\lambda} ,$$

where λ is the odds ratio (sometimes called the cross-product ratio). $U_{12} > 0$ indicates a positive association. Note that U_{12} depends only on the ratio of frequencies, and remains unchanged by multiplying a column or a row by a constant.

We can present the data of Table 1 in another form:

		Wife		
		Smoker	Nonsmoker	
Husband	Same	54	66	120
	Different	36	44	80
		90	110	200

and obtain the parameter estimates

$\hat{U} = -1.4117$, $\hat{U}_1(1) = .2027$, $\hat{U}_2(1) = -.10035$,

$\hat{U}_{12}(1,1) = 0$ (no association) .

By presenting the data in this manner, wife's smoking status and whether or not the husband's status is the same or different appear to be statistically independent. The ensemble of values for subscripted U-terms is the same, but they play different roles. Generally, each subscripted U-term is the "interaction" term for a rearranged table. These rearrangements can produce the analogue of a principal components decomposition into independent factors (see reference 6).

TESTING AND CONFIDENCE INTERVALS (ASYMPTOTIC METHODS)

From the definition of U_{12} in the 2x2 case (using asymptotic theory for logarithms of Poisson variables) with observed frequencies X_{ij}, we can estimate the variance of $\hat{U}_{12}(1,1)$ by

$$(S.E.)^2 = 1/16 \sum_{ij}\sum \frac{1}{X_{ij}+.5} .$$

Therefore, $Z = \hat{U}_{12}/S.E.$ can be used to test H_0: $U_{12}=0$, and produce a confidence interval (95%, say):

$$\hat{U}_{12} \pm 1.96 \ S.E.$$

A confidence interval for the odds ratio is obtained by transforming back to the original scale $[\lambda=\exp(4U)]$. For example, consider the original data from the previous section. The standard error is estimated by .0722, and we obtain a Z-score of 2.81 (.2027/.0722), significant at $P\cong.005$ for a two-sided test. This analysis indicates that married couples' smoking habits are positively related. In addition, husband and wife smoking rates are similar (49% versus 45%). Equality of these rates can be tested directly or by comparing the off-diagonal frequencies (36 and 44) under a model where they represent successes and failures in 80 Bernoulli trials with success probability equal to $\frac{1}{2}$. This latter is McNemar's test, and is the analogue of a paired t-test for Gaussian data.

As another example consider these typical data from a case-control study, where the statistical properties of $\hat{U}_{12}$ are the same as before even though the column totals are fixed by the design of the study.

TABLE 2. Case-Control Data (Comparing Two Binomials)

	Controls	Lung cancer
Smoker	32	60
	(74%)	(95%)
Nonsmoker	11	3
	43	63

Here $\hat{U}_{12} = \frac{1}{4} \ln (.1455) = -.482$ (negative association between smoking and <u>lack</u> of lung cancer)

S.E. = .1620, Z = -2.98, P = .003, two-tailed .

Therefore, we obtain the 95% confidence interval for U_{12} and the odds ratio λ:

U_{12}	λ
(-.800,-.164)	(.041,.519)

Note that the confidence interval for λ is asymmetric.

Three additional asymptotically equivalent approaches to inference can be formulated as follows:

1. Set $U_{12}(i,j) \equiv 0$ (independence: $P_{ij} = P_{i+} \cdot P_{+j}$)

2. Estimate the expected frequencies m_{ij} under this model, by

$$m_{ij} = \frac{X_{i+} \cdot X_{+j}}{X_{++}} = \hat{P}_{i+} \cdot \hat{P}_{+j} \cdot X_{++} \; .$$

Note that under independence

$$P_{ij} = \exp[U_1^* + U^*(i) + U_2^*(j)] \; ,$$

where the U*'s do not necessarily equal the U's as defined for the saturated model.

3. Compute a distance between observed and expected.

Pearson: $$\sum\sum \left[\frac{(X_{ij} - m_{ij})}{\sqrt{m_{ij}}} \right]^2$$

Freeman-Tukey: $\sum\sum (\sqrt{X_{ij}} + \sqrt{X_{ij}+1} - \sqrt{4m_{ij}+1})^2$

Likelihood (G^2): $2\sum\sum X_{ij} \cdot \ln (X_{ij}/m_{ij}) \; .$

Under H_0, as the table total goes to infinity and if the data are generated by either Poisson, multi-nomial, or product multinomial models, these statistics all converge in distribution to a chi-square variable with degrees of freedom $(I-1)(J-1)$.

Steps 1, 2, and 3 comprise a general strategy. Usually the expected frequencies must be estimated by numeric iteration (see Appendix). The 3 distance measures all behave identically (asymptotically) under the null hypothesis, and the Pearson and Freeman-Tukey measures are essentially equivalent. The likelihood G^2 is in a logarithmic scale (percentage change) and has different power under models where the two factors are dependent. It is produced by the generalized likelihood ratio test and is recommended for use in the step-up and step-down procedures referenced in the sequel.

For our example, the m_{ij} are

	Controls	Lung cancer
Smoker	37.3	54.7
Nonsmoker	5.7	8.3

and we have 5 chi-square tests of the null hypothesis of no association:

Test statistic	χ^2	P-value
Pearson	9.58	.002
Pearson (Yates correction)	7.85	.005
Freeman-Tukey	9.36	.002
G^2	9.65	.002
$[\hat{U}_{12}(1,1)/S.E.]^2$	8.85	.003
Fisher's exact	–	.002

One should remember that the value of the chi-square statistic is affected both by the pattern of observed relative frequencies and the total sample size. In fact, for a given pattern, the statistic is proportional to the sample size and will go up by a factor of 10, for example, if all frequencies are multiplied by 10.

Exact Tests

The Fisher exact test for a 2x2 table is derived by conditioning on the row and column margins. This conditioning, whether for the exact or asymptotic tests, is a consequence of the mathematical model for the data. Similar conditioning on so-called reference sets occurs in more complicated settings (4,21).

To derive the 2x2 exact test, consider a case where the column totals N_1, N_2 are fixed (the derivation is similar if only the table total is fixed):

Data		True column probabilities		
X_{11}	X_{12}	P_{11}	P_{12}	
X_{21}	X_{22}	P_{21}	P_{22}	$P_{i+} = 1$
N_1	N_2			

Then, using standard conditioning arguments we have

$$P(X_{11}=x \mid N_1, N_2, X_{11}+X_{12}=S)$$

$$= \frac{\binom{N_1}{x}\binom{N_2}{S-x}\lambda^x}{\sum_\nu \binom{N_1}{\nu}\binom{N_2}{S-\nu}\lambda^\nu} \quad , \quad \lambda = \frac{P_{11}P_{22}}{P_{12}P_{21}} \quad ,$$

$$\max (0, S-N_2) \le x \le \min (N_1, S) \quad ,$$

with these same limits on the summation in the denominator. When the parameter λ, the odds ratio, equals
1 ($P_{11}=P_{12}$) we obtain the hypergeometric distribution,
used in Fisher's exact test:

$$\frac{\binom{N_1}{x}\binom{N_2}{S-x}}{\binom{N_1+N_2}{S}} .$$

The P-value is computed by summing these probabilities
for all X_{11}-values producing a smaller probability
than the observed X_{11}, adding over tables that are
more extreme.

This development provides another justification for
log-linear models, which are based on the odds ratio.

Exact tests are important in many applications, for
if cell frequencies are small and generate small expected values under a model, the P-values produced by
chi-square statistics can be deceptive. To see this,

412   Louis

consider Tables 3A and 3B summarizing the results of
an antacid (A) versus control (C) treatment study,
stratified by risk factors.

TABLE 3A. Results of Antacid vs. Control Treatments[a]

No. of risk factors	Therapy	Relapse Yes	No	Percent relapse
0-1	A	0	24	0
	C	1	13	7
2	A	0	8	0
	C	3	12	20
3-6	A	2	17	11
	C	8	12	40
Total	A	2	49	4
	C	12	37	24

[a]Data from Hastings et al. (11). Reprinted, by permission of The New England Journal of Medicine, 298:
1043 (1978).

The chi-square tests are very misleading for the
individual strata, but not for the pooled data. This
anticonservatism occurs when expected cell frequencies
are small and is especially influential when the likelihood G^2 is used (14,15).

While the pooled data can be handled nicely by a
chi-square test, such pooling can be dangerous. It
is quite possible to find that A is preferred over C
in each stratum, but not in the pooled data. Such a
flip-flop is called Simpson's paradox and will be discussed in the sequel.

We can safely combine the evidence in this experiment mathematically, however. Such a combination is

TABLE 3B. Chi-Square and Exact Test Results of
H_0:   No Treatment Differences ($U_{23} \equiv 0$)[a]

Stratum	Likelihood (G^2)	Pearson	Exact
0-1	.150	.184	.368
2	.095	.177	.526
3-6	.031	.035	.065
Total	.002	.003	.006

[a]Data from Gregory and Brown (9). Reprinted, by
permission of The New England Journal of Medicine, 299: 831 (1978).

provided by the 3-way log-linear model, with variable
1 the number of risk factors, variable 2 the therapy,
and variable 3 the relapse status:

$$\ln P_{ijk} = U+U_1(i)+U_2(j)+U_3(k)+U_{12}(i,j)+U_{13}(i,k)$$

$$+U_{23}(j,k)+U_{123}(i,j,k) \; ;$$

U_{23} represents the relationship between treatment
and relapse and

U_{123} measures how much U_{23} changes from stratum to
stratum;

$U_{123} \equiv 0$ implies that U_{23} does not change.

Setting $U_{123} \equiv 0$ gives a model where the relationship between the treatments (as measured by the odds
ratio) is constant over strata. This model can be
compared with the model with $U_{23} \equiv U_{123} \equiv 0$, to see
if one treatment is better, since U_{23} measures the
association between treatment and relapse rate. In
the model containing all terms but U_{123}, U_{23} is the

treatment effect adjusted for strata. Exact methods of analysis are available (7,19,21) but here we use the chi-square approach based on comparing nested models.

(I)   Fit [12], [13], [23]; there are no closed form estimates. If the fit is good (G_I^2 not significant) then the constant odds ratio assumption is supported.
(II)   Fit [12], [13].
(III) Compare G_I^2 with G_{II}^2.

The notation [12], [13], [23] indicates that U_{12}, U_{13}, and U_{23} plus all lower-order terms (U, U_1, U_2, and U_3) are in the model. G_I^2 is the likelihood chi-square for model I. If model I is a bad fit, then the odds ratio varies among strata and no uniform treatment relationship holds. Even here, however, if A always dominates C, a powerful test is provided by the constant odds ratio assumption (7). If, however, the treatment of choice switches from stratum to stratum, the constant odds ratio assumption is scientifically inappropriate.

For our data, we obtain:

1. G_I^2 = 1.03 on 2 df, $\hat{U}_{23}(1,1)$ = -.5177 .

2. G_{II}^2 = 9.54 on 3 df,

   $\Delta G^2 = G_{II}^2 - G_I^2$ = 8.51 on 1 df, $P \cong .0036$,
   exact test P=.0056 .

These nested hypotheses, where one model is a special case of the other, are tested by taking differences of G^2 statistics and degrees of freedom. To find the degrees of freedom for a chi-square statistic, subtract those for the model from those in the entire table (2=12-10). Equivalently, the degrees of freedom equal those associated with U-terms set to 0.

The pooled 2x2 table can be tested for no association without collapsing the 3-way data by testing

[12], [23] versus [12], [3],

giving $\Delta G^2 = 9.56$, $P \cong .002$ and $\hat{U}_{23}(1,1) = -.5182$. Notice that in this example the pooled and unpooled analyses give similar $\hat{U}_{23}(1,1)$'s, but the pooled analysis produces a smaller P-value.

U_{13} describes the effect of risk factors on the outcome, adjusted for treatment effect. In the model [12], [13], [23], we obtain

$$\frac{\hat{U}_{13}(1,1)}{-.628} \quad \frac{\hat{U}_{13}(2,1)}{.024} \quad \frac{\hat{U}_{13}(3,1)}{.604} \quad ,$$

indicating a statistically and clinically significant influence. For example, the odds ratio of the 3-6 risk factor group to the 0-1 risk factor group is 137. We do, however, need to consider the risk factor effect on the actual probabilities of relapse.

This analysis is similar to the Mantel-Haenszel test (2). We note that in general the exact test might produce a P-value far different from .0036, but in this case it is similar. Our expected values satisfy the Lawal and Upton (15) criteria, and U_{12} is about the same in the collapsed table (the total) and the full table under the constant odds ratio model. If the P-value for the stratified table had been much lower than the .002 from the collapsed table, we would have cause for concern and should check the exact level.

Computer programs (19) are available to perform a wide class of exact tests. In certain contexts, they consume considerable amounts of computer and real time.

SIMPSON'S PARADOX

In unbalanced treatment studies we can find that a treatment can be apparently good for men and good for

women, but bad for people. This relationship is an
example of Simpson's paradox. In log-linear model
notation the problem is that [12], [13], [23] is not
collapsible, in that U_{23} will not necessarily be the
same as in the model [12], [23]. This latter model
is equivalent to estimating U_{23} from the table collapsed on variable 1. For example, consider these
results for two treatments, A and B:

		Men				Women	
		Alive	Dead			Alive	Dead
	A	150	50		A	240	560
Treatment							
	B	400	400		B	25	175
		$\lambda = 3$				$\lambda = 3$	

		Total	
		Alive	Dead
	A	390	610
Treatment			
	B	425	575
		$\lambda = .86$	

The odds ratio comparing treatments is 3 (favoring
A) for both men and women. The odds ratio in the total table is .86, favoring B. Such data can be properly analyzed using the [12], [13], [23] model, but
not the pooled data.

A PROBLEM WITH LOG-LINEAR MODELS

Although log-linear models seem justified by the
exact test and their treatment of independence, they
do represent probabilities in a transformed scale.
This transformation produces some nonintuitive

relationships. Consider the following hypothetical
2x2 tables of true probabilities where in each the
odds ratio is 4. Let $P_{11}-P_{12}=\Delta$, and let $\hat{\Delta}$ be the estimate of Δ based on N observations in each column.

	.667	.333	.9900	.9612	.999	.996
	.333	.667	.0100	.0388	.001	.004

	$\hat{\Delta}$:	.334	.0288	.003
$N \cdot 10^3$ var $\hat{\Delta}$:		440	47	1.4
$N \cdot$var $\hat{U}_{12}$:		9/16	8.0	78

In these tables, the same odds ratio produces varying differences in probabilities. From the other
viewpoint, the log of the odds ratio (or the U_{12}-term)
stretches distances between probabilities that are
near 0 or 1 as compared with those near .5. At the
same time, the variance of the estimated U_{12}-term is
larger for probabilities near 0 or 1 as compared with
those near .5. Therefore, this stretching does not
create statistical information; it does provide a convenient modeling framework.

The odds ratio of 4 has a very different influence
if the P_{ij}'s are near $\frac{1}{2}$ than if they are near 0 or 1.
The 4-fold increase in odds may always have scientific
significance ("something is going on"), but clinical
significance in some cases and not in others. Therefore, it is important to transform models back to the
original scale, to see what is actually happening to
probabilities. Figure 1 displays the lines of constant odds ratio for a pair of probabilities showing
this nonlinear relationship.

RESIDUALS AND PARSIMONIOUS MODELS

In any statistical analysis, goodness of fit statistics and graphical displays provide important

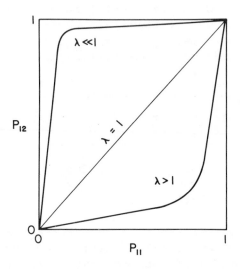

Figure 1. Lines of constant odds ratio.
$\lambda = P_{11}P_{22}/P_{12}P_{21}$; $P_{12}=P_{11}/(\lambda P_{21}+P_{11})$.

information. In regression and ANOVA, plots of residuals versus predicted values, histograms of residuals,
and normal probability plots can be used to select new
terms for a model, identify outliers, and determine
if a data transformation would help the analysis.
These techniques play the same roles in log-linear
analyses.

Consider, for example, Tables 4A and 4B, providing
information on the relationship between aptitude and
education in a random sample of 4353 individuals. We
would all be surprised if the two variables were not
related. The chi-square statistic of 175 on 12 degrees of freedom [5x4-1-(5-1)-(4-1)] is highly significant. What we want is information on where the association is high, low, and moderate, and the pattern
of association. The U_{12} terms in a saturated model
provide such information as do residuals defined by
the unsquared components of the Freeman-Tukey chi-
square statistic (Pearson will do nicely too):

TABLE 4A. The Relationship between Aptitude
and Education: Model [1], [2]; χ^2 = 175
on 12 df (N=4353); P<.001

Aptitude	Education Low	•	•	High
Low	215	208	138	83
•	281	285	284	197
•	372	386	446	385
•	128	176	238	186
High	44	53	131	117

TABLE 4B. Freeman-Tukey Deviates from [1],
[2]. (The Sum of Their Squares Equals 175)

Aptitude	Education Low	•	•	High
Low	5.1	3.1	-3.7	-5.9
•	-0.4	1.9	0.0	-1.7
•	0.5	-1.2	-0.6	1.4
•	-3.1	-0.9	1.9	1.7
High	-4.4	-4.3	3.0	4.0

$$\text{Residual} = \sqrt{X_{ij}} + \sqrt{X_{ij}+1} - \sqrt{4m_{ij}+1} \ .$$

The m_{ij} are computed based on the independence model.
These residuals, under the further assumption of
Poisson sampling, are approximately normal (0,1).
They are correlated, however, as there are only 12
degrees of freedom in this set of 20 values. Never-
theless, we can see that the high association, both

negative and positive, is for the low and high aptitude individuals, and in the middle residuals are
relatively small. Further, the pattern of signs indicates that we might be able to fit a dependency model that does not use up all remaining 12 degrees of
freedom, as would be required in the "all or nothing"
approach as implemented in BMDP3F (5). We can try a
model where, in addition to independence, we include a
term

C in cells (1,1), (1,2), (5,3), (5,4),
-C in cells (1,3), (1,4), (5,1), (5,2).

Properly chosen, this value can reduce the chi-square
statistic by 121 units to 54, accommodating much of
the structure in the data. The remaining chi-square
of 54 on 9 degrees of freedom is large, but we are
dealing with a large sample size where even small differences in probabilities produce large chi-square
values.

MODEL SELECTION

In situations with more than 3 variables, there are
a great many candidate models. Stepwise and other
procedures are useful tools in getting started and are
described in detail in Bishop et al. (2) and Fienberg
(6). These step-up and step-down methods are implemented in BMDP3F. All should be coupled with user-
supplied insights, diagnostic plots, and some method
of assessing the stability of findings in a future
sample. These latter cross-validation methods are
fairly well developed for regression models, but their
properties in the discrete-data context are not yet
well understood.
One interesting method for getting started in a
model building process is to fit the saturated model
(this fit depends on non-zero cell entries and "½" can
be added to each frequency before fitting) and then

standardizing the U-terms to be approximately normal (0,1). Dependency among U-terms needs to be removed by a reparametrization, but for tables with only binary factors, use of the $U_1(1)$, $U_2(1)$,...,$U_{12}(1,1)$, etc., terms only gives the right number of values. Since the sign on $U_1(1)$, for example, depends only on labeling, the absolute values are used. Under the global null hypothesis that only U is needed (all cells have equal probability), the standardized, absolute U-terms (evaluated at level 1 of each coordinate) are distributed approximately as the absolute value of standard normal deviates. A half-normal plot will show which U's are candidates for including in a model.

For an example, consider data from Dyke and Patterson, cited by Fienberg (6), relating various information gathering activities to knowledge about cancer. The variables are binary indicators of newspaper reading, radio listening, solid reading, attendance at lectures, and good or poor knowledge about cancer. There are $2^5-1 = 31$ degrees of freedom associated with subscripted U-terms. From Figure 2, we see that a first model might include U, U_1, U_2, U_3, U_4, U_5, U_{12}, U_{13}, U_{15}, and U_{24}. The absolute standardized values for U_1, U_2, U_4, and U_{13} are all greater than 5 and are not plotted. The model fits poorly and so U_{345}, U_{34}, U_{35}, and U_{45} are added, producing an acceptable model. Including U_{345} automatically spawns the lower-order offspring, due to the hierarchy principle discussed in the Appendix on iterative proportional fitting.

RANDOM EFFECTS MODELS

As in regression and ANOVA, analyses can be performed based on the assumption that model parameters are themselves random variables. These random effects (sometimes called Bayes or empirical Bayes) models are used for both conceptual and empirical reasons. They can smooth out a sparse table, and provide generaliza-

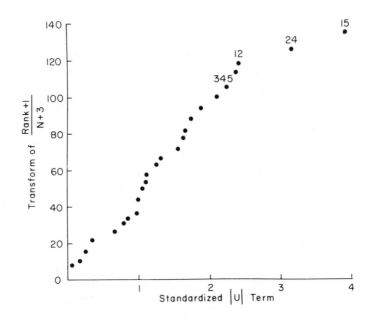

Figure 2. Half-normal probability plot of the Dyke-
Patterson data.

tions to the assumption that the data are Poisson or
multinomial. Brier (3) and Laird (12) provide examples and references for these topics.

Here we consider assessment of the institution component of variance in observed operative rates. With
20,000 patients per hospital, assume the following
data in Tables 5A and 5B that have been ordered for
ease of presentation. For each operation we have put
the data in a 2x5 array where each column totals
20,000 and the overall rates are 134/100,000 and 565/
100,000 respectively. Total variation is estimated
by computing a sample variance of observed rates or
their transforms. Even if all underlying rates are
equal, some variation is induced by sampling and must
be removed to produce a fair comparison. Otherwise,
rates with relatively small denominators can appear
more variable than those based on relatively large

TABLE 5A. Procedure A

	Institution					
	1	2	3	4	5	Total
Procedures performed	15	20	25	30	44	134
Other patients	19,985	19,980	19,975	19,970	19,956	99,866
Total	20,000	20,000	20,000	20,000	20,000	100,000

TABLE 5B. Procedure B

	Institution					
	1	2	3	4	5	Total
Procedures performed	80	100	110	130	145	565
Other patients	19,920	19,990	19,890	19,870	19,855	99,435
Total	20,000	20,000	20,000	20,000	20,000	100,000

denominators. We consider two methods of subtracting out this sampling component.

First, the expectation of the Pearson chi-square statistic testing for independence (equal rates) is

$$E(\text{Pearson } \chi^2) \cong (J-1)(1+N\sigma^2) \ ,$$

where

$$\sigma^2 = \frac{1}{J-1} \sum_j W_j \frac{(P_j-\bar{P})^2}{\bar{P}(1-\bar{P})} \ .$$

N is the table total, P_j is the true operative rate for institution j, $\bar{P} = \sum W_j P_j$, and W_j = fraction of total patients treated in institution j. The (J-1) is the expectation of a chi-square variable on (J-1) degrees of freedom. The parameter σ^2 represents a weighted variance computed from the true underlying rates in the square-root scale. We can estimate σ^2 by

$$\hat{\sigma}^2 = \frac{\text{Pearson } \chi^2}{N(J-1)} - \frac{1}{N} \ .$$

The same approach can be used with the G^2 and Freeman-Tukey statistics. If the P's are considered random, a further expectation shows that the above formula estimates τ^2, the variance of the distribution generating transformed probabilities.

For another approach, consider the $\hat{U}_{12}(i,j)$'s estimated from the saturated model in a two-way table. The sum

$$\sum_{j=1}^{J} \hat{U}_{12}(1,j)^2$$

has expectation

$$(J-1)\tau^2 + \sum_j \text{Var}[\hat{U}_{12}(1,j)] \ ,$$

where we think of the true $U_{12}(1,j)$ as coming from a

distribution with variance τ^2. Notice that variation is being measured in a log odds scale.

Now, we estimate τ^2 by

$$\tau^2 = \frac{\Sigma\hat{U}_{12}(1,j)^2 - \Sigma\text{Var}[\hat{U}_{12}(1,j)]}{J-1} .$$

The second term in the numerator can be estimated (16). We obtain

Prior Variance Components

Operative procedure	Pearson basis x 10^5	U_{12} basis x 10^3
A	13.8	26.0
B	19.3	7.0

We should not compare across rows. Using the Pearson approach A is less variable than B, while using the U_{12} method gives the opposite conclusion. This difference is produced by the different transforms used before a variance computation (square root versus log odds). The desired transform depends on both statistical and subject-matter considerations. It will have a strong influence on comparisons of variance if the rates are near 0 or 1, and results will be relatively insensitive to its form, if rates are near 0.5.

BRADLEY-TERRY MODEL

The Bradley-Terry model of paired comparisons provides an example where log-linear models apply in a nonstandard context. Here, pairs of contenders (treatments, baseball teams) compete and a winner of each contest is determined. Such data can arise in a clinical context in a crossover design. In each contest, we have:

P(contender i beats contender j) $= \pi_{ij}$

and the Bradley-Terry model imposes $\pi_{ij} = \pi_i/(\pi_i+\pi_j)$, where the π_i can be thought of as relative efficacies. These efficacies can be estimated from data of the following sort, taken from Fienberg (5).

	Baltimore	Boston	New York
Baltimore	-	9	8
Boston	9	-	11
New York	10	5	-

Rows = wins in baseball games

For example, Boston beat New York 11 times, while New York beat Boston only 5 times.

To fit the Bradley-Terry model, rearrange these data to

	Pairing 1	2	3
Baltimore	9	8	-
Boston	9	-	11
New York	-	10	5
Total games	18	18	16

where the columns index pairs of teams and "-" represents a zero frequency (i.e., New York did not play in the Boston-Baltimore pair). These hyphens indicate structural zeros, zeros that are inherent in the design.

Now, the Bradley-Terry structure is represented by the independence model

$$\ln P_{ij} = U + U_1(i) + U_2(j)$$

fit only to the nonempty cells. (This is a model of quasi-independence.) There are only 6 df in total (due to 3 structural zeros) and this model uses 5, leaving one for lack of fit.
When we fit the model,

$$G^2 = 1.41 \text{ on 1 df (a good fit)}$$

and $U_1(i)$ gives the basis for the π_i .

Team	$U_1(i)$	$\exp[U_1(i)]$	π_i(normalized)
Baltimore	-.07	.93	30.5
Boston	+.24	1.27	41.6
New York	-.16	.85	27.9

The π_i have been normalized to add to 100, but are in the same proportions as the middle column. Of course, Boston is shown to be the best team.

ADDITIONAL TOPICS

This presentation has omitted more than it has covered. The relationship of these methods to survival analysis can be found in Laird and Oliver (15). Agresti (1) and McCullagh (17) discuss the treatment of ordinal data. Although logistic regression has not been discussed explicitly, its structure is obtainable by writing conditional probabilities from log-linear models. The details of the relationship may be found in Bishop et al. (2) and Fienberg (6).

APPENDIX. FITTING MODELS

Once a model is specified, parameter values must be estimated. Minimum chi-square and maximum likelihood are the most popular methods for finding the "best" parameter values. The former is implemented in PROC FUNCAT of the SAS (20) system, and is asymptotically equivalent to maximum likelihood as long as the frequencies in each category of the table go to infinity.

The most common and flexible approach to fitting log-linear and other models is maximum likelihood where the likelihood of the observed table under Poisson, multinomial, product multinomial, or hypergeometric sampling is maximized. The same estimates result in each case. General purpose programs such as BMDPAR and BMDP3R can be used, and produce the covariance matrix of the parameters as well as the point estimates.

An attractive and intriguing method of finding MLEs is available for a pure contingency table using linear models with full degrees of freedom for each U-term included. The method, iterative proportional fitting (IPF), goes as follows:

1. Start with a table of 1's in each nonstructural zero cell, 0's elsewhere.
2. Adjust the entries so their sum matches a marginal table associated with a U-term model.
3. Take these values and match another marginal.
4. Continue matching margins associated with the model, until the entries converge.
5. These convergent values will be the MLE expected values.

The marginals to match are those associated with the highest-order U-terms for each subscript. For example, in a 4-variable model, [12], [13], [234], the 12, 13, and 234 margins would be matched in sequence.

Detailed discussion of the method and its properties is in Bishop et al. (2) and Fienberg (6). Its

virtues are simplicity and guaranteed convergence,
but it cannot handle models using part of a U-term's
degrees of freedom, continuous data with slopes, or
models that do not satisfy the hierarchy principle.
This principle dictates that if a certain U-term is
included, so must be all lower-order offspring. IPF
does not deliver the variances and covariances of parameter estimates. These are available from other
fitting methods or when the parameters can be estimated in closed form (16). Computer programs using IPF
must approximate variances by those associated with a
closed form model containing the one actually fit.
This approximation can be quite coarse.

Historically, IPF was used to fit internal structure to a given set of marginals. Whatever cross-
product ratios (and therefore U-terms) values exist
in the array starting IPF that are not associated with
a margin being matched are preserved throughout.
Mosteller (18) makes use of this preservation of
structure to match a table to uniform marginals. At
convergence, dependency patterns in a table are quite
apparent.

REFERENCES

1. Agresti, A. (1980), Generalized odds ratios for
   ordinal data, Biometrics 36: 59-67.

2. Bishop, Y., Fienberg, S. E., and Holland, P. W.
   (1975), Discrete Multivariate Analysis, MIT Press,
   Cambridge, Massachusetts.

3. Brier, S. S. (1980), The analysis of contingency
   tables under cluster sampling, Biometrika 67: 591-
   596.

4. Cox, D. R. (1970), Analysis of Binary Data,
   Methuen, London.

5. Dixon, W. J., and Brown, M. B., eds. (1979), BMDP
   Biomedical Computer Programs P-Series, University
   of California Press, Berkeley, California.

6. Fienberg, S. E. (1980), The Analysis of Cross-
   Classified Categorical Data (2nd ed.), MIT Press,
   Cambridge, Massachusetts.

7. Gart, J. (1971), The comparison of proportions:
   A review of significance tests, confidence intervals, and adjustments for stratification, International Statistical Institute Review 39: 148-169.

8. Goodman, L. A. (1978), Analysing Qualitative Categorical Data: Log Linear Models and Latent-
   Structure Analysis, Abt Books, Cambridge, Massachusetts.

9. Gregory, P. B., and Brown, B. W., Jr. (1978), Letter to the editor, The New England Journal of
   Medicine 299: 830-831.

10. Haberman, S. J. (1974), The Analysis of Frequency
    Data, University of Chicago Press.

11. Hastings, P. R., Skillman, J. J., Bushnell, L. S.,
    and Silen, W. S. (1978), Antacid titration in the
    prevention of acute gastrointestinal bleeding: A
    controlled, randomized trial in 100 critically ill
    patients, The New England Journal of Medicine 298:
    1041-1045.

12. Laird, N. M. (1978), Empirical Bayes methods for
    two-way contingency tables, Biometrika 65: 581-
    590.

13. Laird, N. M., and Olivier, D. (1981), Covariance
    analysis of censored survival data using log-
    linear analysis techniques, Journal of the Ameri-
    can Statistical Association 76: 231-240.

14. Larntz, K. (1978), Small-sample comparisons of exact levels for chi-squared goodness-of-fit statistics, Journal of the American Statistical Association 73: 253-263.

15. Lawal, H. B., and Upton, G. J. G. (1980), An approximation to the distribution of the goodness-of-fit statistic for use with small expectations, Biometrika 67: 447-454.

16. Lee, Y. J. (1977), On the asymptotic variances of u-terms in log-linear models, Journal of the American Statistical Association 72: 412-419.

17. McCullagh, P. (1980), Regression models for ordinal data, Journal of the Royal Statistical Society B42: 109-142.

18. Mosteller, F. M. (1968), Association and estimation in contingency tables, Journal of the American Statistical Association 65: 35-48.

19. Pagano, M., and Tritchler, D. (1982), Algorithms for the analysis of several 2x2 contingency tables, Journal of Scientific and Statistical Computing. (In press.)

20. SAS Manual, (1979), and Supplements, (1980), SAS Institute, Cary, North Carolina.

21. Zelen, M. (1971), The analysis of several 2x2 contingency tables, Biometrika 58: 129-137.

CHAPTER 14

Analysis of Categorical Data: Logistic Models

DAVID A. SCHOENFELD

INTRODUCTION

In many clinical trials, response to therapy is measured by a dichotomous variable. For instance, in chemotherapy studies a patient is said to respond to therapy if his tumor shrinks by more than 50%. Often response is affected by patient characteristics such as sex, disease stage, and patient age. The logistic model can be used to determine the effect of these covariates on response and to test for a treatment effect. The first section of this chapter describes small sample, exact tests for determining whether there is a treatment effect.

Large sample methods for testing for a treatment effect and estimating covariate effects are presented next. Methods for interpreting and reporting these estimates are discussed as are methods for recoding and selecting covariates that are used in the model. The model selection in the analysis of a clinical

---

This work was supported by National Cancer Institute Grant CA-25162.

trial of patients with soft tissue sarcoma is given
as an example to illustrate the procedures.

All too often goodness of fit of these models is
ignored. Methods of testing the hypotheses of a constant odds ratio are described.

In some clinical trials a response to therapy is
measured by a polychotomous ordinal variable. For instance, a clinical trial may have complete response,
partial response, and disease progression as outcomes.
Complete response is better than a partial response,
which is better than progression. Other trials may
grade pain or toxicity as mild, moderate, severe, and
life-threatening. Methods of analyzing ordinal response are discussed.

EXACT TEST FOR TREATMENT OR COVARIATE EFFECTS

Let y_i be a binary variable indicating response of
the ith patient, i=1,...,n. Suppose further that
there is a (p+1)-vector $\underline{x}_i=(x_{i0},x_{i1},...,x_{ip})'$ of variables in which $x_{i1},...,x_{ip}$ indicate treatment and patient characteristics and $x_{i0} = 1$. To simplify the
exposition assume that x_{i1} is a treatment variable
with $x_{i1} = 1$ or 0 depending on the patient's treatment
group. The logistic model specifies that the probability that $y_i = 1$ is

$$p_i = \exp(\underline{\beta}'\underline{x}_i)/[1+\exp(\underline{\beta}'\underline{x}_i)] , \qquad (1)$$

where the (p+1)-vector $(\beta_0,\beta_1,...,\beta_p)$ represents unknown parameters. This model has the property that
it is monotonic in the linear function $\beta'\underline{x}$. Furthermore, unlike in the log-linear model, all parameter
values are allowed.

The likelihood function is simply that of a sequence of Bernoulli variables, each with a different
parameter p_i and is given by

$$\prod_i p_i^{y_i}(1-p_i)^{1-y_i} \ . \tag{2}$$

Substituting in equation 1 for p_i gives

$$\exp[\Sigma y_i(\underline{\beta}'\underline{x}_i)] \ \prod_i [1+\exp(\underline{\beta}'\underline{x}_i)]^{-1} \ . \tag{3}$$

Since the x_i's are assumed to be known, formula 3 shows that the logistic model is a member of the (p+1)-parameter exponential family with sufficient statistics defined by

$$s_0 = \Sigma y_i, \ s_1 = \Sigma y_i x_{i1}, \ \dots, \ s_p = \Sigma y_i x_{ip} \ . \tag{4}$$

This fact can be exploited to construct optimal tests for treatment or covariate effects using the methods of Lehmann (9).

Suppose there are two treatments indicated by $x_{i1} = 1$ and $x_{i1} = 0$. The hypothesis of no treatment effect is given by $H_0: \beta_1 = 0$. To perform the uniformly most powerful unbiased test of this hypothesis against a one-sided alternative, one rejects the null hypothesis when s_1 is larger than a critical value k which depends on $s_0, s_2, \dots, s_p$. This constant is chosen so that

$$P(s_1 > k \mid s_0, s_2, \dots, s_p) \leq \alpha \tag{5}$$

under H_0. To perform this computation let m_x be the number of ways that $s_1 = x$ when $s_0, s_2, \dots, s_p$ are fixed. Then

$$P(s_1 \geq k \mid s_0, s_2, \dots, s_p) = \sum_{x \geq k} m_x / \Sigma m_x . \tag{6}$$

As an example, consider the data in Table 1 and suppose we wish to test whether patients without the rare characteristic have a higher response rate than patients with the characteristic. Let $x_{i1} = 1$ if the

TABLE 1. Analysis of 2x2 Table

		Rare characteristic		
		Yes	No	Total
Response	Yes	1	36	37
	No	9	64	73
	Total	10	100	110

One-sided test statistic	P-value
Exact test	.09
Wald's test	.07
Score test	.05
Likelihood ratio test	.03

patient does not have the rare characteristic and let y_i be the response indicator. To find k, we first note that there are 37 responses so the maximum value of s_1 is 37. To compute $P(s_1=37)$ note that there are 100!/37!63! ways that the 37 responses could occur among the 100 patients without the rare characteristic. There are 110!/37!73! ways that the 37 responses could occur among all patients so

$$P(s_1=37) = \frac{\binom{100}{37}}{\binom{110}{37}} = .013 \ .$$

Similarly,

$$P(s_1=36) = \frac{\binom{100}{36}\binom{10}{1}}{\binom{110}{37}} = .076 \ .$$

Thus, to achieve a 5% significance level k would be chosen to be 37. The P-value of the data in Table 1 is .013 + .076 = .089.

As another example, suppose there are 3 different drug doses given to patients, say, 1, 2, and $3mg/m^2$. Suppose there are 5 responses among 10 patients and the doses of the 5 responders are $(2,2,3,3,3)$ while the doses of the 5 nonresponders are $(1,1,1,2,3)$. Let y_i be the response indicator and x_{i1} be the dose level. Assuming that s_0 and the values of x_{i1} are fixed, s_1 can take any value between 7 and 14. Since 3 patients receive a dose of $1mg/m^2$, 3 receive $2mg/m^2$, and 4 receive $3mg/m^2$, there are $10!/3!3!4!$ ways of assigning doses to patients. To compute the probability that $s_1 = 14$, note that there must be 4 doses equal to $3mg/m^2$ and one equal to $2mg/m^2$ among the responders and 2 doses equal to $2mg/m^2$ and 3 equal to $1mg/m^2$ among the nonresponders. Thus, there are $5!5!/4!3!2!$ assignments with $s_1 = 14$ and therefore $P(s_1=14) = .012$. Similarly, it can be shown that $P(s_1=13) = .06$; thus for a 5% significance level test k should be set equal to 14.

This procedure is especially easy to implement when the patient characteristics divide the patient group into k mutually exclusive classes or there are very few patients. In other situations, the computation is more difficult and asymptotic methods must be used to test for treatment or covariate effects.

For further discussion of exact methods see reference 3.

ASYMPTOTIC TESTS FOR TREATMENT EFFECT

Since many clinical trials involve large samples, asymptotic methods are often appropriate for testing for treatment effects. There are 3 commonly used methods (12): the likelihood ratio test, the score test, and Wald's test. These tests are all asymptotically efficient. To perform the likelihood ratio test, first estimate $\beta_0, \beta_1, \ldots, \beta_p$ by maximum likelihood. Calculate the log likelihood, denoted by $LL(\hat{\underline{\beta}})$, at these parameter estimates. Then estimate $\beta_0, \beta_2,$ $\ldots, \beta_p$ by maximum likelihood, assuming that $\beta_1 = 0$, that is, fit a model with no treatment variable. Similarly, compute $LL(\hat{\underline{\beta}}^\circ)$, the log likelihood at these estimates. The test statistic is given by

$$-2[LL(\hat{\underline{\beta}}^\circ) - LL(\hat{\underline{\beta}})] . \tag{7}$$

This statistic is asymptotically χ_1^2 under the null hypothesis.

An alternative procedure is to use the score statistic given by

$$(\partial\ LL/\partial\beta_1)^2/\text{Var}(\partial\ LL/\partial\beta_1) \tag{8}$$

evaluated at the estimates of $\beta_0, \beta_2, \ldots, \beta_p$, when $\beta_1 = 0$. The denominator of formula 8 is $1/(M^{-1})_{11}$, where M is the information matrix evaluated at these estimates. This statistic is also χ_1^2 and is asymptotically equivalent to formula 7. The advantage of this test is that it only requires one parameter estimation. Another equivalent test is Wald's test, which is based on

$$\hat{\beta}_1^2/\text{Var}(\hat{\beta}_1) . \tag{9}$$

This test also requires only one estimation, but in this case the estimation is performed under the assumption that $\beta_1 = 0$.

The maximum likelihood estimates $\hat{\beta}_0, \hat{\beta}_1, \hat{\beta}_2, \ldots, \hat{\beta}_p$ are those values for which $\partial\ LL/\partial\beta = 0$.

The first derivative of the log likelihood function with respect to β_j can be shown to equal

$$V_j(\underline{\beta}) = s_j - \sum_i x_{ij} \exp(\underline{\beta}'\underline{x}_i)/[1+\exp(\underline{\beta}'\underline{x}_i)]$$

which is simply the observed value of s_j minus its

expected value. Thus, as in any member of the exponential family, $\underline{\beta}$ is estimated by the vector that equates the observed values of the sufficient statistics to their expected values.

The covariance matrix of $\underline{\beta}$ is estimated by the inverse of the information matrix given by

$$M_{jk}(\underline{\beta}) = \sum_i x_{ij}x_{ik}\exp(\underline{\beta}'\underline{x}_i)/[1+\exp(\underline{\beta}'\underline{x}_i)]^2 ,$$

where $j=0,\ldots,p$ and $k=0,\ldots,p$. The estimates $\beta_0,\ldots,\beta_p$ can be found iteratively using the Newton-Raphson algorithm (8). Start with an initial estimate $\underline{\beta}^*$, defined by $\beta_0^* = \ln[s_0/(n-s_0)]$ and $\beta_1^*,\ldots,\beta_p^* = 0$. Find an improved estimate given by

$$\underline{\beta}^* + [M(\underline{\beta}^*)]^{-1}\underline{v}(\underline{\beta}^*) .$$

Repeat this process until the change with each iteration is negligible.

For example, suppose response is affected by treatment (x_{i1}) and stage (x_{i2}), which has values 1-4. (Stage is coded in this manner to simplify the example; the coding of covariates is discussed in more detail in a later section.) Let Table 2 represent the results of a hypothetical study with these covariates.

For this study $s_0 = \sum y_i = 14$, $s_1 = \sum y_i x_{i1} = 10$, and $s_2 = \sum y_i x_{i2} = 7\cdot1+4\cdot2+3\cdot3+0\cdot4 = 24$. Set $\beta_0^* = \ln(14/34) = -.89$ and $\beta_1^* = \beta_2^* = 0$; $p_i = 14/48 = .29$ and $V(\underline{\beta}^*)$ is given by:

$$V_0(\underline{\beta}^*) = 0 ,$$

$$V_1(\underline{\beta}^*) = 10-.29\cdot28 = 1.88 , \text{ and}$$

$$V_2(\underline{\beta}^*) = 24-.29(19\cdot1+13\cdot2+11\cdot3+5\cdot4) = -4.42 .$$

Finally,

TABLE 2. Example of Study in which Response is Affected by Treatment and a Covariate (Stage)

Stage	Treatment 0 Response		Treatment 1 Response		Total Response		Total
	Yes	No	Yes	No	Yes	No	
1	2	6	5	6	7	12	19
2	1	4	3	5	4	9	13
3	1	4	2	4	3	8	11
4	0	2	0	3	0	5	5
Total	4	16	10	18	14	34	48

$$M_1 = \begin{pmatrix} 9.9 & 5.8 & 20.2 \\ 5.8 & 5.8 & 11.7 \\ 20.2 & 11.7 & 51.5 \end{pmatrix} .$$

Thus, the new estimates are $(-.42, .76, -.44)$. Repeating this process yields estimates $(-.44, .82, -.50)$ and then the estimates $(-.44, .83, -.50)$. Further iterations do not change these values. The covariance matrix of the final estimates by M^{-1} is

$$M^{-1} = \begin{pmatrix} .71 & -.30 & -.22 \\ -.30 & .49 & -.015 \\ -.22 & -.015 & .13 \end{pmatrix} .$$

Thus, Wald's criterion to test for a treatment effect is $\hat{\beta}_1^2/\text{Var}(\hat{\beta}_1) = 1.41$, which is not significant. The maximized log likelihood is -27.16. If we estimate β_0, β_2 in a model without treatment, $\hat{\beta}_0 = .054$ and $\hat{\beta}_2 = -.49$, and the maximized log likelihood is -27.9. The likelihood ratio criterion to test for a treatment effect is 1.48, which is similar to Wald's criterion.

To compute the score test note that the variance of ∂ LL/$\partial\beta_1$ is $1/(M^{-1})_{11}$ with $\hat{\underline{\beta}} = (.054, 0, -.49)$. Thus, the score statistic is $(1.818)^2/2.305 = 1.43$, very similar to the other two criteria.

INTERPRETING THE MODEL

The parameter β_1, which measures treatment effect, has the following interpretation. Suppose the covariates $x_{i2}, \ldots, x_{ip}$ are held fixed. Then the parameter β_1 is the log of the ratio of the odds of response on treatment 1 to the odds of response on treatment 0. The major assumption of the logistic model is that this odds ratio is constant no matter what the values of the covariates. Thus, the treatment effect should be reported using the odds ratio, $\exp(\beta_1)$. One should not report "adjusted" response rates with covariates set at their average value. Consider the hypothetical example given in Table 3. In this example there are roughly the same numbers of males and females randomized to each treatment. Among males and females the odds ratio of response on the two treatments in 10/1; however, the roles of response and nonresponse are reversed in males and females. When we combine the data for males and females there is not a great difference between the treatments and the odds ratio is merely 1.21. If we fit a logistic model with x_{i1} indicating treatment and x_{i2} indicating sex, then $\hat{\beta}_0 = 2.2$, $\hat{\beta}_1 = 2.3$, and $\hat{\beta}_2 = -6.7$. The effect of a logistic model in this example was to increase the odds ratio between the treatments. If, in an attempt to report "adjusted" response rates the covariates are set at their average values, the "adjusted" response rates will be $\exp(2.2-6.7/2)/[1+\exp(2.2-6.7/2)] = .24$ and $\exp(2.2+2.3-6.7/2)/[1+\exp(2.2+2.3-6.7/2] = .76$, which are quite different from the actual response rates of .48 and .52. This does not indicate either misfit of the model or imbalance in the prognostic factors. Rather

TABLE 3. Example of the Effect of "Adjusted" Response Rates

Males ($x_{i2}=0$)		Treatment (x_{i1})		
		0	1	Total
Response (y_i)	yes (1)	1	10	11
	no (0)	90	90	180
	Total	91	100	191

Females ($x_{i2}=1$)		Treatment (x_{i1})		
		0	1	Total
Response (y_i)	yes (1)	90	90	180
	no (0)	10	1	11
	Total	100	91	191

Total		Treatment (x_{i1})		
		0	1	Total
Response (y_i)	yes (1)	91	100	191
	no (0)	100	91	191
	Total	191	191	382

it is a consequence of the shape of the function that relates p_i to $\underline{\beta}'\underline{x}_i$.

CODING VARIABLES

Coding is the process of transforming data on patient characteristics into numerical covariates.

Patient characteristics may be categorical, ordinal, or continuous. To code categorical variables one needs J-1 covariates for a variable with J values. The first covariate is set to one if the categorical variable has its first value and is set to zero otherwise. Similarly, the second covariate indicates whether the variable has its second value. The last value of the variable does not need an indicator covariate. If $x_{i1}, \ldots, x_{iJ-1}$ are the resulting covariates, then $\hat{\beta}_k$ estimates the log odds ratio of response of patients with the kth value to patients with the Jth value and $\hat{\beta}_k - \hat{\beta}_m$ estimates the log odds ratio of response of patients with the kth value to patients with the mth value.

Ordinal variables have values which indicate increasing strength of a characteristic. For instance, cell differentiation is classified as well differentiated, moderately differentiated, and poorly differentiated. These variables may be coded in the same manner as categorical variables as long as all of the covariates that are generated are used in the model. Alternatively, one can obtain a more parsimonious model by coding ordinal variables as if they were continuous. That is, if z is the ordinal covariate, let $x_{i1} = (z-\bar{z})$, $x_{i2} = (z-\bar{z})^2$. The linear term gives the extent to which the probability of response increases with the variable z and x_{i2} allows this to be quadratic.

If a step-up algorithm will be used to select covariates, ordinal variables should be coded by dichotomizing their range. Suppose the ordinal variable, z, has 4 values, namely 1, 2, 3, and 4, representing initial symptom levels of none, mild, moderate, and severe, respectively. We code 3 covariates as follows:

$$x_{i1} = 1 \text{ if } z \geq 2, \quad x_{i1} = 0 \text{ otherwise,}$$

$$x_{i2} = 1 \text{ if } z \geq 3, \quad x_{i2} = 0 \text{ otherwise,}$$

$$x_{i3} = 1 \text{ if } z = 4, \quad x_{i3} = 0 \text{ otherwise.}$$

If we use a step-up procedure to choose covariates then the first covariate to be selected will be the most important cut point of the ordinal variable. That is, if x_{i_2} were chosen it would imply that the most important characterization of z was 1, 2 versus 3, 4. If this is the only covariate chosen, then the difference between moderate and severe and between none and mild is unimportant. If x_{i_1} is chosen as well, then the difference between none and mild is also important. In this manner, the final coding used in the model is determined by the data.

VARIABLE SELECTION TECHNIQUES

Suppose $x_{i_1}, \ldots, x_{i_p}$ are patient covariates. Choosing a subset of these to use in a logistic model is equivalent to estimating the parameters of a logistic model using a technique which forces some of the β_j to be estimated by 0. This method of estimation has several advantages. It provides information about the disease being studied. Variables that are not included in the model are probably not independently important in determining prognosis. It allows the data to determine the coding of ordinal variables as discussed previously. Most importantly, if all the covariates are included, the estimation of $\underline{\beta}$ becomes extremely unstable. Forcing estimates to be zero by a variable selection algorithm may be the only way to simultaneously consider all the possible covariates.

There are several methods of variable selection. However, all of them are based on a similar principle. At any step of these algorithms there are k covariates $x_{i_1}, \ldots, x_{i_k}$ included in the model and a candidate covariate $x_{i_{k+1}}$ which is to be included or excluded on the basis of a hypothesis test. The hypothesis H_{k+1} is the hypothesis that $\beta_{k+1} = 0$, given a model with $x_{i_1}, \ldots, x_{i_k}$. If this hypothesis is rejected then one concludes that $x_{i_{k+1}}$ is useful in predicting response when $x_{i_1}, \ldots, x_{i_k}$ are known, and $x_{i_{k+1}}$ will be included in the model. Different algorithms test these hypotheses in different sequences with different test statistics. They all terminate at a point where all the covariates that are excluded from the model have been found to be not significantly prognostic. If $\beta_j \neq 0$, then for large samples the jth covariate will be included in the model. Furthermore, if $\beta_j = 0$ then, depending on the algorithm, x_j will either be excluded or the estimate of β_j will approach 0. Thus, all the common algorithms will arrive at the same model for large samples.

The following algorithm is suggested because it requires a minimal amount of computer time. It appears to be similar to the algorithm used by BMDPLR (4) when "Method = ACE" is specified. Define the following sets: IN_k are the variables in the model at step k; OUT_k is the set of variables not in the model at step k. Initialize the algorithm by letting IN_1 be treatment and prognostic variables that are known to be important. Let OUT_1 be all other variables. Figure 1 shows a flow chart of the stepwise algorithm, modeled after the algorithm given by Peduzzi, Hardy, and Holford (11). Note that different tests are used for including and excluding variables from the model.

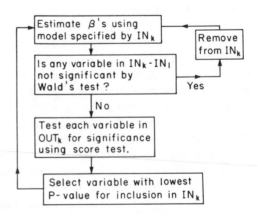

Figure 1. Algorithm for stepwise variable selection.

Wald's test is used to exclude variables because once
parameters have been estimated, Wald's test can be
used to test whether an included covariate is significantly prognostic without additional estimation. On
the other hand, the score test is used to include variables since it requires no parameter estimation to
test whether a variable should be included. Thus, at
each iteration of the algorithm, only one parameter
estimation is performed.

Care must be taken in interpreting the results of
a variable selection algorithm. One must distinguish
between biologic and clinical variables. Biologic
variables indicate underlying facts about the patient's disease while clinical variables indicate the
patient's condition. For instance, cell type is a
biologic variable while ambulatory status is a clinical variable. One might find that cell type is significantly prognostic alone, but when ambulatory status is included in the model, cell type plays an in-
significant role. This implies that with the knowledge of ambulatory status, cell type is not useful in
predicting response. This fact might be used to save
the patient the expense of histologic diagnosis. However, this does not imply that cell type is not bio-
logically important. Cell type probably determines
ambulatory status.

When treatment is confounded with a prognostic variable the results of a logistic model may be difficult
to interpret. Treatment may be significant when cell
type is not in the model. However, with cell type in
the model, treatment is no longer significant. The
fact that the uncorrected treatment comparison is significant indicates that the probability of seeing the
observed or greater treatment effect by chance was
less than 5%. However, the fact that the corrected
comparison is not significant indicates that this rare
event may actually have occurred!

Finally, characteristics may be included in the
model because of a failure in the asymptotic methods
of estimation. Even in large data sets some charac-

teristics will be extremely rare. In this case asymptotic theory is not entirely valid. Table 1 shows an
example of this problem. The rare characteristic
occurs 10 times in a sample of 110. Even though the
sample size is large the asymptotic tests do not give
the correct P-value. Depending on the test used, the
P-value varies from .03 to .09. To prevent this problem one should remove from a model covariates indicating a patient characteristic that occurs less than
perhaps 10 times in the patient population. Furthermore, items included by a variable selection procedure
that are marginally significant should be interpreted
with caution since many statistical tests are being
conducted by the algorithm and some null hypotheses
will be rejected by chance alone.

As an example of a variable selection technique, a
logistic regression was performed to analyze the effect of 3 treatments for soft tissue sarcoma (13).
Table 4 shows the result of this analysis. The variables are presented as well as the proportion of patients with the characteristic and the P-values for
inclusion in the model. At step 1 the model contained
only treatment. The P-value for each variable not included in the model was computed and the variable with
the lowest P-value added to the model. The parameters
were recomputed and the process was repeated. An un-
derlined value denotes a variable included in the model. P-values > 0.1 are not shown. Each P-value shown
is the two-sided significance level of the test that
the variable is prognostic, with adjustment for other
variables in the model. The P-values of covariates
included in the model were computed using Wald's criterion. The other P-values were computed using the
score test. The first variable included was the presence of diabetes, which occurred in 3% of the patient
population. This covariate is probably spurious due
to the failure of the asymptotic test statistic. The
next variable included was the presence of respiratory
metastatic disease symptoms. This is an example of a
clinical variable being included rather than a

TABLE 4. Example of a Stepwise Logistic Regression

Variable	% of Patients	P-Values by step								
		1	2	3	4	5	6	7	8	9
Treatment A	10	.02	.02	.02	.01	.01	.01	.01	.01	.01
Age (<30)	16	.04	.05	.02	.04					
Age (30-45)	40		.06	.05	.02					
Age (45-65)	53	.02	.01	.01	.01	.01	.01	.01	.01	.01
Surgery alone	14	.09	.08							
Performance status			.08							
Respiratory metastatic disease symptoms	34	.01	.01	.01	.01	.01	.01	.01	.01	.01
Reduced appetite	33	.04	.04	.04	.07	.01	.01	.01	.01	.01
Phenothiazines	4		.09	.01	.02	.01	.01	.01	.01	.01
Steroids	1				.06					
Other chronic medications	14	.08								
Diabetes	3	.01	.01	.02	.02	.01	.01	.01	.01	.01
Adjacent anatomic involvement	44						.08			
Liposarcoma	12	.04	.08	.08						
Mixed mesodermal sarcoma	2	.05	.10			.09		.06	.08	.07
Rhabdomyosarcoma	4									
Neurofibrosarcoma	2							.08	.08	.08
Malignant Schwannoma	2			.09	.06					
Nausea	20				.08	.02	.03	.01	.01	.01

biologic one. The presence of lung metastases was a possible covariate but was not included in the model because the presence of symptomatic lung metastases was more prognostic than the presence of lung metastases. Next, use of phenothiazines was included in the model. The final model also included age, reduced appetite, mixed mesodermal sarcoma, neurofibrosarcoma, and the presence of nausea. In each model, treatment was significant.

TESTING GOODNESS OF FIT

Suppose that our primary purpose is to test for treatment effect in a randomized study. The probability of a Type I error is probably not severely affected by a misfitting logistic model to control for covariates. However, if the logistic model does not fit then the power of the treatment comparison may be compromised. Furthermore, the interpretation of the treatment effect will depend on whether the logistic model fits the data. The results of misfitting a logistic model need further research and are currently under investigation by the author.

The logistic model specifies that the odds ratio for two treatments is constant for any combination of the covariates. If the odds ratio varies but always is on the same side of unity, then treatment is said to have a quantitative interaction with covariate value. In this case a different model may give a more powerful test for a treatment effect but otherwise the logistic analysis is adequate. If the odds ratio is sometimes greater and sometimes less than unity the interaction is said to be qualitative and one treatment is better for some patients and worse for others.

If there are few covariates, goodness of fit can be tested by forming k 2x2 tables. Each 2x2 table tabulates treatment by response for patients with the same covariate values. The hypothesis of a constant odd ratio is tested using the method of Halperin

et al. (7). Efficient exact tests are also available
(10). When there are many covariates, patients should
be grouped into k risk groups. In this case, the hypothesis of a constant odds ratio may be tested by the
chi-square test of Tsiatis (14).

We can use the data in Table 2 to illustrate how
goodness of fit might be tested. We divide the covariate space into 4 categories, based on the value of
x_{i1} and whether or not $x_{i2} \geq 3$. It is preferable to
reduce the number of categories as much as possible
since this yields a more powerful test and insures
that the actual distribution of the resulting statistic is closer to its asymptotic distribution. Following the notation in Tsiatis (14), A is the diagonal
matrix with entries $A_{jj} = \Sigma p_i(1-p_i)$, where the summation is over the patients in the jth category. Thus,
A = diag (2.4, .7, 4.6, 1.5). Similarly $B_{jk} = \Sigma x_{ik} p_i(1-p_i)$. Thus,

$$
B = \begin{pmatrix}
2.4 & 0 & 3.2 \\
.7 & 0 & 2.2 \\
4.6 & 4.6 & 6.4 \\
1.5 & 1.5 & 5.0
\end{pmatrix} .
$$

Finally $O = \Sigma y_i$, $E = \Sigma p_i$ and C = M. All vectors and
matrices are evaluated at $\hat{\beta}$.

The goodness of fit statistic is $(O-E)'H(O-E)$
where H is the pseudo inverse of $A-BC^{-1}B'$. This statistic has an approximate chi-square distribution with
degrees of freedom equal to the rank of H. To find
this pseudo inverse, one finds the singular value decomposition of $A-BC^{-1}B' = UDU'$. Then one forms the
diagonal matrix D^- by

$$D_{ii}^- = 1/D_{ii} , \text{ if } D_{ii} > .0001; \ D_{ii}^- = 0 \text{ otherwise } .$$

Then $H = UD^-U'$. The rank of H is the number of non-
zero diagonal elements of D_{ii}^-. In this example, the
rank of H is 2 and $(O-E)'H(O-E) = 0.11$. Thus, the
data are consistent with the logistic model.

ORDINAL RESPONSE DATA

Many end points in clinical trials have more than
two values, and these values are often ordered. For
example: Patients may have a complete response, a
partial response, stable disease, or progression; they
may have none, mild, moderate, severe, or life-
threatening toxicity. To test for a treatment effect
it is inappropriate to use the usual rx2 chi-square
test. This test essentially determines whether the
proportion of patients in each category is the same
in each treatment. It has power against the general
alternative hypothesis but low power against the alternative that one treatment is superior to the other.
An example of the difference between these two alternative hypotheses is shown in Tables 5 and 6. In Table 5 treatment 1 has a higher complete response rate

TABLE 5. Example of Superiority of Treatment 1

	Treatment 1	Treatment 2
Complete response	10%	5%
Partial response	6%	7%
Progression	84%	88%

TABLE 6. Example of an Ambiguous Difference Between Treatments

	Treatment 1	Treatment 2
Complete response	10%	5%
Partial response	2%	11%
Progression	88%	84%

than treatment 2. Furthermore, although the partial response rate on treatment 1 is less than that on treatment 2, the total response rate on treatment 1 is better than that on treatment 2. Thus, patients on treatment 1 have uniformly better outcome than those on treatment 2. A test of treatment effect should be sensitive to this alternative. In Table 6 there is an ambiguous treatment difference. The complete response rate is higher on treatment 1 but the overall response rate is lower. We do not require a test to be sensitive to an ambiguous treatment difference because if the null hypothesis is rejected we would still not know which treatment to prefer.

Treatment effect on an ordinal response variable should be tested using the binary regression test (3). Table 7 gives the 3x2 table that would result if 2 treatments with 3 ordinal categories were being compared. One assigns a score, a_i, to each category, with $a_1 \geq a_2 \geq a_3$. The test statistic is then given by

$$T_1 = \sum_{i=1}^{3} a_i M_{i1} .$$

An exact P-value may be found in the same manner as

TABLE 7. Binary Regression Test

Category	Score	Treatment 1	Treatment 2	Total
1	a_1	M_{11}	M_{12}	$M_{1\cdot}$
2	a_2	M_{21}	M_{22}	$M_{2\cdot}$
3	a_3	M_{31}	M_{32}	$M_{3\cdot}$
	Total	$M_{\cdot 1}$	$M_{\cdot 2}$	n

used in equation 6 and its formula is given by

$$P(T_1 \geq k \mid M_{.1}, M_{.2}, M_{1.}, M_{2.}, M_3.) \quad .$$

In fact, this test is equivalent to the test that
would result if treatment group were considered as a
dependent variable with the ordinal response as the
independent variable. The computation of this test
was discussed in the second example of the section on
the exact test for treatment effects. Alternatively,
in large samples the asymptotic distribution of T_1 can
be used (5). Although the test statistic depends on
the choice of scores, this choice is not as important
as it might seem. Define $F_i(x)$ as the empirical distribution function of the response to treatment i,

$$F_i(x) = M._i^{-1} \sum_{j \leq x} M_{ji} \quad .$$

A test based on T_1 is equivalent to

$$\sum_{x=1}^{3} w(x)[F_1(x) - F_2(x)] \quad ,$$

where $w_1 = a_1 - a_2$, $w_2 = a_2 - a_3$, and $w_3 = a_3$. This is
the familiar one-sided Cramer-von Mises statistic for
comparing distribution functions. Thus, evenly spaced
scores which give a constant weight function are appropriate for most situations.

The logistic model is one of the statistical techniques that has been increasingly used due to the
widespread availability of the digital computer. The
computer allows rapid estimation of parameters and
test construction. Programs for performing this analysis are available in most statistical computer programming packages. (See Chapter 9.) Useful books
which include discussion of logistic regression are
references 1, 2, 3, and 6.

REFERENCES

1. Anderson, A., Auquier, A., Hauck, W. W., Oakes, D., Vandaele, W., and Weisberg, H. (1980), Statistical Methods for Comparative Studies, Wiley, New York.

2. Bishop, Y. M. M., Fienberg, S. E., and Holland, P. W. (1975), Discrete Multivariate Analysis, MIT Press, Cambridge, Massachusetts.

3. Cox, D. R. (1970), Analysis of Binary Data, Chapman and Hall, London.

4. Dixon, W. J., and Brown, M. B., eds. (1979), BMDP Biomedical Computer Programs P-Series, University of California Press, Berkeley, California.

5. Gail, M. (1974), Value systems for comparing 2 independent multinomial trials, Biometrika 61: 71-100.

6. Haberman, S. J. (1974), The Analysis of Frequency Data, University of Chicago Press, Chicago.

7. Halperin, M., Ware, J. H., Byar, D. P., Mantel, N., Brown, C. C., Koziol, J., Gail, M., and Green, S. B. (1977), Testing for interaction in an IxJxK contingency table, Biometrika 64: 271-273.

8. Kalbfleisch, J. D., and Prentice, R. L. (1980), The Statistical Analysis of Failure Time Data, Wiley, New York.

9. Lehmann, E. L. (1959), Testing Statistical Hypotheses, Wiley, New York.

10. Pagano, M., and Tritchler, D. (1982), Algorithms for the analysis of several 2x2 contingency tables, Journal of Scientific and Statistical Computing. (In press.)

11. Peduzzi, P. N., Hardy, R. J., and Holford, T. R.
    (1980), A stepwise variable selection procedure
    for nonlinear regression models, Biometrics 36:
    511-516.

12. Rao, C. R. (1973), Linear Statistical Inference
    and its Applications, Wiley, New York.

13. Schoenfeld, D. (1980), A comparison of Adriamycin
    versus Adriamycin, Vincristine and Cyclophospha-
    mide versus Actinomycin-D, Vincristine and Cyclo-
    phosphamide for advanced sarcoma, Division of Bio-
    statistics Technical Report No. 190E, Sidney
    Farber Cancer Institute, Boston.

14. Tsiatis, A. A. (1980), A note on the goodness-of-
    fit test for the logistic regression model, Bio-
    metrika 67: 250-251.

15. Zelen, M. (1971), The analysis of several 2x2 con-
    tingency tables, Biometrika 58: 129-137.

CHAPTER 15

Monitoring and Stopping Clinical Trials
MITCHELL H. GAIL

INTRODUCTION

This discussion is confined to methods for monitoring accumulating data on a single major end point, such as time to death. It is usually unrealistic to ignore other end points such as toxicity, or administrative factors such as failure of patient accrual, in making a decision to stop a clinical trial. We shall discuss some of the limitations of available formal methods, which have a very restricted focus.

We are not including important related topics such as adaptive treatment assignment methods, in which the treatment allocation probabilities are allowed to depend on accumulating end point information. Such methods have been reviewed by Hoel, Sobel, and Weiss (40) and Simon (62). Nor do we discuss adaptive randomization to achieve a balance on prognostic factors as in Efron (33), Pocock and Simon (57) and Wei (66). We consider only the case of two treatments with equal allocation fractions.

Those who monitor clinical trials must make two important decisions: (a) when to stop accrual, and (b) when to publish scientific results. The formal theory reviewed here does not make this distinction, and a decision to "stop the trial" is usually taken

as synonymous with a decision to publish an estimate
of treatment effect and P-value. Rubinstein and Gail
(58) have shown how one can advantageously separate
these two decisions in survival studies. In some situations one can monitor accumulating data solely to
terminate accrual early, and then one can rely on the
reservoir of patients still at risk to provide the required information to test for a treatment effect when
enough deaths have subsequently occurred. In the rest
of this chapter, however, we assume that the purpose
of monitoring the trial is solely to come to a treatment decision and publish.

Of course the reason why monitoring a trial is so
difficult is that a balance must be struck between the
need for convincing scientific evidence and the desire
to minimize the number of experimental subjects who
are given the inferior treatment. Convincing scientific evidence generally requires that sufficient patients be studied (a) to obtain an unbiased estimate
of treatment effect with good precision (small variance), (b) to adjust the analysis for imbalances in
important prognostic factors, (c) to look for consistency of treatment effect in subgroups, and (d) to obtain reliable information on toxicity and side effects. Such information is likely to influence the
thinking and behavior of medical opinion makers and
practitioners. Conflicting with the need for strong
scientific evidence are the desires (a) to use as few
patients as possible in the experiment, (b) to make
the data available to the outside community as soon
as possible, and (c) never to "knowingly" assign a patient to an inferior experimental treatment. These
latter considerations suggest the need to monitor the
accumulating end point data and to stop accruing patients and publish the results as soon as possible.

In view of these conflicting objectives it is
hardly surprising that there are several statistical
approaches to monitoring clinical trials. We shall
discuss 4 formulations of the problem: (a) frequentist, (b) Bayesian, (c) decision theoretic, and (d)

selection theory. These formulations differ in how
they measure the strength of evidence and in what is
to be emphasized as the central purpose of the trial.
In the section entitled "Monitoring Data on Pairwise Treatment Differences," we review these 4 approaches as applied to the problem of accumulating data on normally distributed pairwise treatment differences. The section entitled "Criticisms and Comparisons of Proposed Boundaries" contains a discussion of
limitations of this theory, and accumulating survival
data is discussed in the section entitled "Monitoring
Time to Response Data."

MONITORING DATA ON PAIRWISE TREATMENT DIFFERENCES

Statement of the Problem

The following problem has been considered by Armitage (5, Chap. 5), Anscombe (4), Colton (18) and others. One observes the differences $D_i = X_{1i} - X_{2i}$ for
the n patient pairs i=1,2,...,n, where X_{1i} and X_{2i} are
the responses for treatments 1 and 2 in pair i.
These differences are assumed to be made available
sequentially. The D_i are normal $N(\delta, \sigma^2)$ variates.
The variance σ^2 is assumed known. We study this problem in some detail because it has been the focus of
attention in the literature and because solutions to
this problem seem to apply, at least approximately,
to monitoring time to response data.

Frequentist Approaches

The most familiar method for planning and analyzing
such data is to use a __fixed sample__ design. Such a design requires that we observe

$$n = (Z_{\alpha/2} + Z_\beta)^2 (\sigma/\delta)^2 \qquad (1)$$

treatment pairs and then reject the null hypothesis

δ = 0 in favor of a two-sided alternative $|\delta| \neq 0$ whenever

$$|S(n)/\sigma| > 1.96n^{\frac{1}{2}} \qquad (2)$$

where

$$S(n) = \sum_{i=1}^{n} D_i \ . \qquad (3)$$

In equation 1, Z_β and $Z_{\alpha/2}$ are standard normal deviates corresponding to power 1-β and two-tailed size α. We shall require size α = 0.05 and power 0.95 against the alternative $|\delta/\sigma|$ = 0.5. (For comparison, all frequentist boundaries discussed below will have the same size and power parameters.) Thus, $Z_{\alpha/2}$ = 1.96, Z_β = 1.645, and equation 1 yields n = 52 required pairs.

Of course the fixed sample design specifically prohibits early stopping based on accumulating evidence in the cumulative sum S(i), i=1,2,...,n. However, this fixed sample design has several attractive features. It is easy to plan and execute. The analysis is straightforward. In particular, the estimate $\hat{\delta}$ = S(n)/n is unbiased with variance σ^2/n, and confidence intervals, such as the 95% confidence interval $\hat{\delta}\pm1.96\sigma n^{-\frac{1}{2}}$, are easily constructed. By contrast, estimation in sequential designs can be quite complicated as illustrated in Siegmund (61). For the fixed sample design, the evidence against the null hypothesis, as measured by the observed significance level P, has a simple correspondence with a more satisfactory measure of evidence, the observed likelihood ratio r for values δ = 0 and δ = $\hat{\delta}$. Indeed, r = exp($-\hat{\delta}^2 n/2\sigma^2$) = exp$[-S(n)^2/2n\sigma^2]$, which shows that large values of $|S(n)|$ give evidence against the null hypothesis. But the observed two-sided P-value is P=P(χ_1^2>-2·ln r), which exhibits the correspondence between small P-values and small likelihood ratios. For example, P= 0.05 and P=0.01 correspond respectively to r = 0.147

and r = 0.035. This concordance between evidence as
measured by P-value and evidence as measured by likelihood ratio does not hold for most sequential designs.

A simple modification of the fixed sample design
is to examine the data a few times as the data accumu-
late and to stop the trial if early evidence against
the null hypothesis is strong. Wetherill (67, Chap.
11) reviews double sampling plans and refers to the
early work of Dodge and Romig (29). Pocock (55) emphasizes the practical advantages of monitoring a
clinical trial after successive groups of observations
are obtained and uses the term "group sequential" to
describe such designs. To be explicit, suppose it is
desired to examine the data at most L times, once after each batch of m patient pairs has been observed.
The Pocock (55) rule is to continue to enter batches
of m patient pairs as long as

$$\left| S(n)/\sigma \right| < k(L,\alpha)n^{\frac{1}{2}} \tag{4}$$

where $n = im$, $i=1,2,\ldots,$ L-1, and $k(L,\alpha)$ is a constant
determined to assure overall size α. If the inequality 4 is satisfied for all $i=1,2,\ldots,L$, accept the null
hypothesis. If i^* is the smallest $i \leq L$ such that the
inequality 4 is violated, reject the null hypothesis
and stop sampling after $n^* = i^*m$ patient pairs. For
example, if there are to be at most L = 5 groups of
patients, then, for $\alpha = 0.05$, $\beta = 0.05$ and $\left| \delta/\sigma \right| =$
0.5, the boundary 4 requires $k(5,0.05) = 2.413$ and m =
13. The parameters $k(L,\alpha)$ and m are computed from tables in Pocock (55), who relies on the methods of
Armitage, McPherson, and Row (7) and McPherson and
Armitage (47).

Note that $k(5,0.05) = 2.413$ is greater than 1.96.
If the value 1.96 were used instead, the multiple
looks at the data would increase the chance of rejection, under the null hypothesis, to 0.14. The value
$k(L,\alpha)$ must be calculated to compensate for repeated
looks and to yield a true size α test.

The boundary 4 is said to be parabolic because if $S(n)/\sigma$ is plotted against n, the boundary points satisfy $S(n)^2/\sigma^2 = k^2(L,\alpha)n$. Figure 1 depicts the group sequential boundary discussed here, together with 3 other boundaries we shall discuss. One can monitor accumulating data by plotting the points $[n,S(n)/\sigma]$ and stopping whenever they infringe the boundaries indicated in Figure 1.

Nonparabolic group sequential boundaries have also been proposed. Haybittle (39) and Peto et al. (54) suggested using constants 3.00 in place of $k(L,\alpha)$ for $i=1,2,\ldots,L-1$ and 1.96 for $i = L$. Such a boundary has a size which for moderate L only slightly exceeds 0.05 (for L=5, the true size is 0.053). This boundary

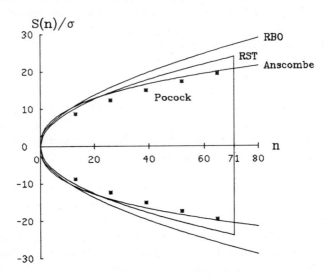

Figure 1. The Pocock boundary is given by equation 4 with L = 5, m = 13, and k(5,0.05) = 2.413, and the repeated significance test (RST) boundary is given by equation 4 with L = 71, m = 1, and k(71,0.05) = 2.84. The Bayesian RBO and decision theoretic Anscombe boundaries come from equation 7, with $\tau=\sigma=1$, and equation 9, respectively.

rarely causes the trial to stop early, but it does offer the possibility to stop if early estimates of
treatment effect are very large. Another conservative
rule is the horizontal boundary $|S(n)/\sigma|$ = (CmL) for
n = im, i=1,2,...,L with C chosen to assure proper
size as in O'Brien and Fleming (52).

Rather than use a fixed sample rule or group sequential plan, the frequentist may choose to monitor
the data after each patient pair enters. Such a
scheme is termed purely sequential. Armitage (5,
Chap. 5) reviews several such plans, which can be represented as boundaries in Figure 1. One of these, the
repeated significance test (RST) boundary, is illustrated in Figure 1 and is really a special case of the
Pocock boundary (inequality 4) with batch size m = 1,
maximum looks L = 71, and $k(L,\alpha)$ = k(71,0.05) = 2.84.
It is seen in Figure 1 that the RST boundary is parabolic and that it encloses the Pocock boundary with
L = 5 discussed before. The larger boundary width is
required to assure proper size in the face of 71 looks
instead of only 5 looks. The methods for constructing
RST boundaries were published by Armitage et al. (7)
and McPherson and Armitage (47).

The first purely sequential boundaries were developed by Wald (65). The continuation region consists
of two channels bounded by the straight lines labeled
"rejection" and "open acceptance" in Figure 2. The
null hypothesis is accepted if the inner wedge is infringed, and the null hypothesis is rejected if the
outer lines are infringed. Details are in Armitage
(5, Chap. 5). The main aim of this design is to
reduce the number of pairs required to make a decision
while retaining the specified size α = 0.05 and power
$1-\beta$ = 0.95 against $|\delta/\sigma|$ = 0.5.

A troublesome feature of the Wald boundary is that
the continuation region extends indefinitely. Thus,
although the test is known to have probability one of
stopping eventually, the researcher cannot specify in
advance how many patient pairs will actually be needed
or even set an upper limit on this number. Armitage

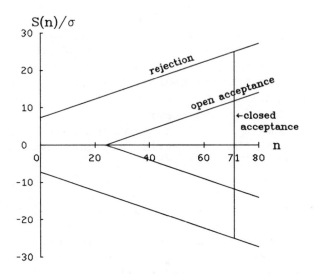

Figure 2. The Wald boundary has rejection lines
$S(n)/\sigma = 7.28 + n/4$ and $S(n)/\sigma = -7.28 - n/4$. The inner wedge defining the acceptance region for the Wald
boundary is formed by the intersection of $S(n)/\sigma =$
$-5.94 + n/4$ with $S(n)/\sigma = 5.94 - n/4$. The closed Wald
boundary uses the same rejection lines as above, but
the null hypothesis is accepted if the line $n = 71$ is
reached prior to rejection. The inner open acceptance
lines play no role in the closed Wald boundary. These
boundaries were chosen to have size 0.05 and power
0.95 against $|\delta/\sigma| = 0.5$

(5, Chap. 5) restricted the Wald design by imposing an
upper limit (for our example n=71) as shown in the
closed Wald plan in Figure 2. The continuation region
is bounded by the previous rejection lines of the Wald
boundary and by the vertical line $n = 71$. The inner
open acceptance lines play no role. If the Wald rejection lines are crossed, the null hypothesis is rejected, and otherwise the null hypothesis is accepted
at $n = 71$.

Some comparisons among frequentist boundaries are

indicated in Table 1. These boundaries are all intended to have size α = 0.05 and power 1-β = 0.95
against the alternative $|\delta/\sigma|$ = 0.5. Armitage (5,
Chap. 5) finds that the closed Wald boundary has actual α = 0.04 and β = 0.06. The fixed sample design
never requires more than max(n) = 52 patient pairs,
and, of course the average number of patient pairs re-
quired is 52 if $|\delta/\sigma|$ = 0 and 52 if $|\delta/\sigma|$ = 0.5. No-
tice that, in terms of the maximum number of pairs
that might be required, the fixed sample design is

TABLE 1. Comparisons of Frequentist Boundaries[a]

| | Maxi-mum n | Average n | | α | β |
		$(\delta/\sigma)=0$	$(\delta/\sigma)=1/2$		
Fixed sample	52	52	52	0.05	0.05
Pocock (L=5)	65	65	33	0.05	0.05
Wald (open)	∞	33	26	0.05	0.05
Wald (closed)	71	69	30	0.04	0.06
Repeated signifi-cance test	71	68	30	0.05	0.05

[a]The Type II error β is calculated for $|\delta/\sigma|$ = 0.5.

best, and the open Wald boundary is intolerable. Un-
der the alternative $|\delta/\sigma|$ = 0.5, the average number
of pairs needed is only 33 for the Pocock boundary,
so that monitoring the data only L = 5 times captures
most of the savings obtainable with purely sequential

methods. Under the null hypothesis $|\delta/\sigma| = 0$, the average sample number for the fixed sample design is smaller than for any of the other boundaries except the open Wald boundary.

It is sometimes overlooked that the chief benefit of sequential plans, early stopping, also results in loss of precision in estimates of treatment effect. Moreover, naive estimates such as $\hat{\delta} = S(n)/n$ are biased, and more complicated methods are required to obtain reliable estimates as discussed by Cox (23), Anscombe (3), and Siegmund (61).

The purely sequential designs above by no means exhaust the possible boundaries. Triangular continuation regions with base on the vertical line $n = 0$ have been discussed by Anderson (2) and Jones and Whitehead (41,42). Several means of closing the Wald boundaries are considered by Schneiderman and Armitage (59). Nonetheless, the repeated significance test boundary in Figure 1 is taken as representative of the class of purely sequential frequentist boundaries and is used for comparison with nonfrequentist boundaries. This seems reasonable, especially because Armitage (5, Figure 5.3) shows the repeated significance test boundary and closed Wald boundary are nearly superimposable.

Stopping Based on Relative Betting Odds:
A Bayesian Approach

Cornfield (21) reviewed certain problems with the frequentist approach and objected especially to the notion that the observed α level could be taken as a measure of the evidence against the null hypothesis (see next section). Instead he proposed that one monitor the relative betting odds, RBO, defined by

$$RBO = \frac{P(\text{null hypothesis}|\text{data})}{P(\text{alternative hypothesis}|\text{data})} \times \frac{(1-p)}{(p)} , \quad (5)$$

where p is the prior probability that the null hypothesis is true. For continuous variables such as we are discussing, it is important to assign nonzero prior probability to the null hypothesis. Indeed, for our problem, the prior distribution of δ, given by Cornfield (20,22) is the mixed density

$$P(\delta=0) = p>0 \qquad (6)$$

and

$$(1-p)(2\pi\tau^2)^{-\frac{1}{2}}\exp(-\delta^2/2\tau^2) \quad \text{for } \delta \neq 0 .$$

Thus, nonzero values of δ have a $N(0,\tau^2)$ distribution. The conditional distribution of $S(n)$, given δ, is normal with known variance $n\sigma^2$. It follows that

$$\left| RBO \right| = \left(1 + \frac{n\tau^2}{\sigma^2} \right)^{\frac{1}{2}} \exp\left[-\frac{S(n)^2}{2n\sigma^2} \cdot \frac{n\tau^2}{(\sigma^2+n\tau^2)} \right] . \qquad (7)$$

It would seem reasonable to use the RBO as a summary measure of evidence for or against the null hypothesis and to reject the null hypothesis whenever RBO gets too small. For $\tau=\sigma=1$, the boundary $\left| RBO \right|$ = 1/20 is shown in Figure 1. One might stop an experiment and reject the null hypothesis as soon as the cumulative sum $S(n)/\sigma$ crosses this boundary.

Decision Theoretic Stopping

Anscombe (4) and Colton (18) consider the following decision theoretic model:

1. There are N patients who may potentially be affected by a clinical trial, either because they are experimental participants or because their therapies will be influenced by the outcome of the trial.
2. Whenever a patient receives the inferior treatment, an amount $\left| \delta \right|$ is lost. There are no other losses and only two possible treatments.

3. The parameter δ has a diffuse normal prior distribution.
4. Given δ, D_i has a normal $N(\delta,\sigma^2)$ distribution,
with σ^2 known.
After n patient pairs have entered such an experiment, the expected loss is

$$nE|\delta|+(N-2n)E\{\max[0,-\delta\,\text{sgn}(S(n))]\} . \qquad (8)$$

The first term represents the n experimental individuals who got the inferior treatment, and
the second term corresponds to the remaining
(N-2n) patients who will receive the inferior
treatment if the sign of S(n), denoted
sgn(S(n)), is misleading.

Anscombe (4) gave an approximate boundary to minimize the expected loss (formula 8) as

$$|S(n)/\sigma| = -n^{\frac{1}{2}}\Phi^{-1}(n/N) \qquad (9)$$

where Φ is the standard normal distribution function.
This solution has been shown to be nearly optimal for
large N by Lai et al. (45) and by Chernoff and Petkau
(17). Day (25) gives an exact method of solution
which is feasible for small N. Begg and Mehta (10)
also consider this problem, but Petkau (53) finds
their solution inferior to equation 9.
   The boundary 9 is shown in Figure 1 for the "patient horizon" N = 10,000. If this boundary is
crossed, theory would dictate that the experiment stop
and the remaining (N-2n) patients be given the treatment which appears better.
   The boundary 9 represents a purely sequential solution to this problem. Colton (18,19) and Day (26)
have discussed one stage and multistage solutions, and
Colton (18) argues that the boundary $|S(n)/\sigma| = (N/6)^{\frac{1}{2}}$
is nearly optimal among horizontal boundaries. Fur-
ther work related to this decision theoretic model is

reported by Donner (30) and Mendoza and Iglewicz (49, 50).

Selection Theory

This survey of methods for monitoring and stopping clinical trials would be incomplete without a discussion of selection theory, which has been reviewed recently by Gibbons, Olkin, and Sobel (36) and Dudewicz (31). The object of selection theory is to select the superior treatment with probability exceeding γ = 0.95, say, whenever the true treatment difference $|\delta/\sigma|$ exceeds a specified "indifference" value $(\delta*/\sigma)>0$. For only two treatments, the selection will be based on the sign of $S(n)$. Bechhofer (8) treats the general case, but it is easy to show for only two treatments that the fixed sample size n required to assure P(better treatment selected) $\geq \gamma$ for all $|\delta/\sigma| \geq \delta*/\sigma > 0$ is given by

$$n = (\sigma/\delta*)^2 z_\gamma^2 \qquad (10)$$

with Z_γ the γth percentile of a standard normal deviate. For $(\delta*/\sigma) = 0.5$ and $\gamma = 0.95$, we obtain $Z_\gamma = 1.645$ and n = 11 pairs.

That only n = 11 pairs are required indicates that it is much easier to select the better treatment with high probability [if the treatment difference is known to exceed the "indifference" value $(\delta*/\sigma) = 0.5$] than it is to convince others with classical hypothesis tests that one treatment is better than the other. Clearly, if one studies only 11 pairs, the precision of the estimated treatment effect will be low in cases of practical interest. Sequential selection procedures reduce sample size even further, as discussed in Bechhofer, Kiefer, and Sobel (9).

CRITICISMS AND COMPARISONS OF PROPOSED BOUNDARIES

General Criticisms of These Methods

Before describing criticisms that have been leveled at the 4 basic approaches (frequentist, Bayesian, decision theoretic, and selection) outlined earlier, we shall mention certain features which may be unrealistic and which apply to each of the methods discussed. These points are illustrated in accounts of the decision to stop real trials, as in the University Group Diabetes Program (64), Gilbert et al. (37), Pocock (56), Ederer (32), Canner (15), and DeMets, Williams, and Brown (28).

Logistic problems hamper purely sequential approaches. Even if the pair response is instantaneous, which is seldom the case, accurate data are sometimes not available when needed. DeMets et al. (28) illustrate how the final data set can give different results for interim analyses from those performed in real time. It is often not feasible to perform continous up-to-date statistical surveillance. The nature of the patients accruing or the treatments may change subtly during the course of the trial, so that the variables D_i are not truly identically distributed. Such change may affect the performance of sequential methods more than fixed sample methods. Certain details of the model are open to question, such as entry in matched pairs and the assumptions of normality with known variance. However, in monitoring time to response data (see section below), there is no pairing and the normality and known variance assumptions appear to be reasonable.

Perhaps the overriding inadequacy of all the methods in the previous section is that, in focusing only on the main study end point, they fail to take into account a variety of other factors. For studies having multiple end points, the framework presented above is clearly inadequate. Toxicity data are often a powerful determinant of whether or not to continue a

study. Limitations of financial and medical resources, including inadequate accrual, may end a
study. New treatments or evidence presented in the
literature may influence the decision to stop a trial.
Unexpected results, such as adverse treatment effects
in a subgroup of patients, may bring the trial to a
halt. In addition, there is the issue of how convincing the data would be if the trial were stopped. In
part, this is determined by following the main end
point as in the section above. Other aspects include
consistency within subgroups, critical examination of
the control arm, and a consideration of the possibility that continued study would lead to a reversal of
the present conclusions. The decision to stop a clinical trial is more complicated than the simple stopping boundaries in Figure 1.

Technical Criticisms of the Frequentist, Bayesian, Decision Theoretic, and Selection Methods

Anscombe (4) and Cornfield (20,21) criticize frequentist approaches to sequential monitoring of clinical trial data. A central concern is whether the
level associated with a sequential trial is a reasonable measure of the evidence against the null hypothesis. Cornfield coins the term "α-postulate," namely,
"All hypotheses rejected at the same critical level
have the same amounts of evidence against them." He
argues that the α-postulate is not true. If at one
point in the monitoring the null hypothesis is not rejected at the 0.05 level, then no matter how much evidence against the null hypothesis subsequently devel-
ops, the overall critical level must exceed 0.05. For
this and other reasons, Cornfield and Anscombe reject
the α-postulate and prefer to base their inferences
on the likelihood function. Because the observed
likelihood does not depend on sequential boundaries,
likelihood based inference is not affected by the
stopping rules. Such inference is based solely on
what was observed, rather than on what might have been

observed in hypothetical repetitions of the entire experiment with the same stopping rules. Indeed, Anscombe insists that it is inappropriate to use methods of inference, such as Neyman-Pearson hypothesis testing, which might be entirely appropriate for repeated sampling inspection, for analysis of a complicated clinical trial that is unlikely to be repeated. Other criticisms of frequentist methods include the artificiality of the parameter space (20), and the arbitrary specification of parameters α and β and the alternative hypothesis of interest, which determine the rejection region.

The Bayesian relative betting odds approach might be criticized for the arbitrary choice of prior distribution on δ. Cornfield (20) emphasizes that non-zero prior probability must be placed on the null hypotheses to avoid "sampling to a foregone conclusion." Otherwise, likelihood based inference will lead to rejecting the null hypothesis with probability one if monitoring continues long enough. This difficulty is avoided by use of a prior distribution such as formula 6. More realistic null hypotheses, such as $|\delta| \leq \Delta$ rather than $\delta = 0$, have been treated by Lachin (44). Nonetheless, the need to specify a prior, as typified by the parameters p and τ in formula 6, must be considered a weakness of this methodology.

The decision theoretic method discussed above is based on an oversimplified view of the loss structure. As already mentioned, many other factors would enter into a realistic assessment of losses. Even the notion that the loss is symmetric is questionable, especially if one is comparing a new treatment against a widely accepted conventional therapy. In that case it may be that mistakenly selecting the new treatment entails more loss than mistakenly selecting the conventional treatment. Except for minimax solutions, the decision theoretic approach also requires specification of a prior distribution on δ. An especially disturbing feature of this model is the assumption that there is a fixed "patient horizon," N, of

patients who may be influenced by the trial. As Anscombe (4) pointed out, a dramatic trial result will
likely cause more people to receive the recommended
treatment than a less dramatic result. Thus, N is not
fixed, but depends on the trial data. The mathematics
are altered by such a relationship between N and S(n).
Even if N is fixed, the choice of N has an important
impact on the boundary 9, as illustrated in Anscombe
(4, Table 1).

The selection methodology can be faulted for yielding too few data to estimate δ with precision. Furthermore, an indifference interval [0,δ*] must be
specified as well as a required probability of correct
selection γ. Thus, this method is no more free of the
requirement to specify arbitrary design parameters
than are the other methods discussed.

Comparison of Frequentist, Bayesian, Decision Theoretic, and Selection Boundaries

For reasons already mentioned, we shall not consider purely sequential selection boundaries. Figure 1
contains 3 representative purely sequential boundaries, a repeated significance test (frequentist)
boundary, a Bayesian relative betting odds boundary,
and a decision theoretic Anscombe boundary. It is
striking how similar the shapes of the boundaries are,
despite the very different considerations going into
their constructions. An expositor of each approach
could interpret the other boundaries in his own terms.
For example, the decision theorist might say that the
repeated significance test boundary is just a decision
theoretic boundary with N about 12,000, and the Bayesian might regard the repeated significance test
boundary as appropriate behavior for a relative betting odds limit of say RBO≤1/16 instead of RBO≤1/20.
Thus, these boundaries are approximately commensura-
ble. While these comments do not apply to all frequentist boundaries, it should be recalled that the

repeated significance test boundary and closed Wald
boundary (Figure 2) are nearly superimposable.

MONITORING TIME TO RESPONSE DATA

Introductory Comments

Time to response data, such as time to death or
time to recurrence, are the major end points of many
clinical studies. If all patients enter simultaneously, with N/2 assigned to each group, and if there
are no losses to follow-up, observations are said to
exhibit "progressive censorship." The theory of progressive censorship is well understood, because the
progressive revelation of new death rank information
does not alter earlier rank orderings. Although progressively censored data are common in industrial reliability tests, they seldom arise in clinical trials.
Rather, in clinical trials patients arrive haphaz-
ardly, and the entry is said to be "staggered." The
analysis of staggered entry experiments is complicated
by the fact that a patient who enters late and dies
shortly thereafter can alter the death ranks of those
who entered earlier. For this reason, we shall review
available methods for progressive censoring and staggered entry separately.

We shall see that many of the boundaries discussed
earlier can be applied to monitoring time to response
data.

Progressive Censoring

If all N patients enter simultaneously, it may be
possible to monitor the data until a point is reached
at which the monitoring statistic cannot possibly
change enough in the final phase of observation to alter the final decision. At this point, the experiment
is "curtailed," and a decision is reached. Alling (1)
and Halperin and Ware (38) discuss curtailment in

connection with the Wilcoxon statistic. Canner (13) uses Monte Carlo methods to develop critical values for repeated tests of equality of the proportions surviving in two treatment groups. These tests are performed at fixed intervals in real time, which makes the results analogous to group sequential tests.

Chatterjee and Sen (16) establish a sound theory for monitoring progressively censored life data using rank statistics modified for such censorship. They show that the increments of such rank statistics are uncorrelated, and, further, that such rank statistics may be normalized to converge to a Wiener process. To be specific, consider the log-rank statistic discussed by Mantel (48) and Cox (24). Let $t_1 < t_2 \ldots < t_N$ be times of death of the N patients, and, assuming there are no ties, let $Z_i = 1$ if the death at t_i is in group 1 and $Z_i = 0$ otherwise. Further, let p_i denote the proportion of those at risk at t_i who are in group 1. Then, the log-rank score after d deaths is

$$U(d) = \sum_{i=1}^{d} (Z_i - p_i) \qquad (11)$$

and an associated variance is

$$V(d) = \sum_{i=1}^{d} p_i (1 - p_i) . \qquad (12)$$

The results of Chatterjee and Sen (16) and Koziol and Petkau (43) demonstrate that increments of $U(d)$ are uncorrelated, and that under the null hypothesis $U(d)(N/4)^{-\frac{1}{2}}$ converges to a Wiener process $W(\tau)$ on $[0,1]$ with $\tau = V(d)/(n/4)$. The log-rank score $U(d)$ thus behaves much like $S(n)$, because $S(n)(\sigma^2 N)^{-\frac{1}{2}}$ also converges to $W(\tau)$ on $[0,1]$ with $\tau = n/N$. Indeed, a plot of $2U(d)$ against $4V(d)$, as suggested by Armitage (6, p. 143), is entirely analogous to plots of $S(n)/\sigma$ against n as in Figures 1 and 2. Chatterjee and Sen

(16) and Koziol and Petkau (43) recommend horizontal boundaries like $|U(d)| = k$, whereas Muenz, Green, and Byar (51) obtain approximately parabolic boundaries of the form $|U(d)| = kd^{\frac{1}{2}}$.

The theory of Chatterjee and Sen (16) covers a wide range of rank statistics, modified for progressive censoring. In the case of simultaneous entry, such a modified rank statistic behaves approximately like the cumulative sum of independent normal variates. Thus, boundaries like those in Figures 1 and 2 may be used, and the properties of such boundaries can be determined, at least approximately.

Staggered Entry

The problem of staggered entry is still an area of active research. Until rather recently, the only available sequential methodology relied on the assumption of exponential lifetimes, as outlined by Breslow and Haug (11). They showed that the quantities $Y(d) = (d/2)\ln(\hat{\lambda}_1/\hat{\lambda}_2)$ and d were analogous, respectively, to $S(n)/\sigma$ and n in Figures 1 and 2. Here $\hat{\lambda}_1$ and $\hat{\lambda}_2$ are the observed death rates (per person year exposure) in treatment groups 1 and 2, respectively, at the time of death d. The variate $Y(d)$ behaves approximately like the cumulative sum of d independent $N(\delta,1)$ variables with expectation $\delta = (\frac{1}{2})\ln(\lambda_1/\lambda_2)$. Thus, boundaries like those discussed earlier are applicable. Canner (14), who also assumes exponentiality, obtains approximate critical values for repeated significance tests performed at fixed time intervals.

Armitage (6, p. 143) credits Richard Peto for suggesting that, even in the case of staggered entry with random loss to follow-up, the boundaries appropriate to a cumulative sum like $S(d)/\sigma$ in Figures 1 and 2 could be applied to a plot of $2U(d)$ versus $4V(d)$. With staggered entry, the summations in equations 11 and 12 are only over death times, not censorship times. It is suggested the quantity $2U(d)$ be regarded as the cumulative sum of d deviations, $2(Z_i - p_i)$, each corresponding to an independent Bernoulli trial with null expectation $EZ_i = p_i$ and variance $p_i(1-p_i)$. Under the proportional hazard alternative $h_1(t) = h_2(t)\exp(\theta)$, for θ near the null value 0, the expectation of the deviate $2(Z_i-p_i)$ is approximately $2\theta(p_i)(1-p_i) \doteq \theta/2$, and the corresponding variance is $4p_i(1-p_i) \doteq 1$. Thus, one can design boundaries as before by using the parameters $\delta = \theta/2$ and $\sigma^2 = 1$ for local proportional hazards alternatives. This result appears in Armitage (6, p. 143), and is obtained by Schoenfeld (60). It is essentially identical to the standard power calculation given by George and Desu (35) for use with a parametric test for comparing two exponential distributions. This approximation to the power of the log-rank test is known to be quite accurate for relative hazards $\exp(\theta)$ ranging from $\frac{1}{2}$ to 2 (46).

Jones and Whitehead (41,42) justify the use of the approximations above by formal treatment of the partial likelihood of Cox (24), and by supporting simulations. But in essence, the partial likelihood asserts that the survival information relevant to treatment effects is to be found in a sequence of independent Bernoulli trials with parameters $\exp(\theta)p_i/(\exp(\theta)p_i + 1-p_i)$. Further, it is assumed that survival information obtained later in an experiment does not appreciably alter the partial likelihood formed previously. If one is willing to accept this representation of the experiment, one is naturally led to monitoring $U(d)$ [or $2U(d)$] against $V(d)$ [or $4V(d)$]. Jones and Whitehead (41) give approximate calculations of expected sample size for horizontal boundaries $|U(d)| = k$, and Whitehead and Jones (68) discuss estimation of θ and expected sample size for linear boundaries such as the Wald boundary.

One is tempted, therefore, to monitor time to response data simply by regarding $2U(d)$ as a cumulative sum and using the boundaries discussed earlier. For example, one could use the Pocock group sequential boundaries in Figure 1 by computing $2U(d)$ at the times

of deaths 13, 26, 39,..., which correspond roughly to
equal increments of 4V(d) so long as the p_i are near
½. Further methodologic work is required, however.
No rigorous weak convergence results on 2U(d), computed at times of deaths, are as yet available, though
Tsiatis (63) has recently shown that increments of
U(d), computed at fixed real times (rather than at
fixed numbers of deaths), are asymptotically uncorrelated and jointly normal. Further simulations or theoretical developments are needed to define the small
sample behavior of such tests. Simulations of Gail,
DeMets, and Slud (34) show that group sequential procedures are less robust to trends in the types of patients entering the study than is the fixed sample approach. In this regard it is reassuring to note, however, that in an experiment in which those last entering lived twice as long on average as those first entering, the Pocock boundary size was 0.071 compared
with the fixed sample test size of 0.040 and nominal
size 0.05.

Even when the theory of staggered entry is fully
developed, there will be a special need for caution
in applying sequential methods to survival data. If
the two survival curves cross, a sequential procedure
may declare an early winner, but further follow-up may
reveal that there is no clear treatment preference.
Thus, early reports based on sequential monitoring of
time to response data should be suitably qualified.

DISCUSSION

We have not discussed certain important end points,
such as binomial responses, as considered by Bross
(12) and Armitage (6, Chaps. 3 and 4). Also, the
boundaries presented are appropriate for two-sided
testing only. Often one-sided procedures are more appropriate, as discussed by DeMets and Ware (27). Emphasis has been placed on sequential decision making

or hypothesis testing rather than sequential estimation of a treatment effect. The latter topic is more
in tune with the work of Rubinstein and Gail (58), who
propose testing the null hypothesis only after a fixed
number of deaths (and hence a fixed degree of precision on the estimated relative hazard) has been observed.

It is clear from the variety of approaches to monitoring a single end point, and from a consideration
of the many other factors that go into determining
when to stop a clinical trial, that it is inappropriate to reach such a decision mechanically on the basis
of a predetermined boundary such as in Figures 1 or 2.
Nonetheless, a study of such boundaries is a useful
aid to interpreting the evidence, and may assist those
monitoring trials in their difficult deliberations.

REFERENCES

1. Alling, D. W. (1963), Early decision in the Wilcoxon two-sample test, Journal of the American
   Statistical Association 58: 713-720.

2. Anderson, T. W. (1960), A modificatin of the sequential probability ratio test to reduce sample
   size, Annals of Mathematical Statistics 31: 165-
   197.

3. Anscombe, F. J. (1952), Large sample theory of sequential estimation, Proceedings of the Cambridge
   Philosophical Society, 48: 600-607.

4. Anscombe, F. J. (1963), Sequential medical trials,
   Journal of the American Statistical Association
   58: 365-383.

5. Armitage, P. (1960), Sequential Medical Trials,
   Blackwell, Oxford.

6. Armitage, P. (1975), Sequential Medical Trials, Wiley, New York.

7. Armitage, P., McPherson, C. K., and Rowe, B. C. (1969), Repeated significance tests on accumulating data, Journal of the Royal Statistical Society A132: 235-244.

8. Bechhofer, R. E. (1954), A single-sample multiple decision procedure for ranking means of normal populations with known variances, Annals of Mathematical Statistics 25: 16-39.

9. Bechhofer, R. E., Kiefer, J., and Sobel, M. (1968), Sequential Identification and Ranking Procedures, University of Chicago Press, Chicago.

10. Begg, C. B., and Mehta, C. R. (1979), Sequential analysis of comparative clinical trials, Biometrika 66: 97-103.

11. Breslow, N., and Haug, C. (1972), Sequential comparison of exponential survival curves, Journal of the American Statistical Association 67: 691-697.

12. Bross, I. (1952), Sequential medical plans, Biometrics, 8 188-205.

13. Canner, P. L. (1976), Repeated analysis of clinical trial data, in: Proceedings of the Ninth International Biometric Conference, Vol. 1, The Biometric Society, Boston.

14. Canner, P. L. (1977), Monitoring treatment differences in long-term clinical trials, Biometrics 33: 603-615.

15. Canner, P. L, The Coronary Drug Project Research Group (1981), Practical aspects of decision making in clinical trials: The Coronary Drug Project as

a case study, Controlled Clinical Trials 1: 363–376.

16. Chatterjee, S. K., and Sen, P. K. (1973), Nonparametric testing under progressive censorship, Calcutta Statistical Association Bulletin 22: 13–50.

17. Chernoff, H., and Petkau, A. J. (1981), Sequential medical trials involving paired data, Biometrika 68: 119–132.

18. Colton, T. (1963), A model for selecting one of two medical treatments, Journal of the American Statistical Association 58: 388–400.

19. Colton, T. (1965), A two-stage model for selecting one of two treatments, Biometrics 21: 169–180.

20. Cornfield, J. (1966), A Bayesian test of some classical hypotheses with applications to sequential clinical trials, Journal of the American Statistical Association 61: 577–594.

21. Cornfield, J. (1966), Sequential trials, sequential analysis, and the likelihood principle, American Statistician 20: 18–23.

22. Cornfield, J. (1969), The Bayesian outlook and its application, Biometrics 25: 617–657.

23. Cox, D. R. (1952), A note on the sequential estimation of means, Proceedings of the Cambridge Philosophical Society 48: 447–450.

24. Cox, D. R. (1972), Regression models and life tables (with discussion), Journal of the Royal Statistical Society B34: 187–202.

25. Day, N. E. (1969), A comparison of some sequential designs, Biometrika 56: 301-311.

26. Day, N. E. (1969), Two-stage designs for clinical trials, Biometrics 25: 111-118.

27. DeMets, D. L., and Ware, J. H. (1980), Group sequential methods in clinical trials with a one-sided hypothesis, Biometrika 67: 651-660.

28. DeMets, D. L., Williams, G. W., Brown, B. W., Jr., and the NOTT Research Group (1982), A case report of data monitoring experience: The nocturnal oxygen therapy trial, Controlled Clinical Trials 3: 113-124.

29. Dodge, H. F., and Romig, H. G. (1929), A method of sampling inspection, Bell System Technical Journal 8: 613-631.

30. Donner, A. (1977), The use of auxiliary information in the design of a clinical trial, Biometrics 33: 305-314.

31. Dudewicz, E. J. (1980), Ranking (ordering) and selection: An overview of how to select the best, Technometrics 22: 113-119.

32. Ederer, F. (1980), Monitoring for treatment effects: An inexact science, Presented at the Annual Meeting of the Society for Epidemiological Research, June 19, Minneapolis, Minnesota.

33. Efron, B. (1971), Forcing a sequential experiment to be balanced, Biometrika 58: 403-417.

34. Gail, M. H., DeMets, D. L., and Slud, E. V. (1982), Simulation studies on increments of the two-sample logrank score test for survival time data, with application to group sequential bound-

aries, in: Crowley, J., and Johnson, R., eds., Institute of Mathematical Statistics Monograph on
Survival Analysis. (In press.)

35. George, S., and Desu, M. (1974), Planning the size
and duration of a clinical trial studying the time
to some critical event, Journal of Chronic Diseases 27: 15-24.

36. Gibbons, J. D., Olkin, I., and Sobel, M. (1979),
An introduction to ranking and selection, American
Statistician 33: 185-195.

37. Gilbert, J. P., Meier, P., Rumke, C. L.,
Saracci, R., Zelen, M., and White, C. (1975), Report of the committee for the assessment of biometric aspects of controlled trials of hypoglycemic agents, Journal of the American Medical Association 231: 583-608.

38. Halperin, M., and Ware, J. (1974), Early decision
in a censored Wilcoxon two-sample test for accumulating survival data, Journal of the American Statistical Association 69: 414-422.

39. Haybittle, J. L. (1971), Repeated assessment of
results in clinical trials of cancer treatment,
British Journal of Radiology 44: 793-797.

40. Hoel, D. G., Sobel, M., and Weiss, G. H. (1975), A
survey of adaptive sampling for clinical trials,
in: Elashoff, R. M., ed., Perspectives in Biometrics, Academic Press, New York, pp. 29-61.

41. Jones, D., and Whitehead, J. (1979), Sequential
forms of the log rank and modified Wilcoxon tests
for censored data, Biometrika 66: 105-113.

42. Jones, D., and Whitehead, J. (1979), Applications
of large-sample sequential tests to the analysis

of survival data, in: Tagnon, H. J., and Staquet, M. J., eds., Controversies in Cancer, Masson, New York, pp. 1-5.

43. Koziol, J. A., and Petkau, A. J. (1978), Sequential testing of the equality of two survival distributions using the modified Savage statistic, Biometrika 65: 615-623.

44. Lachin, J. M. (1981), Sequential clinical trials for normal variates using interval composite hypotheses, Biometrics 37: 87-101.

45. Lai, T. L., Levin, B., Robbins, H., and Siegmund, D. (1980), Sequential medical trials, Proceedings of the National Academy of Sciences 77: 3135-3138.

46. Lininger, L., Gail, M. H., Green, S. B., and Byar, D. P. (1979), Comparison of four tests for equality of survival curves in the presence of stratification and censoring, Biometrika 66: 419-428.

47. McPherson, C. K., and Armitage, P. (1971), Repeated significance tests on accumulating data when the null hypothesis is not true, Journal of the Royal Statistical Society A134: 15-25.

48. Mantel, N. (1966), Evaluation of survival data and two new rank tests arising in its consideration, Cancer Chemotherapy Reports 50: 163-170.

49. Mendoza, G., and Iglewicz, B. (1977), A three-phase sequential model for clinical trials, Biometrika 64: 201-205.

50. Mendoza, G., and Iglewicz, B. (1978), An extension of Colton's model for comparing two treatments,

Journal of the American Statistical Association
73: 646-649.

51. Muenz, L. R., Green, S. B., and Byar, D. P.
(1977), Applications of the Mantel-Haenszel statistic to the comparison of survival distributions, Biometrics 33: 617-626.

52. O'Brien, P. C., and Fleming, T. R. (1979), A multiple testing procedure for clinical trials, Biometrics 35: 549-556.

53. Petkau, A. J. (1980), Frequentist properties of
three stopping rules for comparative clinical trials, Biometrika 67: 690-692.

54. Peto, R., Pike, P., Armitage, P., Breslow, N. E.,
Cox, D. R., Howard, S. V., Mantel, N.,
McPherson, K., Peto, J., and Smith, P. G. (1976),
Design and analysis of randomized clinical trials
requiring prolonged observation of each patient,
British Journal of Cancer 35: 585-611.

55. Pocock, S. J. (1977), Group sequential methods in
the design and analysis of clinical trials, Biometrika 64: 191-199.

56. Pocock, S. J. (1979), Can sequential methods be
used for the analysis of cancer clinical trials?
in: Tagnon, H. J., and Staquet, M. J., eds., Controversies in Cancer, Masson, New York, pp. 63-74.

57. Pocock, S., and Simon, R. (1975), Sequential
treatment assignment with balancing for prognostic
factors in the controlled clinical trial, Biometrics 31: 103-115.

58. Rubinstein, L. V., and Gail, M. H. (1982), Monitoring rules for stopping accrual in comparative
clinical survival studies, Controlled Clinical

Trials. (In press.)

59. Schneiderman, M. A., and Armitage, P. (1962), A family of closed sequential procedures, Biometrika 49: 41-56.

60. Schoenfeld, D. (1981), The asymptotic properties of nonparametric tests for comparing survival distributions, Biometrika 68: 316-319.

61. Siegmund, D. (1978), Estimation following sequential tests, Biometrika 65: 341-349.

62. Simon, R. (1977), Adaptive treatment assignment methods and clinical trials, Biometrics 33: 743-749.

63. Tsiatis, A. A. (1981), The asymptotic joint distribution of the efficient scores tests for the proportional hazards model calculated over time, Biometrika 68: 311-315.

64. University Group Diabetes Program (1970), A study of the effects of hypoglycemic agents on vascular complications in patients with adult-onset diabetes, Diabetes 19, Supplement 2, 789-815.

65. Wald, A. (1947), Sequential Analysis, Wiley, New York.

66. Wei, L. (1977), A class of designs for clinical trials, Journal of the American Statistical Association 72: 382-386.

67. Wetherill, G. B. (1975), Sequential Methods in Statistics, Wiley, New York.

68. Whitehead, J., and Jones, D. (1979), The analysis of sequential clinical trials, Biometrika 66: 443-452.

Part VI

Communication

CHAPTER 16

Interacting with the Medical Community: Consulting, Collaboration, Teaching

Panel Discussion
THEODORE COLTON, *Chairman*
EDMUND A. GEHAN
LAWRENCE E. HINKLE, Jr.
CARL M. PINSKY
KENNETH E. STANLEY

T. Colton: I view this panel as dealing with two major questions. First, with regard to consultation and collaboration, what do the biostatistician and physician have to bring to provide a fruitful and productive collaborative arrangement? Once defined, the second question is: What is the best method to get this training? How does the biostatistician get the training he needs to enter this collaboration and how does the physician get the training he needs to deal effectively with the biostatistician?

ROLE OF THE BIOSTATISTICIAN

K. E. Stanley: The first issue I would like to address is consulting versus collaboration. Virtually all statistical textbooks and exams in undergraduate and graduate school focus on problem solving. Two or three sentences describe a particular situation, the data appear, and the student conducts the analysis

---

This work was supported in part by National Cancer Institute Grants CA-12014 and CA-30138.

without the possibility of exploring the problem in greater depth. This aspect of the training of statisticians is not the best preparation for working in a biomedical environment. Although many professional contacts involve short-term consultation on a well-defined problem, the goal in medical research should be collaboration. I define collaboration as being part of a research team in all steps of an investigation, from the initial planning to the final publication.

In the initial contact on a new medical problem the statistician should not enter a situation cold, but should spend some time learning about the disease being studied. He should have access to books such as a physiology text and The Merck Manual of Diagnosis and Therapy (1), which describes current standard medical therapies. He should review a copy of the protocol document or similar research plan, if available. The statistician has the responsibility to acquire a modest background in the medical subject, in order to interact more efficiently with the clinical investigator. Specialization in a particular aspect of medical science is an advantage.

I suggest the following order of topics and strategies in the initial personal contact session. First, discuss with the investigator the overall objectives of the research project. Often, an investigator comes with a particular problem and after a thorough discussion one finds that his real interest is with an objective quite different from that initially stated. This is simply a matter of looking at the proposed objective from different perspectives and deciding which is the best approach. Part of this also involves a discussion on the quantification of the research goals. The end points used to measure outcome should be clear in everyone's mind. Next, review the procedures for data collection. Before such procedures are finalized the statistician might find it helpful to walk around the research site, looking over the shoulder of the technicians to see how they count the cultures, and so on. One should identify the source, understand the purpose, and know the individual responsible for each item of information collected. As the last step in this initial meeting, discuss the proposed analysis. I suggest generating this discussion by having the investigator describe the abstract that is likely to appear for the eventual publication. This should include the 4 or 5 key sentences with the various anticipated conclusions and one or two tables or figures that would justify the major conclusions.

The biostatistician should next conduct a short literature search on the statistical methodology appropriate for the research undertaken. In almost all circumstances research builds on previous results. Someone may have done previous work with analysis of prognostic factors, for example, and one must understand many literature traditions. Even if the biostatistician has developed or used a statistical technique that he has shown to be superior to a traditional procedure, the new technique may not be readily accepted in that particular medical field. One should not compromise the quality of the analysis, but often one will need to simplify the analysis or follow the standard technique so that the final publication constitutes an effective medical statement that is accepted by the appropriate audience. Also, the biostatistician should be aware of the necessity to collect and analyze traditional end points so that the study results will assimilate into the existing medical literature. The desired result is an effective final publication.

The last item is the data analysis. There is no such thing as a single final report of a study. New points that need clarification or further analyses always arise during the presentation to the investigators, in the preparation of the manuscript, or in the process of editorial review for publication.

WORKING AS EQUALS

<u>C. M. Pinsky</u>: My background is one of studying immu-
nology in the cancer patient and involvement in a number of immunotherapy trials. As a result of this
work, almost as a means of self-defense, I became familiar with various biostatistical techniques and have
begun to work closely with biostatisticians. I am
also a member of one of the National Institutes of
Health study sections and, as such, look at a number
of grant proposals from around the world. For the
most part, statistical considerations in these proposals are poorly prepared. Very frequently, insufficient attention has been paid to how the data are to
be collected and how they will be analyzed, due to the
fact that no biostatistician has participated in the
planning of the study.

   With regard to collaboration and consulting, one
should be guided mainly by the complexity of the study
and the knowledge of the biomedical investigator with
whom the biostatistician is working. In certain cases
I think a single consultation may be sufficient. If
the study is relatively simple and if the statistical
techniques are either available from the literature or
already known from prior collaboration, then it may
only be necessary to provide rather limited assistance
to ensure that the study is well designed and well executed. In other situations, more extensive collaboration may be necessary. The biomedical investigator,
clinical investigator, and biostatistician have to
plan the study from day one, and they are collaborat-
ing more or less as equals because each contributes
relatively similar amounts to the overall study design, the aims of the study, and how best to satisfy
these.

ASPECTS OF CONSULTING

<u>E. A. Gehan</u>: I agree with everything that has been
said. Some key questions that we need to address are:

How can the biostatistician become a good consultant
in clinical trials? In interrelating with an investigator how much should he assume the investigator knows
about statistical and computing concepts? How should
statisticians deal with clinician clients, especially
the difficult ones? My remarks will review some of
the points made in the 3 papers on training of biostatisticians for clinical trials that recently appeared in Biometrics (2,3,5).

The biostatistician has to have adequate knowledge
of the medical specialty involved. He must make a
commitment to read the literature and regularly attend
seminars. He needs to know a lot about the particular
disease before he can collaborate effectively with a
clinician. He also should be familiar with the theory
and application of statistical concepts, the capabilities of computing machines, the availability of statistical packages and data base management systems,
and he should have an ability to communicate. Communication is not taught in school but is of fundamental
importance, especially in a cooperative group situation. There may be a wide-ranging discussion on some
issues with differing viewpoints expressed by the participants. The study chairman often turns to the
statistician and says, "Now we have heard these different points of view, what do you think we should
do?" The statistician should be ready to rise to the
occasion and speak to these issues. His role is to
present the statistical options for various viewpoints. That is, if a particular experimental design
is adopted, what does it mean in terms of the number
of patients required, approximate length of study, and
the consequences of that line of action? It is up to
the physicians to make the final decision, but if the
biostatistician can delineate the consequences of the
various decisions, he will have done his part.

Another role for the statistician is understanding
what the clinicians wish to achieve in a particular
study. Clinicians often say that they wish to study
a particular drug in a specific disease. The precise

form of the research design, however, may not be evident. The biostatistician should assist in formulating a general idea into a particular clinical trial with specific objectives, end points, and a data collection plan. Many of these issues may not be resolved in the clinician's mind and the biostatistician can help him a lot in their resolution. For example, I was working with a clinician interested in the effect of bone marrow transplantation on the prognosis of lung cancer patients. At least in the initial sessions, he did not appreciate the importance of also studying the patients who did not receive a bone marrow transplant. Those patients should be part of the study as well to serve as a control group.

A biostatistician should be sensitive to sources of bias and as statisticians we naturally tend to be skeptical. What this entails, in many cases, is multiple analyses. If there are nonevaluable cases or patients who did not quite adhere to the protocol, the biostatistician should be prepared to analyze the study both including and excluding such cases to determine the effect on the conclusions. If they do not have an effect, these biases are not important; if they do, the results of the study are questionable.

With respect to ethical issues, the primary feature of clinical trials is that the patient is the experimental unit. A biostatistician should not be involved in planning a study for others that he would not be willing to participate in himself, if he happened to be suffering from that particular disease. I myself have had bone marrows taken. I participated in discussions where people said that it was impossible to get a bone marrow every week because it is too painful. It is not too bad, really.

It does not take long for a consulting statistician to be overwhelmed with problems and have a lengthy list of things to do each day. No one knocks on his door and says that he should be undertaking theoretical research, unless it is the department chairman. But there are clients who have abstracts to be

finished, or reports to be prepared or grants that
have to be submitted. I do not have any good answer
for the problem of setting priorities but I do have
some prescriptions that I have developed over the
years.

Avoid investigators with a "gold mine of data."
Often the investigator has studied some disease for a
long period of time, but with no particular hypotheses
to be tested. The investigator should be the one to
try to mine these data rather than the biostatistician.

Be wary of investigators who ask for 5 minutes of
your time. First, if it is only going to take 5 minutes, it cannot be too important. Even if you are
able to solve the problem, the investigator will not
give you much credit for it, since it only took 5 minutes. Sometimes an investigator has applied some
statistical test of his own to the data and he asks if
it is correct. Of course, there is no answer to that
question until you understand the full problem. Often
that takes at least one hour to describe. Sometimes
it is clear that he does not understand the particular
problem and he wishes you to explain it to him.
Again, it is going to take a lot of time. My pre-
scription is that the first time someone comes, see
him and spend the necessary time. If the same person,
however, returns on another occasion, give him the 5
minutes and no more. You really will not have lost
much, because that investigator does not have a good
appreciation of what a biostatistician can contribute.

In my initial consulting experience I learned much
about short-cut methods from Nathan Mantel in my work
at the National Cancer Institute. I would go out as
a consultant and end up trying to make sense out of
piles of data from the investigator. Mantel always
seemed to have plenty of time for research and discussions because he used graphical and short-cut methods
and had the investigator do his own analyses. For example, he had a paper in 1951 on the standard error of
the mean being approximately the range divided by the

number of observations up to a sample size of 15 (4).
This is a very useful formula when evaluating many
small data sets. Another useful number is 75. Often
people ask how large a study is needed. Without further information I say 75 patients in each group and
usually I am not too far off. Seventy-five patients
in each group will approximately test for a one-sided
difference of 20% in effectiveness between two treatments at a 5% significance level and 80% power.

The statistician should be aware of a situation
that frequently arises at committee meetings. Following a discussion of differing viewpoints on a particular study, the chairman of the group determines the
consensus and asks if anyone objects to the compromise
proposal. The statistician should be the first to
stand and object because that is not the proper question. Frequently, a compromise is really not satisfactory to anyone and the study may not proceed at
all. Few will object to a compromise, but most will
not give it their full support. The statistician
should try to find out which investigators support the
study and whether it is feasible.

Equal collaboration is important. I am glad that
the physicians at this conference feel that biostatisticians should be equal collaborators.

I am concerned about situations where the statistician is responsible for the data managers. I think
the clinician should be responsible for the quality
of his data and that it should be a junior clinician
or similar person who supervises the data managers.

The statistician should try to write reports of all
consulting meetings, especially those that have taken
only 5 minutes, for several reasons. One is to document what really was accomplished. He should summarize the main points of the project, the agreements
reached, and the consequences of the proposal in statistical terms. It is important both in communication
and in collaboration on the final paper to have documentation of the sequence of events that took place
in the consulting relationship.

With respect to the final publication, the biostatistician should write a large part of the "Results" section in addition to the statistical aspects within the "Materials and Methods" section. When writing, he will find it helpful to have reports previously prepared on these analyses as well as his notes from the consulting sessions.

We have to give as well as take in collaborative activities. For example, I have occasionally been berated by people who say, "How could you ever have cooperated in such a clinical trial? There were a lot of flaws in that particular design and it really did not work very well." A cooperative clinical trial is a group responsibility and, in some cases, the statistician may have argued against a particular design but was overruled by the group. He should be an equal collaborator and have equal responsibility with the clinicians. If there happens to be a poor design, he should feel badly about it only if he had not earlier argued for a better design and expressed the various statistical consequences of the particular study undertaken. One should be willing to accept one's responsibility. If the study does not work out well, not all the fault, however, should be put on the statistician.

The work of a biostatistician can be very rewarding, since one is exposed to real medical as well as statistical problems. The difficult task is to find time to work on them all and set priorities appropriately.

PROFESSIONAL INTERCHANGE

L. E. Hinkle: I have listened to the discussion with interest because it seems to me that, in a university setting, consultation is archaic. The investigator and the statistician should be collaborators. Together they jointly seek the truth. I am an investigator who has some knowledge of how to measure phenomena of a cardiovascular nature, and the biostatistician has

some knowledge of how to evaluate these phenomena
mathematically. Together we can make a better estimate of the probability that my findings are not the
result of chance or bias, and of the extent to which
my conclusions might be applicable to a broader population.

Many of the studies in which I have been involved
include a good many people and cost a great deal of
time and money. Before one undertakes such a study,
it is essential that he have in mind the goal that he
is seeking and the specific hypothesis that he wishes
to investigate. He should know what kinds of counts
or measurements he may be able to make that will yield
data that support or negate his hypothesis. He must
collaborate with a biostatistician from the very beginning. The investigator and the statistician should
consider these matters together in advance in order to
come to an agreement, not only about the hypothesis
that is being tested and the methods that will be
used, but also about the sampling procedure, sample
size, and methods of analysis of the data.

The biostatistician should expect from me, as an
investigator, that I have some understanding of his
concerns, methods, and the logic behind them. The investigator and statistician should not be hesitant to
ask each other about what they propose to do, and what
is the logic behind it. You notice that I do not expect this to be a one-way street. It is essential
that the statistician be able to ask the investigator
what he is doing and why he does it, but it is equally
important that the statistician be able to explain to
the investigator what he is doing and why he does it.

The biostatistician, it seems to me, has to be
aware of the limitations of the concepts and methods
of the clinical investigator, and he should have an
understanding of the limitations and implications of
the entire task in which he and the investigator are
jointly engaged. The limitations of measurements, especially, pose great problems. Many commonly used
measures can be notably inaccurate. The biostatisti-

cian must be aware of the possibility of this if he
is to provide a realistic analysis of the data.

I am quite beyond the stage of believing that I
need a biostatistician simply for a consultant.   I
need him for much more than that.   I cannot carry out
an investigation without having him as a collaborator
on whom I rely very heavily.   I expect to have the
kind of interchange between us and the kind of collab-
orations that university scientists should have.

RESPONSIBILITY AND COLLABORATION

K. E. Stanley: I disagree with Dr. Gehan with regard
to supervision of data management.   This probably reflects differences between our two major cooperative
groups.   The point I wish to make concerns the idea
that the physician is solely responsible for the
study.   When the physician conceives the study, designs it, collects the data, analyzes them, and reports results, it is entirely his responsibility.   I
believe, however, that there are few studies that fit
this model.   In most cases it is a collaborative effort where each person on the team contributes his
particular expertise.   I believe that the biostatistician, whose training is in research logic, should su-
pervise the data management once the purely medical
issues have been resolved.   My concern here is primarily with potential bias in the judgment of case evaluability and eligibility.   There is certainly the medical component but there is also a very important logical component in the decision to include or exclude a
case.

I would like to mention what I feel is the most en-
joyable situation arising from a long-term collaboration: statistician-initiated medical research.   In
some circumstances the statistician has worked with
the investigator for many years and together they have
developed an extensive data base.   The major clinical
findings comparing various treatments have been reported.   The statistician may then explore the data

in further research; he may perhaps investigate prognostic factors, patterns of failure, or long-term survivors. The initiative for this work is essentially the statistician's.

C. M. Pinsky: In an on-going collaborative arrangement, one should not be too dogmatic about the dangers of the 5-minute consultation. Even when the biostatisticians and clinicians have worked together in planning and running the study, there are problems that continually arise. There are difficulties in following the protocol; there are patients who have not been entered; there are patients who are unevaluable for reasons that were not considered in the study design. Questions such as these often take only a few minutes to resolve. Whereas 5 minutes in a single consultation could be disastrous, 5 minutes in on-going relationships may be extremely useful.

WHO SHOULD PAY?

Participant: In collaboration or consultation with physicians, how do you determine who pays and what they pay for?

K. E. Stanley: This is one of the toughest questions consultants face. I do not believe there is any way we would want to charge for a meeting with an investigator of one hour or less. In terms of grant development, I think that the statistician should take a gamble. He invests his time and, unless the grant is approved, he will never see any remuneration. The truly difficult situations are those moderate to long-term projects where, after one hour or so of working with the investigator, the statistician finds that he needs additional time. He must then estimate the future costs for the investigator and ask if there are grant, department, or core resource funds available. Often, unfortunately, there are not. In these circumstances he must stop even though collaboration looks interesting. The statistician cannot take on unfunded activities and ignore the specific research projects that provide his salary support. However, he must make sure that the investigator is fully aware that funds for statistical collaboration should be a part of future research budgets. One must necessarily take a long-term view of this problem.

T. Colton: I would like to add my concern with costs. Earlier it was said that the biostatistician should learn about the disease and visit the clinic or laboratory to view the data collection process. This takes time and such a level of collaboration is expensive. Who pays for it? If one has a core grant or support for general statistical activities, then it might be used. But such thoroughness in the biostatistician's education can be very expensive.

C. M. Pinsky: One has to be aware that one cannot have it both ways. Collaboration means full collaboration. The writing of grants involves risk; some will be funded and some will not. Biostatisticians take the risk, just like the clinicians. The better written the grant proposal, the better its chances of being funded. If this means consultation without a fee, so be it.

V. Miké: The problem I frequently encounter on site visits around the country is a lack of strong support for biostatistical activities on the part of some medical center administrators. If the institution does not have a large biostatistics group there may not be a developed structure of funding. Statisticians and clinical investigators must work together to convince their administration of the necessity of making available part of a core grant, or equivalent resources, to cover the cost of short-term statistical consultation, the assessment of research problems, and the writing of grant applications. The important point is that the statistician must take the initiative in asking for financial support. He should not be expected to do all this work in addition to a full-time commitment in other areas.

AUTHORSHIP

T. Colton: The end product of both 5-minute consultations and much more extensive collaboration is usually a published paper. I would like to have the statisticians comment on the circumstances in which they feel they should become a coauthor of a paper.

K. E. Stanley: The issue of authorship is always sensitive but many consider it the bottom line for academic promotion. Ideally, the expenditure of intellectual capital should be the measure and those who do the work should get the credit. The biostatistician is a partner in the team and authorship is a natural development relative to his contribution.

Many cooperative groups have a more structured plan such as the study chairman first, the statistician second, then, depending on their case entry down to 10% of the study total, the other principal investigators. Those who entered fewer than 10% appear in a footnote. This structured system is useful in a situation where many papers are written and authorship is repeatedly decided. In many cooperative groups this order is close to the actual relative contributions.

E. A. Gehan: I agree, but one should not be an author on a paper where the contribution is merely a t- or χ^2-test. Occasionally I have been asked to be an author when I really had almost no involvement, or what is worse, made an author without my knowledge. Authorship should result from a significant degree of involvement in the study during its conduct. One danger that has not been mentioned is that of authorship on projects in which one does not wish such designation. If the biostatistician disagrees with a number of the major conclusions expressed in a paper, he

should ask to have his name removed from authorship.
There is the danger not often mentioned of publishing
and perishing.

EVALUATING THE WORK OF OTHERS

T. Colton: How should a biostatistician respond when
he is asked to evaluate another statistician's work?

E. A. Gehan: Evaluation of another statistician's
work depends on the extent to which you are interested
in that particular subject. Clinicians should be
aware that statisticians, like clinicians, may hold a
variety of different opinions about any one particular
problem. Biostatisticians may propose different designs or different methods of analysis, and there is
nothing inherently wrong with that. There is a certain art, as well as science, to data analysis. Clinicians should understand that conclusions can depend
on the particular model chosen or the particular approach that an individual biostatistician might take.
Different statistical viewpoints can be helpful in
many circumstances.

PHYSICIANS' VIEW OF A GOOD STATISTICIAN

T. Colton: I have a question for the physicians:
When you enter into a collaborative or consulting arrangement with a biostatistician, how do you know that
you are getting good advice?

C. M. Pinsky: I know I have a good biostatistician
when: he is available, he attempts to understand the
clinical problem, he is realistic about what is possible, he attempts to make me aware of pitfalls, he is
kind, he has a good sense of humor, and, most important, he guarantees a positive trial.

L. E. Hinkle: Well, I generally agree. I would say
that he should be kind but firm. A statistician who

helps you ahead of time is much better than one who consoles you after you have had a bad review. In general, investigators must depend on the good judgment of biostatisticians. On the positive side, let me say that the likelihood of running into a good biostatistician is probably greater than the likelihood of running into a good clinical investigator.

THE NEED FOR SPECIALIZED ASSISTANCE

T. Colton: What does the biostatistician do if the physician investigator expects more from him than his technical biostatistical acumen can provide? For example, the biostatistician may be assigned the task of evaluation of a cancer control community program or the analysis of an epidemiologic study.

E. A. Gehan: My solution to that problem is to be honest at the outset. Tell the investigators that you do not have the expertise in this area and that they should find or request funding for a biostatistician or other research scientist who would be an expert in that particular area.

V. Miké: The practice of statistics is analogous to the practice of medicine. You are really a good statistician, just as you are really a good doctor, if you tell your client or patient when your knowledge about a subject is limited and refer him to specialists in the area. What may be helpful to biostatisticians who are alone at medical centers is to develop a group of consultants who are willing to assist. If it is a grant application, one should suggest that in addition to your own time, perhaps a fixed sum be added for consultation assistance in some particular area. In reviews of grant applications this is usually taken as an indication that you know what you are doing.

PHYSICAL PROXIMITY: PROS AND CONS

Participant: One point that has not been discussed
yet is the benefit of proximity between biostatistician and clinician.

K. E. Stanley: I feel that the biostatistician should
not be in close proximity to the clinician.   There is
certainly a need for the biostatistician initially to
spend a few days getting to know what the clinician
does, but it need not be a situation where offices are
adjacent.   I think that is counterproductive.   With
close proximity, the clinician will call on the biostatistician to provide frequent updates of the study
results or projected patient entry.   The major analysis decision points are best conducted quite apart in
time, every 6 months or so, for a typical clinical
trial.   Another problem with close proximity is that
investigators tend to get too close to the data.   They
see patient results as being deterministic.   It is
difficult to see variations in patients when the records are in front of you all the time and you continue
to analyze the study every few days.   You cannot
really step back and see that there are prognostic
factor differences and that there is a great deal of
variation.   With a bit of distance between the statistician and the clinician the variation in the clinical
findings comes into more proper perspective.

E. A. Gehan: I agree and I think that close proximity
encourages those 5-minute consultations, which I spoke
against earlier.   In the close proximity situation,
the biostatistician can be called on at any moment.
It is better to have an appointment, either in the
physician's office or occasionally in the biostatistician's office, but the meeting should be a formal af-
fair with objectives, an outcome, and so forth.

J. R. O'Fallon: There are advantages and disadvantages with close proximity.   In the area of clinical

trials, if there is a lot going on, it is helpful to
have the statistician available. Scheduled meetings
with physicians pose difficulties because the physician's first responsibility is patient care. Often,
however, it is possible to sit down over a cup of coffee for 20 minutes and sort out an idea for a new
study. Close proximity is very hard on the statisticians because they are being consulted virtually every
hour of the day. It is a trade-off, however, and I
think that the benefits outweigh the disadvantages.

Participant: I am an in-house biostatistician at a
university hospital with the belief that there are a
lot of advantages to being in-house as opposed to being off-site. First, I have a better appreciation of
the day-to-day problems involved in a study because I
hear and see many of the problems and complaints that
arise before things get out of hand. I also see and
hear exactly what is going on, not what the protocol
says is supposed to be going on. If a biostatistician
knows a project well, a 5-minute consultation can save
many times that in wasted effort. A clinician is not
likely to walk to another building for what he thinks
is a very small point. But if you meet him in the
hallway, he is likely to ask. Another advantage is
that one can establish personal as well as professional relationships. The two physicians on the panel indicated the characteristics they would like to see in
biostatisticians. Most of these, such as availability
and being realistic and kind, are favorable for in-
house biostatisticians. All too often I have seen and
heard that a grant paid thousands of dollars for a
sophisticated analysis that had absolutely no relevance to the question asked, or that the technique was
too complicated for the physician to understand. A
number of times I have received analyses and computer
printouts from physicians with a request to explain
the results. I am sure it was a good analysis but it
was not what was needed. I think that one finds such
insensitivity more frequently in an off-site biostat-

istician. Due to the nature of being in-house, one is busier because people drop in constantly. But I feel that it is an advantage to be involved in all the current activities. I have never really been hounded for frequent updates of ongoing studies.

K. E. Stanley: Many of the problems that you mention exist, but I would not necessarily attribute them to being on-site or off-site. If one is off-site, one still has the responsibility to be closely involved in the activities of the clinical center. I feel that a biostatistician should be involved with an activity, but not to the extent of his being in the middle of it.

E. A. Gehan: I am concerned about what is happening to the discipline of biostatistics. Statisticians are being challenged on the computing side because there are many computer scientists who can apply all the statistical tests and produce results. Biostatisticians need to be able to collaborate and communicate effectively. The working relationship described as the role of an on-site biostatistician is fine, but it makes it difficult to assume the full role of a biostatistician in which one has responsibilities to one's field as well as to the particular research project. It is a difficulty that each person has to resolve for himself.

Participant: It seems that we need both types of biostatisticians. We need people in the field, and people off-site. There are advantages to both approaches and real needs for both types.

J. R. O'Fallon: It is not necessary to make a choice, though. Some talented biostatisticians live on-site but have developed a number of protective mechanisms to get off-site for research.

MEETING DEADLINES

V. Miké: How does one provide the physician with an appreciation for how long it takes to get the data cleaned up, edited, and analyzed?

K. E. Stanley: The best means is an established working relationship over a period of time. If that is impossible, one might take the clinician to the data management or the computing area during the consultation visit and show him what will be done.

E. A. Gehan: Physicians can also participate in the analysis of their own data. By learning some of the short-cut methods and some graphical methods, they can get a reasonably quick answer. But it will not be the full answer.

C. M. Pinsky: The biostatistician is probably as well aware as the clinician of deadlines for abstracts and reports. The biostatistician should point out to the clinician that he needs a specific lead time in order to have things run smoothly. This type of planning in collaborative projects will jog the clinical investigator's memory the next time he needs statistical assistance.

FACING TRADITION

Participant: How do you handle the difficult situation where the best analysis of a particular problem is not well referenced and the physician prefers a more traditional analysis?

E. A. Gehan: If he insists on a particular technique that is not optimal, the biostatistician always has the option to withdraw his name from the paper. An alternative is to write to several other biostatisticians and obtain their views and support in the matter.

T. Colton: I disagree with your first answer and take
a more pragmatic view. If the conventional, but less
than optimal, method does not lead to a misleading result, I would use the conventional method in the paper
for the medical journal. I would, however, write up
my preferred and optimal analysis technique and submit
it for publication in a statistical methods journal.

EDUCATING PHYSICIANS

C. M. Pinsky: We all come up against a situation
where we are asked to work with a clinical investigator who needs to be taught from the start, just what
can be done, what about the study is possible, why he
has to determine the number of patients he expects to
see, why sample size is important, and so forth. Even
though one would think today that this teaching of the
biomedical investigator is less necessary, as I said
earlier, it is pretty obvious to me from reviewing a
number of grants, that such instruction is indeed
still necessary. I think that a reasonable amount of
resources of a biostatistical department should be set
aside to teach investigators.

L. E. Hinkle: In the past we have relied on what
might be called "on-the-job training." If one wanted
to learn about the pitfalls in a clinical trial or in
an epidemiologic study, one worked with the data analysts and the investigators. I think we have reached
the point at which it should be possible to give brief
introductory courses for people who are going to be
involved in various kinds of investigations. These
should include the clinical investigators as well as
the biostatisticians. In the sessions they should
learn to talk to each other and be impressed with the
necessity of having a mutual understanding of the research in which they are engaged and the methods that
they will use before they embark on their investigation.

<u>Participant</u>: An M.D. degree provides a license not only to practice medicine but also to undertake clinical investigation. Society makes sure that physicians who commence practicing medicine have suitable training: an internship, residency, and so on. But a typical medical school will have only a very short statistics course, often only one hour a week for 10 weeks. I wish to ask whether the statistical training in most medical schools is sufficient?

<u>L. E. Hinkle</u>: It seems to me essential that the administration of a medical school realize that adequate medical research cannot be carried out unless there is adequate biostatistical assistance. If you expect that graduates of your medical school may become involved in clinical investigations, then clearly it is desirable that they have some understanding of the basis of biostatistics as it is applied to such investigation.

<u>T. Colton</u>: For the future physician-researcher, I am not so sure that medical school is the right place to learn statistical methods. Those of us who teach statistics to medical students should realize that most of our students will be practitioners and not researchers. I feel our students should know how to read and evaluate the research of others and understand someone else's use of statistical methods. However, for those who anticipate a research career, as part of their research training later on they should have further statistical training with greater emphasis on research methodology. One should not attempt to teach a medical school statistics course in the same manner one would teach physician-investigators at a major research center.

<u>V. Miké</u>: It may take a great deal of negotiation with the curriculum committee to get a statistics course of even 10 hours into the very heavy curriculum of a medical school. But further courses should be made

available to medical students on an elective basis.
We should do the best we can to provide appropriate
modes of learning for all young people whether they
are going into research or will become mainly readers
of the literature.

EDUCATING STATISTICIANS

Participant: The panel has addressed a number of the
issues involved with the statistical training of clinicians. Would anyone care to address the clinical
training of biostatisticians who may or may not know
what a hematocrit is when they graduate with their
Ph.D.?

C. M. Pinsky: We have heard that there are biostatistics hours in medical school and I was tempted to suggest that the graduate courses for Ph.D. biostatisticians contain 40 or 50 hours of medicine. I really
do not think that either one is necessarily the right
way to accomplish what we want to do. Much education
happens on the job when one is involved in active collaboration. The biostatistician will, I hope, with
the aid of a patient and interested physician, learn
all he needs to know about the hematocrit and the
problems of measurement of clinical phenomena. This
is not necessarily something that will work in a for-
malized educational sense except for learning the
principles, as has already been mentioned. Simply
learning how to talk to each other sets the groundwork
for this type of interchange.

E. A. Gehan: I have always been impressed how people
learn in different ways. Some learn from reading the
literature or conducting research but I think there
has to be some learning by doing as well. Working as
an apprentice in a clinical trials group or assisting
an experienced consulting biostatistician can be a
definite help. I believe a biostatistician has to be
involved in different situations from which he

can profit. Unfortunately, many statisticians' first
exposure to medical research is a sink-or-swim situation. Conferences such as this are essential, particularly when a useful workbook results which can be
used to motivate those who teach biostatisticians.

K. E. Stanley: I propose that more schools move away
from the traditional problem-solving approach of the
training of biostatisticians and move toward a minia-
turization of the entire collaborative process. For
example, the student could be presented with a problem, just a short description, and then be sent out
into the research environment. His task would be to
become familiar with that particular area of medical
science, review the medical background, and then work
out, with the investigators, the project design, protocol, and research plan. Following that, data could
be collected and quality controlled, the results analyzed, and presented for discussion in front of the
investigators and faculty of the biostatistics department.

A DIFFERENCE IN PERSPECTIVE

Participant: I am a biostatistician in a community
hospital and have found in dealing with physicians
that some problems seem to arise from a fundamental
difference in the way physicians and statisticians are
trained. Physicians are trained in a deductive manner
and statisticians in inductive logic.

K. E. Stanley: I agree that there is a difference.
But rather than describe it entirely as inductive versus deductive, I would say that physicians are trained
to treat patients on a one-at-a-time basis using all
the resources that are needed for each individual patient. This approach is to be contrasted with the
public health perspective where the goal is to dis-
tribute society's limited resources in a manner that
will benefit the greatest portion of the population.

T. Colton: This difference is not necessarily public health, but rather a difference in perspective: From the point of view of a single patient as opposed to a group of patients. It is a difficult concept for the physician to translate group phenomena, such as the results of a clinical trial, into how he handles an individual patient. Clinicians have to realize that not every patient treated a specific way will have the same degree of benefit or will necessarily benefit at all from the treatment prescribed.

THE INSTITUTIONAL REVIEW BOARD

K. E. Stanley: I have a recommendation for biostatisticians associated with medical centers. One of the most important things you can do is to ensure that there are statistical reviews of all clinical trials before they start. One way to achieve this is to be aggressive and perhaps see if you can work with the Institutional Review Board as a consultant or preferably as a member. Since this committee reviews all clinical research studies, it is an excellent place to intercept studies for review and to get an overview of the clinical research at each center.

REFERENCES

1. Berkow, R., ed. (1982), The Merck Manual of Diagnosis and Therapy (14th ed.), Merck Sharp & Dohme Research Laboratories, Rahway, New Jersey.

2. Gehan, E. A. (1980), The training of statisticians for cooperative clinical trials: A working statistician's viewpoint, Biometrics 36: 699-706.

3. Hammond, D. (1980), The training of clinical trials statisticians: A clinician's view, Biometrics 36: 679-685.

4. Mantel, N. (1951), Rapid estimation of standard errors of means for small samples, American Statistician 5: 26-27.

5. Peterson, A. V., Jr., and Fisher, L. D. (1980), Teaching the principles of clinical trials design and management, Biometrics 36: 687-693.

CHAPTER 17

Interpretation and Presentation of Statistical Results

Panel Discussion
KENNETH E. STANLEY, *Chairman*
DAVID P. BYAR
MITCHELL H. GAIL
RICHARD D. GELBER
PAUL P. ROSEN

K. E. Stanley: The interpretation and presentation of statistical results is an issue of major importance because the medical community must rely heavily on the published literature for making therapeutic decisions. The biostatistician plays a major role in both the reporting and evaluation of clinical studies. Each panel member will make a brief introductory statement and then we will return to the various issues at hand.

CONFLICTING GOALS

R. D. Gelber: The topic of interpretation and presentation of statistical results is of particular interest to me because it involves an area where the goals of the physician are often in conflict with those of the biostatistician. For example, in the design of a collaborative study, the participants basically work in their own realm of expertise. The physician poses a medical question and asks for the statistician's

---

This work was supported in part by National Cancer Institute Grant CA-23415.

collaboration on a design that would be appropriate
for answering that question. In the conduct of a
study, again the roles are clearly defined and there
is little opportunity for conflict. But when it comes
to the interpretation and presentation of results, the
statistician desires to analyze the data according to
the initial plan proposed in the design of the trial,
whereas, because of variations in the way patients are
actually treated, the physician may look at the data
from a different point of view. The biostatistician
usually wants to analyze cases according to the treatment assignment regardless of what was given, because
such an analysis would answer questions about the
treatment plan. The physician, on the other hand,
reasons that reporting treatment results for a group
of patients in which many did not receive the planned
treatment does not convey the proper effect of treatment. Hence, a negotiation process must take place.
The resolution of these disagreements affects the
treatment information that gets into the literature.

One could argue that both approaches should be included, following the initial study design as well as
looking at the data retrospectively. The problem is
that most people carry away just one idea from the results of an analysis. One response rate is reported
in the abstract and that is the statistic that gives
the results of the study. Is an agent or therapy effective? The answer is yes or no, based on that one
analysis. But there are multiple ways that the data
could have been analyzed, and there are many factors
that have to be considered. It is very important to
make clear which viewpoint was used in presenting the
statistical results, whether the results presented apply only to patients who complete the therapy as
planned (a conditional statement), or whether the results can be used to predict the chance of responding
to an agent for a new patient prior to the start of
treatment (an unconditional result). These issues
have to be clearly displayed in any report of the results of the study.

THE PATHOLOGIST'S PERSPECTIVE

P. P. Rosen: I was particularly struck by one of the
speakers in the previous panel discussion on consulting (Chapter 16) who gave me the impression that some
biostatisticians view themselves as embattled individuals in the medical community who may be looking for
a friend, or at least somebody who is sympathetic to
the problems that they face when interacting with
their medical colleagues. So the question is, where
do you turn? My suggestion would be that you turn to
your friendly pathologist, since we pathologists have
some of the same problems.

Here are some of the questions mentioned that are
very familiar to me. Should you be a consultant or a
collaborator? That is a question we pathologists face
all the time. Or an investigator may walk into your
office and say, "I've got a really interesting study
and it is only going to take 5 minutes of your time."
Or he may say, "Now we've done this study, and we
would like you to analyze the results." Well, the
equivalent for the pathologist is, "We have already
followed these patients and we would like you to review the slides and tell us whether they really had
cancer or not." These may sound like amusing observations, but actually they reflect the way some clinical
trials and retrospective studies are carried out in
various institutions.

I think a familiarity with what goes into these
studies helps greatly in appreciating the way the results are presented and the conclusions drawn. The
point I would like to make is that, for clinical trials or retrospective studies that involve cancer, most
of the time the diagnosis was made by a pathologist.
The patient came into the hospital with a lump or some
other problem, and eventually some portion of that patient's body was removed and examined, usually in a
pathology laboratory. So one of the most important
pieces of information about patients in an oncology
trial or retrospective study is the diagnosis. And

this raises questions about whether one should use
clinical or pathologic staging. It brings up questions about prognostic factors that are not specifically involved in staging and their relevance for
stratification of patients. And it also brings up
other areas that pathologists are involved in, such
as running biochemistry laboratories and laboratories
that do the radioisotope scans used in staging patients, and so on.

So I think that if there is one message that I as
a pathologist can leave with you, it is that biostatisticians participating in any kind of oncology study
should ask early on in the study, "Where is the pathologist involved in the study, and has he been consulted to be sure that the appropriate pathologic data
are included?" We will come back to some real examples of these points later on in the discussion.

PREPARING THE WRITTEN REPORT

M. H. Gail: When I think of the interpretation and
presentation of clinical trial data, I first think of
writing up a publication because that is what the
process of medical research is all about. It is looking over the experiment, trying to figure out what it
means, and then trying to convey that meaning to other
people. So I would like to discuss the basic structure of a scientific presentation. This structure is
a great help in our thinking about how to present data.

The publication should have an introduction and a
clear statement of purpose, obviously, but perhaps
this purpose should be a bit more refined than usual.
Maybe we should say the purpose of the experiment was
to demonstrate whether or not there is a difference
between treatment plan A and treatment plan B. Therefore the purpose might take into account the fact that
there will be dilution effects if some people do not
get the intended treatment. Clearly, the biostatistician who helps formulate the design of the experiment

has a lot to say about the correct wording of the purpose.

A stringent test of a good "Methods" section is that some other reader could read this section and then presumably be prepared to repeat the experiment. It is obvious that a good treatment description has to be included, but there are other features of the experiment which the biostatistician is uniquely equipped to describe. These include such factors as the stratification, the randomization scheme, whether blocking was used, and if so, what kind of blocking, the description of the end point measurement, how frequently the end point was measured, and whether the observer was blind with respect to treatment. In addition, there should be some detail on the actual methods used to analyze the data. Most of these items are obvious, but it is clear that the biostatistician has an important role in the writing of the "Methods" section.

Concerning the "Results" section, at a minimum the biostatistician should insist on reporting the experiment as originally designed and executed, including an analysis of all patients randomized and all deaths, regardless of cause. This is the experiment that was performed although there are other experiments that we would have much preferred to see. We would obviously prefer that each patient actually accepted the assigned treatment and continued the treatments as prescribed by the protocol, and we would be grateful if all these patients refrained from dying from other causes. Yet, these sorts of things are not always carried out to perfection, and biostatisticians have to analyze the data that the experiment actually presents. This is not to say that other analyses are inappropriate, but rather that they should be carefully qualified because, in general, they are nonrandomized or make some stringent assumptions. Clearly, the biostatistician has a role in adjusting treatment differences to account for imbalances in prognostic factors. He should be able to respond to a particular critic

with statements like, "Well, yes, it's true that initial stage of disease is very important and there was
a slight treatment imbalance on initial stage of disease, but adjustment on initial stage doesn't change
our estimate of treatment effect very much." Other
important components of the "Results" section include
the analysis of toxicity and special analyses.

Finally, there is the "Discussion" section. An important aspect of this section is to give the reader
a feeling for the strengths and weaknesses of the
study and what other work needs to be done. Since
biostatisticians are paid to criticize, they should
be very good at helping point out some of the weaknesses of the study, weaknesses either in the design or
execution, or maybe even weaknesses in the methods of
analysis. This process of self-criticism can also
highlight some of the strengths of the study. In particular, if one can anticipate the criticisms of the
readers and deal with these criticisms by ancillary
analyses and discussion, one can show that maybe the
experiment was even stronger than it appeared at
first. If the biostatistician takes care in addressing these points in the publication, he will earn his
right to coauthorship.

THE STATISTICIAN AS SKEPTIC

D. P. Byar: I agree with everything Dr. Gail said, so
I will not repeat any of that. I think the distinguishing characteristic of the biostatistician is his
skepticism rather than his ability to make fancy calculations on a computer. The statistician is something like the pathologist, in a way, because the
pathologist often plays the role of skeptic in medicine. He is the one who stands back and objectively
looks at things and tells those enthusiastic surgeons
to stop removing normal tissue. Statisticians tell
people not to believe everything that appears to be
true, no matter how much it appears to agree with
their preconceptions. However, as the words in the

title of this panel "interpretation and presentation" suggest, drawing conclusions from statistical results is not an objective process. Interpretation and presentation are selective processes, and one does not usually have the luxury of presenting all the data. Only in some small studies is it both feasible and desirable to present the full data so that other people can do their own analyses.

The art of the statistician resembles that of the pathologist for another reason. Doctors ask pathologists to decide yes or no concerning a particular diagnosis. But pathologists know that the difference between normal and diseased tissue is often a spectrum and that they have to draw a line someplace. Statisticians face a similar problem when asked, "Is it significant or not?" We know that there are various degrees of evidence, but maybe it is a good thing that we are forced to say whether we think something is significant or not. It is not enough to compute a P-value and let someone else decide what it means.

I want to turn now to the problem of bias because this is one of the subjects that concerns me most when I read research reports or try to evaluate medical data. Recently, I was standing in line in a supermarket and ran across an excellent example in an article by Vance Packard in Reader's Digest (11). He describes a marketing research experiment as follows: 200 women were selected and questioned ostensibly about color schemes for furniture. In order to reward them for their time, the company gave them each two jars of cold cream, and told them to take them home, try them out, and decide which one they liked better. When they came back for their second consulting session, they would be given a whole case of the one which they liked better. Both jars were labeled "high quality cold cream," but on the lid of one there were two triangles and on the lid of the other there were two circles. When they came back, fully 80% of the 200 women distinctly preferred the one with two circles on top. Now of course the two jars contained identical cold cream, but they liked the one with the circles on top because it had a better consistency, they found it easier to apply, and it was definitely a finer quality. Well, I submit that if you had told those women that both jars contained the same kind of the cold cream, they would never admit to having believed that the design on the cap could have influenced their judgments of consistency, applicability, or quality. It is just this kind of subtle bias that worries me most, especially when reading historically controlled studies. Such biases can arise with subjective end points or with subjective evaluations of objective end points.

FACTORS AFFECTING QUALITY

K. E. Stanley: We would now like to turn to a discussion of factors that contribute to the quality of a study report. These are the design, conduct, and evaluation, as well as the question of whether some cases should be excluded and the various reasons.

REPORTING DETAILS OF STUDY DESIGN

R. D. Gelber: One thing that deserves attention but is often not presented is a discussion of the original planned sample size. We place a lot of emphasis on designing studies, but then when it comes to writing the study results we often ignore the design considerations. Some report of the initial goal should be included. Further, the reason that the patient entry into the study was stopped is also needed to properly evaluate the results. Was accrual not being met? Was there undue toxicity? Did people become discouraged because new therapies were on the horizon and the ethical considerations forced physicians not to enter any more patients? Was statistical significance reached on an interim report?

One should also describe how patient consent was obtained in a report of a clinical study. But one

also has to be sensitive to the space limitations in
the literature. If all of the methods are well described, there may not be much room to report the results.

One aspect of the topic of counting cases and determining which cases are evaluable I would call denominator determination. An example is the determination of response rate in a study of weekly VM26 in
children with acute lymphocytic leukemia (2). In this
study, 30 patients were entered, 15 were evaluable,
and 4 of the 15 responded. The publication of the
study reports that weekly VM26 is active with a 27%
response rate (4/15). However, if one considers what
happened to the other half of the patients who were
not evaluable, the response rate goes down to 13%.
The investigators were enthusiastic about the weekly
VM26 treatment response rate of 27%, but probably
would not have been as enthusiastic if the response
rate had been 13%. The issue here is about case reporting and the intended use of the statistic generated. With the 27% figure, the physician can say to the
family in his office that if the child manages to get
adequate therapy on this treatment regimen, then he
has an estimated 27% chance of responding. However,
this is not a fair representation of the child's
chance to respond to the therapy because not all children will be able to complete the therapy, that is, be
evaluable, and it is not possible to determine in advance who will complete therapy. For the child sitting in the physician's office prior to the start of
treatment, a proper estimate of the chance of responding to VM26 would be 13%. What is reported should depend on how the information is going to be used.

It is also important to state the criteria for censoring in the analysis of survival-type end points.
Results can differ depending on how the censoring
mechanisms are applied. For example, consider the
evaluation of disease-free interval for patients with
acute leukemia. Some published reports count a patient who dies as a result of toxicity as a censored

case for the evaluation of the relapse of the disease.
Therefore, the relapse-free curves based on that definition of censoring will vary between two treatments
depending on treatment toxicity alone, with the more
toxic treatment tending to show a longer relapse-free
interval.

In reports of clinical studies, one should be careful to make the distinction between formal hypothesis
testing and exploration of the data. It is essential
that exploration of the data take place because unan-
ticipated findings may suggest future research or optimal therapy. However, these efforts should be distinguished from the testing of formal hypotheses when
results are presented.

COMPARABILITY OF DATA SETS

P. P. Rosen: I cannot tell you how to do statistical
analyses, but perhaps some ideas from my point of view
may prove useful.

(Dr. Rosen discussed binocular microscopes and suggested that they could help in reaching agreement between pathologists about diagnoses. He stressed the
fundamental importance of pathology review and reproducibility. He also pointed out that the detailed
records in pathology departments are often more reliable than registry information for confirming diagnoses. Ed.)

Next I would like to review the report of a research study as an example of what to watch for, a recent report of minimal breast cancer (10). The study
was a cancer survey and included 16,894 pathologically
confirmed carcinomas of the female breast, in situ or
infiltrative, with negative or positive nodes. That
is a large number of cases, and one would tend to have
confidence in the results simply by the size of the
study alone. The cases were collected in relatively
short and recent time periods from several hundred
hospitals across the nation, and hence the report suggests that the study data may not have been unduly

influenced by changing diagnostic and therapeutic
techniques. However, if one reads closely, the report
states that because of the interinstitutional nature
of this retrospective study, there was a lack of information on the details of surgical procedures, combinations with other treatments, and completeness of
follow-up. Further, the report indicates that there
are questions about the consistency of the pathologic
diagnoses. Hence, close reading of the report raises
severe doubts as to the reliability of the study results. Such weaknesses are frequently found in retrospective studies but are not evident except on a critical reading of the text.

(Dr. Rosen then described in some detail, by way
of comparison with the American College of Surgeons'
study, a smaller study of minimal breast cancer carried out at his institution. The essential features
were that all cases could be identified from the bound
pathology records available since 1964, and the slides
could be reviewed. Certain patients were excluded
from the final analysis for various reasons, but survival of the excluded group was compared with that of
the patients forming the main study to see whether or
not the results would have been affected by the exclu-
sions. Dr. Rosen suggested that this kind of question
is rarely addressed in the literature and that biostatisticians might find this technique useful for
checking the effects of selection in retrospective
studies. He then described another study designed to
evaluate the risk of later frank breast cancer following an earlier diagnosis of preinvasive cancer or in
situ carcinoma (12). All breast biopsies performed
at his institution between 1940 and 1950 were reviewed
(some 12,000 slides for over 8000 cases) in order to
obtain a correct denominator. The frequency of lobular carcinoma in situ was 1.4%. He noted that because
of changing criteria of diagnosis over the years, only
about half of the 117 cases in the final study would
have been detected by reviewing hospital records as
opposed to reviewing the histologic slides using

modern diagnostic criteria. Of those patients they
were able to follow, 35% subsequently developed cancer, about half in the opposite breast, after an average interval of 15 years. Some patients did not develop cancer until 30 years later. Ed.)

So, I asked my biostatistical colleague, "How can
we best find out whether this risk is equally spread
out over the follow-up period?" He suggested that we
analyze the hazard rate. The results of that analysis
show that the chances of developing subsequent cancer
are increasing with increasing length of follow-up
(Figure 1).

These are some experiences that I have had trying
to carry out studies predominantly of a retrospective
nature, that have raised questions about how one collects and presents the data. One must ensure that the

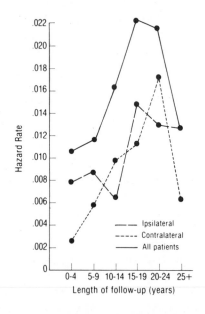

Figure 1. Hazaru rate for subsequent carcinoma related
to length of follow-up. Reproduced from Rosen et al.
(12), Masson Publishing USA, Inc., New York, (1978).

publication represents the actual scientific experience of the investigators and also presents the results to the medical community in a way that will be constructive for future patient management.

OTHER ISSUES: SAMPLE SIZE AND EXCLUSION OF INELIGIBLE CASES

<u>M. H. Gail</u>: I would like to make a few brief remarks. First, I enjoyed Dr. Rosen's presentation, and I would like to point out a connection with Dr. Colton's earlier presentation on epidemiologic studies. Dr. Rosen gave an example of a retrospective cohort study. He had all the data on follow-up essentially in hand, and approached the cases retrospectively. Another interesting issue arises in these very long-term follow-up studies, such as some lung cancer studies with which I am involved. Is the increasing hazard rate due to recurrence of the initial disease, or is it due to second primary cancers? Although clinicians may want to try to make that distinction, I think that an important analysis to be done (since that distinction cannot usually be made with certainty) is to count all cancer occurrences, regardless of how they are classified.

I want to comment on the reporting or stressing of sample size. As several speakers have mentioned, power should be included in a discussion of an experiment. This is especially important for a negative trial since the power measures the strength of evidence for that negative result. If the power is sufficiently high, say 95%, a negative result can be as important as a positive result.

Should we include people in the analysis who were found out later to be ineligible for the study? There are some situations where this might be appropriate, but let me describe one case where I think it might not be appropriate to exclude such patients. Consider a study of operable lung cancer in which only patients with squamous cell carcinoma are eligible. Patients are diagnosed by the local pathologist as having squamous cell carcinoma, and then subsequently entered into the study and assigned a treatment. Now suppose that 6 months later the pathologic review committee examines the slide on a specific patient and determines that the tumor was actually an adenocarcinoma, not a squamous cell carcinoma, and that the patient should not have been included in the study. If the point of view is that every patient who appears to be eligible at the time of randomization should be studied, so as to determine the superior treatment for that set of patients, then it is clear that such a patient should remain in the analysis. Even though the patient did not in fact have a squamous cell carcinoma, he appeared to have one at the time when the clinical decision to treat was made.

There is, of course, a good argument for performing the other analysis, too. If the question is more biologic in nature, then exclusion of the case will permit an uncontaminated analysis. But I would like to stress that, from the point of view of determining therapeutic efficacy, a good argument can be made for including such patients. I do not want to take an extreme position here because there are certain ineligibility criteria so extreme as to warrant excluding patients, but this is an example of interaction with a pathologist where you might want to take a hard stand.

P. P. Rosen: In an abstract sense you have a good point, but you would have to raise the question, "How often is that error going to occur?" If that error is likely to occur frequently, then it seems appropriate to include that error in your analysis. If that error is going to be a relatively infrequent event, then the majority of patients that are said to have squamous cell carcinoma will in fact have squamous cell carcinoma, and it would be more appropriate to present the results of treatment for correctly diagnosed cases.

M. H. Gail: Yes, I think that there is a good case to

be made for doing the alternative analysis, just so
long as both are presented. I can support that position.

REPORTING POWER; PROTOCOL VIOLATIONS AND MISSING DATA

D. P. Byar: Concerning power, Dr. Gail said that if
the power of a negative study approaches 95%, then the
study should be reported because it is as strong as a
positive study. I think it is even more important to
report the power when it is low. If all the people
who report small negative studies based on 20 or 30
patients pointed out that the power for detecting interesting alternatives was only 25%, then our impressions about their conclusions might be considerably
altered. Dr. Chalmers has repeatedly made this point
(6), and I think that when possible, the power ought
to be discussed.

Concerning exclusion of ineligible cases, such as
patients with the wrong pathologic diagnosis, they
certainly should be excluded in some subanalyses, but
I agree with Dr. Gail that the published results
should include one analysis based on all randomized
patients. Then one can selectively exclude some questionable cases, but if the study results change, it
casts serious doubts on the subanalyses.

Concerning protocol violations, it is very hard to
persuade me to omit any of these cases from an analysis. The general rule that I try to follow is only
to exclude patients from an analysis for reasons that
could have been known before they were randomized, but
were not. Otherwise, one is beginning to adjust for
something that possibly happened as a result of therapy. It is relatively easy to get into really silly,
biased situations, and even draw conclusions opposite
from the correct ones.

Missing data pose one of the most pressing and difficult problems that we face in analyzing medical
studies. The first thing to decide about missing data
is not what to do about them, but why the data are

missing. As an illustration, I recently analyzed some pathologic observations made on slides of biopsy material from patients with mycosis fungoides, a type of cutaneous T-cell lymphoma. For every variable, there were a number of patients with missing data. When I tabulated the death rates for those patients with missing data along with rates for those falling in the various known categories, I found that the patients with missing data always had greater death rates. It was therefore quite obvious in this instance that the unknown values were not missing at random.

There are generally 3 things one can do with missing data: (a) try very hard to get the missing data, (b) leave the patients out of the analysis, or (c) use a statistical method that estimates the missing data from the known values. The validity of alternatives (b) and (c) usually depends on the assumption that the data are missing at random, so in this case it seemed that the only sensible thing to do was to try to get the data, even though this delayed completion of the study by a whole year. I think that alternative (a) ought to be pursued more often than it is, especially when pathology data are missing, because with some effort it is often possible to track down histologic slides.

Concerning early withdrawals, I am not quite sure what group of patients this term is intended to include. If this just means censored observations, then one uses methods appropriate for censored observations.

PATIENT REFUSAL AND SELECTION BIAS

K. E. Stanley: We were talking about patients who refused therapy, say after only one dose, or simply leave the hospital to seek treatment elsewhere. If a patient only received one dose and the primary end point of a Phase II study is the response rate, should the patient be included in the denominator, which assumes the worst and essentially makes him a nonre-

sponder, or should the patient be left out, which assumes the best?

D. P. Byar: In Phase III comparative trials, I would
leave the patient in because I would not want to risk
biasing the treatment comparisons. In a Phase II trial where the problem is estimation, that is, to determine whether a drug is active, I think there are important subanalyses in which it would be appropriate
to leave him out.

R. D. Gelber: Rather than trying to state the power
of a study, I prefer this information to be presented
in confidence interval form. If the treatment results
look similar, but the confidence interval on the difference is large, then one can judge the reliability
of the study results for oneself. If, on the other
hand, the confidence intervals are very small, then
one can be assured that there was a fair amount of
power.
     With regard to protocol violations, I would like to
give an example to focus on some of the problems that
can occur (Table 1). This is a complicated study of
head and neck cancer (7) where the two treatments are
radiation followed by surgery versus surgery followed
by radiation, a preop group and a postop group. About
the same number of patients were entered into each
group and about the same number of cases failed to
complete the assigned therapy in both groups. Hence,
one might analyze the study two ways: including all
of the cases randomized or just looking at the results
of the patients who completed the full therapy. One
problem is that the pattern of refusals was quite different for the two treatment groups. Many patients
who were assigned to the treatment where radiation was
given first experienced a shrinkage of the tumor and
relief from the disease, and hence refused the surgery. On the other hand, if surgery was offered
first, patients were more likely to accept that
portion of the study. By excluding patients who did

TABLE 1. Results of a Phase III Study of Head and Neck Cancer[a]

	Radiation followed by surgery	Surgery followed by radiation
Cases	136	141
Treatment not completed	42	41
Reasons:		
Refused surgery	25	10
Refused irradiation	2	10
Deterioration by 2nd modality	11	9
Toxicity by 2nd modality	3	8
Other	1	4
No surgery	35	14
3-year local control		
Treatment completed	70%	72%
All cases	58%	67%

[a]Data from Gelber (7).

not complete the assigned treatment, 35 patients who did not have surgery are excluded from the preop group compared with 14 in the postop group. When we try to decide if one program is better than another program, this example would argue very strongly for including all the randomized patients in the analysis. A report based only on patients who managed to complete the therapy as planned might be very misleading.

M. H. Gail: There is another point to be made from Table 1. Although 70% is similar to 72%, that could

be a very unreliable estimate of the effects of the
two treatments. This is because we have no reason to
believe that the 25 patients who refused surgery on
the preoperative therapy regimen were representative
of all patients on that therapy. Thus, the 70% versus
72% comparison looks similar, but the analysis is not
protected by the randomization, whereas the 58% versus
67% comparison is protected.

R. D. Gelber: Absolutely. Even though this is a randomized study, preop versus postop radiotherapy, the
analysis might be subject to selection biases if we
exclude patients not completing treatment.

The recent increased emphasis on quality control
review raises another issue concerning case exclusion.
The question might arise in pathology review, or modality review in a multimodality study. Consider a
study of radiation therapy versus radiation therapy
plus chemotherapy. Frequently in such a study, two
physicians are assigned to review the quality of the
radiation and chemotherapy, respectively, while only
one review is done on the chemotherapy alone group.
If one uses these quality control reviews of adequate
therapy to selectively exclude patients, one will create a bias by excluding more poorer risk patients on
the radiation plus chemotherapy treatment, simply because there were two opportunities for the patients
to deviate from planned therapy. We randomize to obtain groups that are as alike as possible on the average, and yet we create large mechanisms, such as radiation therapy dose and field review, which can tend
to exclude patients on the basis of the treatment they
were assigned. Hence, the groups that are eventually
analyzed, if one used protocol violations to exclude
patients, are not the groups that are randomized to
be alike on the average.

REPORTING RESULTS

K. E. Stanley: Should more exploratory data analysis

appear in the literature and should the models themselves be reported in the publication of the clinical
trial?

M. H. Gail: I think we should do analyses that are
appropriate and report them fully. Often one can get
a good idea about what will be a meaningful analysis
by looking at the literature and seeing what others
have done. If one uses similar analyses, one will
find it easier to compare one's results with the literature. On the other hand, times have changed and
new methods are available now. It may be unfair to
the experimenter not to give him the benefit of recent
statistical progress. If new methods are used, the
statistician is obliged to describe carefully what he
has done. Exploratory data analysis plays an important role, but I am not certain that analyses of this
type should necessarily be included in the same publication as the summary results of a clinical trial. If
such results are reported they should be specially
highlighted as exploratory in nature, and the discussion should indicate what future observations would
be needed to confirm them.

DESCRIBING ANALYTIC MODELS

R. D. Gelber: I agree that biostatisticians should
include the analytic models in clinical papers and
discuss the characteristics of the models. I am frus-
trated by reading reports where an investigator states
that he has adjusted for various factors and then simply states the results. At a minimum I would like to
see some comment about how the selection of the model
was done, and how the variables have entered the model. I am concerned about reporting spurious conclusions resulting from incorrectly applied models. I
would like to have more information, especially if
conclusions are based on these models, as to exactly
which models were used and how they were constructed.

<u>D. P. Byar</u>:   I pretty much agree with the two previous speakers. I think that when you write, since editors do not give you unlimited space, you should try to write whatever is needed to convince readers of your points in a relatively simple fashion. On the other hand, these days it is certainly all right to use Cox models. I have even had reviewers for medical journals send back articles asking for a Cox analysis!

Certainly, methods of survival analysis for censored data should always be used as opposed to what some clinicians call the "direct method." For the "direct method," a 5-year survival rate is the proportion alive at 5 years of all patients followed 5 years or more. There are actually people who are suspicious of anything other than that method, even though that method may not be very efficient because it may throw away a lot of useful data.

I think that the more we agree on what are the best, strongest methods of analysis and try to stick to them so they become familiar household words, the more we can use them effectively in our studies. But if there is unnecessary proliferation of new methods for the minor variants of standard problems which often arise in clinical data, then unfamiliarity with those methods may hinder the acceptability of study results. Most people use the life table and product limit methods, and many people now use the Cox model in articles. Logistic regression is also getting quite popular. I routinely use these methods of analysis. If space is not too limited, one can present the model in an appendix, state why it was chosen, and give the regression coefficients. Just like my comment that when possible all the data for small studies should be published, I think the more details you can include the better, so long as they are put in a subsidiary place where everyone does not have to read them unless he wants to. There are many details in medical articles that mean little to statisticians, and I suspect that many statistical details would mean little to most medical readers. But if the medical reader has questions, he can at least ask a statistician who can figure out the answer. But if an article just says that the chi-square for an adjusted analysis was 4.2, the statistician would not be able to help him.

P. P. Rosen: I agree with the point about putting in as much data as possible. It always seems unfortunate to me that because of editorial constraints more data cannot be put into papers. But I think one should try to include as much of the information as possible.

RETROSPECTIVE ANALYSES

K. E. Stanley: The final topic for this panel concerns comparisons that are based on characteristics observed after time zero, such as retrospective analyses by dose received.

M. H. Gail: Well, I guess that is a leading question. This question has come up in an important paper on breast cancer where the inference has been made that patients who received a large amount of their chemotherapy were the ones who did well (3). Therefore, you should push the chemotherapy.

POTENTIAL BIAS IN POST HOC COMPARISONS

R. D. Gelber: Table 2 shows the results of the study Dr. Gail is talking about, a study of breast cancer patients where the patients were divided retrospectively according to the dose of CMF received. This is the summary of data from two randomized clinical trials which was reported to show a clear dose-response effect. The total protocol-specific dose was computed and divided into the actual dose received for all patients to create patient groups which were then compared. Apparently, if the doses were reduced on the basis of toxicity or stopped because the patient refused to continue, these patients were included in

TABLE 2. Dose-Response Effect of Adjuvant CMF in
Breast Cancer[a]

Dose of CMF	5-year relapse free survival (%)	Number of patients
≥ 85%	77	78
65-84%	56	222
< 65%	48	149
Control	45	179

[a]Data from Bonadonna and Valagussa (3). Reprinted, by
permission of The New England Journal of Medicine,
304: 10-15, (1981).

the lowest category, <65% of the planned dose.

One can see the relationship between 5-year
relapse-free survival and the dose that was given.
The authors stated that based on this analysis it is
necessary to administer full dose chemotherapy because
it gives the patients the best chance of being
disease-free. Before I comment on the validity of
this conclusion, consider a counterexample that came
out in the same journal only 3 months prior to the
previous example. Table 3 shows the results of an
analysis of the Coronary Drug Project in which groups
were given clofibrate (14) and were divided by adherence to taking the therapy. The same dose response is
seen here as was seen in the CMF example. The group
that received greater than 80% of the dose, as determined by the percentage of capsules that were taken,
had a greater survival at 5 years, 85% versus 75% for
the nonadherence group.

A similar analysis was conducted for the placebo
group in this study. A dose-response relationship
similar to that of the drug was observed for the placebo. The group that had received 80% of the placebo

TABLE 3. Influence of Adherence to Treatment on Mortality -- Coronary Drug Project[a]

Adherence (% of capsules taken)	Clofibrate		Placebo	
	5-year survival	Number of patients	5-year survival	Number of patients
≥ 80	85%	708	85%	1813
< 80	75%	357	72%	882

[a]Data from The Coronary Drug Project Research Group (14). Reprinted by permission of The New England Journal of Medicine, 303: 1038-1041, (1980).

capsules had a much higher 5-year survival rate when compared with those who did not take at least 80% of the placebo capsules. The potential for bias with post hoc comparisons is clearly seen. The dose-response conclusions of the CMF example are subject to similar biases and the statement that higher doses are better may simply reflect the fact that patients with better prognosis are able to get higher doses. One just cannot tell from the data presented.

D. P. Byar: I am familiar with the Bonadonna article. I do not think the authors used the right statistical methods, and because of this, they may have failed to convince many readers. I privately feel, however, that their conclusion is probably correct. In this study full dosages of CMF were deliberately not given to women over age 65 because of fears of toxicity. A well-known result of that study was that adjuvant therapy was not effective in postmenopausal women. The article is an attempt to explain that finding.

Perhaps their analyses were not carried out with as high a level of statistical sophistication as we would like, but the attempt to explain the finding is nevertheless useful and stimulating. So, I think the paper should be regarded as exploratory data analysis that does not firmly establish a conclusion. However, there are some chemotherapists who believe that anticancer drug therapy should be pushed to manageably toxic levels if the greatest success is to be obtained.

TIME-DEPENDENT COVARIATE ANALYSIS

M. H. Gail: I think that we are in danger of getting into problems of this type partly because the technology of time-dependent covariate analysis has become available. In the old days, when one was measuring the yield and the height of cornstalks, one would not even have thought about adjusting the treatment effect on yield for the height of the cornstalks because both of these factors could have easily been influenced by treatment. One might have adjusted on a variable that was known before the treatment was administered in order to reduce variation, but never on a factor that might itself have been influenced by treatment because one could in effect be adjusting away a real treatment difference. Now we are perhaps in a similar situation, although maybe not as stark as in my example. Both of these elements, the amount of dose you receive and, let us say, your survival, are potentially influenced by the treatment itself. There will be a temptation to use time-dependent covariate analysis to perform a variety of adjustments on factors that are potentially influenced by the treatment, and one must therefore consider carefully what one is doing.

CONCLUDING REMARKS

K. E. Stanley: In closing, are there any comments from the floor?

STANDARDIZED REPORTING SCHEME FOR CLINICAL TRIALS

M. L. Lesser: I would just like to comment on the
list of things that should be reported in articles
presenting the results of a clinical trial. I agree
that those items should be reported, and I think most
others would also agree. The biggest problem we face
is that the editors of journals have to limit what is
published because space is limited. I would make the
following proposal. In reporting end results in cancer studies, certain conventions are used such as the
UICC terminology or the TNM system for reporting the
patient's disease stage. Anyone who desires more details of the staging definitions can consult the staging system references. I propose that biostatisticians get together and prepare a concise chart or
standardized reporting scheme that could be put into
the publications of therapeutic clinical trials in oncology. Such a scheme might be acceptable to the editors because it would be easy to read and would not
take up a lot of space.

PUBLISHING RESULTS OF EXPLORATORY DATA ANALYSIS

Participant: I would like to make a couple of brief
points. One point concerns the issue of publishing
the results of exploratory data analysis. I would say
that the primary purpose of exploratory data analysis
is for the person doing the analysis to discover
things in the data, and they are not necessarily meant
to be published. If you find some structure, you
might then fit some models and report on the fitted
models in the usual way. The audience for a lot of
the exploratory data techniques is the researcher himself. A lot of those things, of course, can be used
judiciously to report the results to a wider audience
as well, but you have to be careful and bear in mind
the background of the readers. A second point that
you might discover in exploratory analysis is that,
before you believe something that you have discovered

in a sort of fishing expedition, you should see if it is reproducible in other data sets. Before you publish your new finding, either the finding should be extremely convincing in your data set, it should be explainable after the fact by phenomena that you understand but may have overlooked initially, or else the result should be reproducible in other data sets.

I think it is extremely important that the primary data be published as fully as possible. Not only does it allow other people to make sure that they believe reported results, but also, when new methods of analysis are invented or new results emerge, one can sometimes avoid having to go back to original data sources to apply the new methods or to see if new results are consistent with those reported previously.

REFERENCES

1.* Armitage, P. (1981), Importance of prognostic factors in the analysis of data from clinical trials, Controlled Clinical Trials 1: 347-353.

2. Bleyer, W. A., Krivit, W., Chard, R. L., and Hammond, D. (1979), Phase II study of VM26 in acute leukemia, neuroblastoma, and other refractory childhood malignancies: A report from the Children's Cancer Study Group, Cancer Treatment Reports 63: 977-981.

3. Bonadonna, G., and Valagussa, P. (1981), Dose-response effect of adjuvant chemotherapy in breast cancer, The New England Journal of Medicine 304: 10-15.

4.* Chalmers, T. C., Smith, H., Jr., Blackburn, B., Silverman, B., Schroeder, B., Reitman, D., and Ambroz, A. (1981), A method for assessing the quality of a randomized control trial, Controlled Clinical Trials 2: 31-49.

540   Stanley

540   Stanley
5.* Feinstein, A. R. (1977), Clinical Biostatistics, The C. V. Mosby Co., St. Louis.

6. Freiman, J. A., Chalmers, T. C., Smith, H., and Kuebler, R. R. (1978), The importance of beta, the type II error and sample size in the design and interpretation of the randomized control trial, The New England Journal of Medicine 299: 690-694.

7. Gelber, R. (1980), Analysis of endpoints for RTOG study 73-03: Radiation therapy and surgery in the treatment of head and neck tumors, Technical Report No. 184R, Department of Biostatistics, Sidney Farber Cancer Institute, Boston.

8.* Glantz, S. (1980), Biostatistics: How to detect, correct and prevent errors in the medical literature, Circulation 61: 1-7.

9.* Miller, A. B., Hoogstraten, B., Staquet, M., and Winkler, A. (1981), Reporting results of cancer treatment, Cancer 47: 207-214.

10. Nemoto, T., Vana, J., Bedwani, R. N., Baker, H. W., McGregor, F. H., and Murphy, G. P. (1980), Management and survival of female breast cancer: Results of a national survey by the American College of Surgeons, Cancer 45: 2917-2924.

11. Packard, V. (1981), The new and still hidden persuaders, Reader's Digest February: 120-123.

12. Rosen, P. P., Lieberman, P. H., Braun, D. W., Jr., Kosloff, C., and Adair, F. (1978), Lobular carcinoma in situ of the breast: Detailed analysis of 99 patients with average follow-up of 24 years, American Journal of Surgical Pathology 2: 225-251.

13.* Sackett, D., and Gent, M. (1979), Controversy in counting and attributing events in clinical trials, The New England Journal of Medicine 301: 1410-1412.

14. The Coronary Drug Project Research Group (1980), Influence of adherence to treatment and response of cholesterol on mortality in the coronary drug project, The New England Journal of Medicine 303: 1038-1041.

---

*These are general references not specifically mentioned in the text.

Index